Quantitative Radiobiology for Proton Therapy

Online at: https://doi.org/10.1088/978-0-7503-6209-2

About the Series

The series in Physics and Engineering in Medicine and Biology will allow the Institute of Physics and Engineering in Medicine (IPEM) to enhance its mission to 'advance physics and engineering applied to medicine and biology for the public good'.

It is focused on key areas including, but not limited to:

- clinical engineering
- diagnostic radiology
- informatics and computing
- magnetic resonance imaging
- nuclear medicine
- physiological measurement
- radiation protection
- radiotherapy
- rehabilitation engineering
- ultrasound and non-ionising radiation.

A number of IPEM–IOP titles are being published as part of the EUTEMPE Network Series for Medical Physics Experts.

A full list of titles published in this series can be found here: https://iopscience.iop.org/bookListInfo/physics-engineering-medicine-biology-series.

Quantitative Radiobiology for Proton Therapy

Bleddyn Jones
Gray Institute, University of Oxford Department of Oncology, Old Road Campus, Roosevelt Drive, Oxford OX37DQ

With contribution from
Joshua Moore
University of Oxford Mathematical Institute, Woodstock Road, Oxford OX2 6 GG

IOP Publishing, Bristol, UK

ISBN 978-0-7503-6209-2 (ebook)
ISBN 978-0-7503-6207-8 (print)
ISBN 978-0-7503-6210-8 (myPrint)
ISBN 978-0-7503-6208-5 (mobi)

DOI 10.1088/978-0-7503-6209-2

Version: 20240701

IOP ebooks

British Library Cataloguing-in-Publication Data: A catalogue record for this book is available from the British Library.

Published by IOP Publishing, wholly owned by The Institute of Physics, London

IOP Publishing, No.2 The Distillery, Glassfields, Avon Street, Bristol, BS2 0GR, UK

US Office: IOP Publishing, Inc., 190 North Independence Mall West, Suite 601, Philadelphia, PA 19106, USA

To the late Dr OCA Scott MD (Cantab) FRCR[1]*, who inspired so many scientists and clinicians, gave freely of his ideas and was such a generous benefactor. Also to my mother, Mary Margaret Jones, for her patient care over many years and to my late father, Emlyn John Jones BSc (Wales), CEng for his personalised teaching.*

---

[1] The interesting scientific career of Dr OCA Scott is summarised in two obituaries:

1. Jones B and Hendry J 2017 Professor Jack Fowler and Sir Oliver Scott *Br. J Radiol.* **90** 20160904.
2. Trott K-R 2016 *Radiother. Oncol.* **121** 480–481.

Contents

Preface

The second edition of this book is intended to cover the principles covering the potential advantages and pitfalls of proton therapy, especially its radiobiological modelling applications: for these to be understood, it is essential to present summaries of radiotherapy, radiobiology, clinical radiobiological modelling for conventional radiotherapy techniques as well as for protons and other ion beams. Radiobiological modelling has proved useful in radiotherapy, especially in situations where departures from protocols occur for a variety of reasons such as unintended treatment interruptions, errors in treatment delivery, dose-rate effect applications, comparisons of different techniques, dose-fractionation schedules, re-treatments and even in clinical trial design. These techniques, if suitably adapted, are capable of producing similar insights and practical guidelines in proton and other forms of ion beam therapy. The optimisation of proton and ion beam therapy is essential since there is considerable 'competition' from the more advanced forms of megavoltage photon-based radiotherapy, which allows fewer and highly focussed treatments to be given as well as being more economical.

The use of relatively simple mathematics and some very basic worked examples are included within the text, but has been kept to a minimum, so that *all the relevant disciplines* can understand the principles and then use the historical content and advice provided to develop the subject further. A basic knowledge of radiation biology is assumed, but references have been kept to the minimum necessary. The parameters chosen for exploratory modelling and illustrative purposes may require modification and further input for more specific clinical applications. Any errors are the sole responsibility of the author. There is inevitably some degree of repetition where this is considered essential.

The main approach has been to use the biological effective dose (BED) concept based on the linear quadratic (LQ) model of radiation effect. In recent years it has been possible to assess the BED values of charged-particle therapies such as protons and light ions by incorporation of the maximum and minimum limits of the relative biological effect (RBE), which accounts for the increasing complexity of DNA damage and the increasing proportion of non-repairable damage that occurs when the linear energy transfer (LET) of a radiation is increased. Typically LET increases within the Bragg peak region for charged particles, with resultant increments in RBE, but the RBE reduces with increasing dose and also at very high LET values; and it is important to realise that different biosystems will have quite different RBE values. The topic of RBE remains controversial, although it is being increasingly understood, and there are several models that attempt to link LET with RBE, many of which use formidable mathematics. In contrast, this book addresses how to achieve this by using relatively simple mathematics. Such a simpler approach can be understood by physicians, physicists and biologists. More complex approaches can be limited in their usefulness due to excessive and/or restrictive assumptions and the limits of what can be known. Simpler models, although they must always need caveats, are capable of providing useful qualitative and quantitative understanding of the basic principles which govern clinical outcomes.

This subject is as such multi-disciplinary, and based on a triangular arrangement with physics, medicine and biology forming the apices of an isosceles triangle (figure P.1). The decisive middle ground has to be covered by individuals who have sufficient knowledge and experience of all three disciplines. A basic knowledge of these three subjects and the inter-disciplinary subject of radiation biology is assumed, along with basic aspects of particle therapy such as the Bragg peak effect, the characteristics of the spread-out Bragg peak (SOBP) and how this may be achieved. The author is minded that the text should be reasonably understood by members of all these disciplines, although additional reading will be required from review articles and textbooks to supplement cross-disciplinary understanding. Also, that each primary discipline is divided into a spectrum of further specialisation groups: physicists, split into fundamental particle physicists, accelerator or detector physicists and their medical physicist colleagues; in biology, there are purely molecular biologists (biochemists) concerned with *in vitro* work, biophysicists (physiologists), pharmacologists and zoologists, some concerned with *in vivo* animal testing; and within the faculties of medicine, the knowledge base is spread over anatomy, all forms of pathophysiology, oncology, surgery, patient management as well as a broad interest in epidemiology. Also, many non-biologically trained physicists have had a very significant influence in advancing radiobiology and that, given the added complexities of charged-particle physics, their continued involvement will be essential to understanding particle therapy and its associated radiobiology.

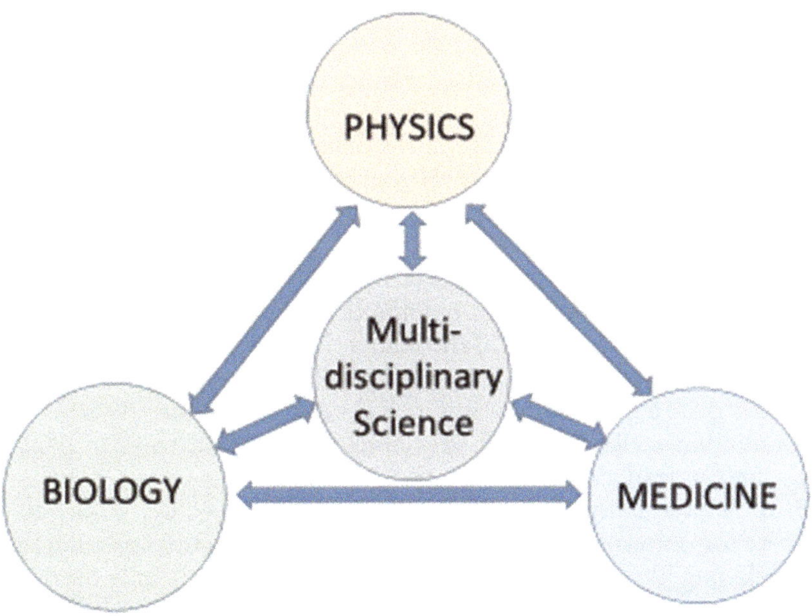

Figure P.1. The central role of multidisciplinary science which must include quantitative radiobiological modelling.

With all these facets in mind, it is necessary to write sympathetically for the non-specialist, but to furnish sufficient detail regarding many necessary fundamental aspects across these topics, while providing more detailed information for the practitioner or researcher in this field. For reasons of space and economy, it has been necessary to omit the classical graphs and diagrams associated with the basic sciences, but which can be found in standard textbooks. In most instances, since most readers of this book will be familiar with these, the brief qualitative descriptions and definitions provided will act as an *aide-mémoire*.

The medical decision-makers of the future in particle therapy will need broad scientific backgrounds, excellent clinical and oncological training, and be able to appreciate the strengths and weaknesses of the available mathematical models that link the clinical, biological and physical parameters, and which can be used to protect the patient against over- or underdosages. Modelling is a necessary way of quantitative communication between the three apices already referred to, in the important multi-disciplinary centre ground, complementing rational verbal or written approaches. In essence, this must be kept sufficiently simple in order for all disciplines to interact.

Considerable practice is necessary to become familiar and competent in this subject. The calculations may appear to be deceptively easy, as only knowledge of some higher school mathematics is necessary, and this can be aided by computer software systems such as Mathematica, Matlab and Maple. However, some of the clinically based calculations are quite protracted, with many more pitfalls (due to RBE, LET, etc.) than for similar calculations in the case of photon-based treatments. To aid the estimation of RBE and isoffective doses, some interactive sections have been introduced to the text by Dr Moore.

There are many who regard particle therapy as just a seamless extension of photon-based radiotherapy. This is certainly useful in terms of departmental organisation within a hospital structure, to ensure good patient access and to capitalise on site-specialist knowledge of the oncologist in terms of detailed regional anatomy and indications for therapy. However, owing to the added complexity of particle therapy, there is an essential need to educate and train all the sub-disciplines involved in treatment delivery and patient management, in order to inform them of the strengths and weaknesses of particle therapy, and by knowing these to continually search for better, highly optimised therapy.

Depending on the background of the reader, it is not necessary to read the whole of the book. Chapter 1 provides the essential physics background, mostly for the benefit of biologists and clinicians, but includes the importance of the choice of the reference radiation in RBE studies as well as the different ways in which LET is expressed, and introduces the potentially important parameter of inter-track distance. In chapter 2, the basis of radiobiological modelling is introduced, with formulations for conventional megavoltage photon radiotherapy and for particle therapy, including low and high dose, dose-rate variations and the useful BED concept. Chapters 3 and 4 have been written for persons who have little or no previous experience of radiotherapy, with discussion of the essential medical aspects of treatment planning, including the influence of surgery and other factors on tissue viability. Some of the key historical developments in radiotherapy are covered in chapter 5, as well as what has been learned from extensive basic and clinical research using fast neutrons for modern applications with charged particles. Chapter 6 considers dose-fractionation effects in photon and particle therapy, with some worked examples.

The rationale for using a variable as opposed to the conventional constant RBE in proton therapy is provided in chapter 7. This is followed by the description of a relatively simple 'energy efficiency' model for estimation of RBE values for any ion beam in chapter 8. More specific applications in proton therapy are given in chapter 9, with some tables that suggest tentative RBE allocations for variable values of LET in different classes of tissues and tumours. Chapter 10 describes a system for estimating risk in the central nervous system and which is designed to be user-friendly in that no RBE-LET models are used, and is considered necessary where the full prescribed proton dose has to be given to a critical normal tissue. Chapter 11 considers the reductions in RBE which have been found in experimental work, where passively scattered beam SOBPs are repositioned from superficial to much deeper positions, whereas no such RBE reductions are found with scanned pencil beams, with important implications.

The correction of unintended treatment interruptions for high-LET treatments, with worked examples, is described in chapter 12, which also includes formulations for assessing re-treatment doses in the central nervous system. Chapter 13 considers the radiobiological correction of Bragg peak placement errors, resulting in deviations in both LET and dose. Chapter 14 contains further possible future developments to improve our overall understanding and especially to obtain more accurate modelling parameters, as well as methods of assessing the potential impact of concomitant drug sensitisation with high-LET radiations.

It is hoped that this book will not only improve the safety and effectiveness of particle therapies, but also inspire further research and enquiry.

Acknowledgements

I am extremely grateful for the help and encouragement provided by the following:

1. Many colleagues who have inspired me over many years to seek solutions to high-LET problems, too large a number to mention individually, but especially Roger Dale, Gillies McKenna, John Hopewell, Oliver Scott, Jack Fowler, Mark Hill, Boris Vojnovic, Ken Peach, Claire Timlin, Herman Suit, Michael Goitein, Tony Lomax, Peter O'Neil, Dudley Goodhead, Kevin Prise, Stuart Green, Alex Carabe-Fernandez, Karen Kirkby, David Colling, Douglas Errington, Andrzej Kacperek, Richard Britten and Hilmar Warenius. Also, to the late Edmund Wilson (CERN) for stimulating discussions.
2. CERN, Geneva for a Visiting Scientist award during 2014, and to the Director General for the award of Guest Professor 2015–2016, with the support of Prof Manjit Dosanjh.
3. The Principals and Fellows of Brasenose College, Oxford 2010–2015, especially Sir Roger Cashmore, and Green Templeton College as from 2017.

B.J. has been an investigator on several UK Research Council and EU FP-7 funded grants concerned with particle therapy, including ENVISION (241851), ENTERVISION (264552), and ULICE (228436), to The Medical Research Council UK for support to study radiobiology (1980–83) and to The Cyclotron Trust (2000–05), and advises the European Particle Therapy Network.

Also, to all the journals which have published my work on this subject, and for reproduction of graphics, some of which are included in this book.

Author biographies

Bleddyn Jones

After studying Medicine at Cambridge, with some mathematics, and developing an interest in cancer topics with Dr Donald Cater ScD FRCS, he underwent clinical and postgraduate training at Guy's, St Thomas's, St Bartholomew's and The Royal London Hospitals. As part of a Medical Research Council Earmarked Fellowship, he studied for a London University Radiobiology MSc and then undertook research in tumour cell kinetics before his clinical oncology training. Consultant and academic appointments were held at Clatterbridge (University of Liverpool), Hammersmith (Imperial College) and Birmingham, before becoming Professor of Clinical Radiation Biology at Oxford University, where his research concentrated on developing new mathematical models of RBE in particle therapy, as well as re-treatments and radiosurgery, all extensions of previous applied research to reduce toxicity in gynaecological brachytherapy and in brain tumour treatments as part of long collaborations with Professor R. G. Dale. He helped design and participated in many teaching courses, such as the Radiobiology MSc at Oxford, on particle therapy at CERN for many years, and held a Guest Professorship there while acting as Secretary to the Medical Applications Committee.

Joshua Moore

Joshua Moore graduated in Mathematics at Cardiff University, followed by a PhD in applied mathematics, supervised by Dr Thomas E. Woolley, primarily focusing on developing multi-scale mathematical models to investigate organoid formation. Whilst at Cardiff he won many academic prizes and worked with Professors Jones and Hopewell on re-treatments using photons, protons and other ions as well as radiosurgery. His additional research interests are in applying mathematics in biological areas of sub-cellular dynamics, pattern formation, virology and oncology. Subsequently, he has been appointed as a post-doctorate Research Associate in the Mathematical Institute at the University of Oxford, where he is primarily interested in unravelling the information contained in the spatial properties of cellular biology to explore questions in cancer detection, optimal treatment planning and cellular self-organisation, intercellular communication and dynamic tissue morphologies. For further information, see https://bit.ly/GoogleScholarJWM.

Glossary of the main terms and symbols used (some others are given in specific chapters)

α, the radiosensitivity coefficient of the LQ model per unit dose, in units of Gy^{-1}.

α_L, refers to α for the low-LET condition when high- and low-LET qualities are being compared.

α_H, refers to α for the high-LET condition when high- and low-LET qualities are being compared.

α_U, the ultimate value of α at the turnover point of the LET–RBE relationship.

β, similarly is the radiosensitivity coefficient of the LQ model per unit dose squared, in units of Gy^{-2}.

β_L, β_H and β_U refer to the same specifications as for α.

α/β, this important ratio, in units of Gy, determines the dose per fraction sensitivity in an inverse sense, such that low values (2–3 Gy) show large dose per fraction sensitivity, but high values denote low dose per fraction sensitivity (those above 7 Gy).

$(\alpha/\beta)_L$, refers to the low-LET ratio in situations where low- and high-LET radiation qualities are being compared.

$(\alpha/\beta)_H$, refers to the high-LET ratio in situations where low- and high-LET radiation qualities are being compared.

ω, the average cellular doubling time during radiation.

μ_F, the DNA repair rate constant for the fast component of repair.

μ_S, the DNA repair rate constant for the slow component of repair.

Absorbed dose, refers to the energy absorbed in a specified mass, in units of $J\ kg^{-1}$.

BED, the biological effective dose, in units of Gy, which expresses the dose required to achieve a specific bioeffect if given in ultra-small dose fractions, and represents a ceiling of dose which can be used for comparative purposes.

d, the dose per fraction, in units of Gy; D is the total dose (or $n \cdot d$).

E, the negative logarithm of the surviving fraction, often referred to as the log cell kill, which is proportional to the surviving fraction

Fluence, refers to the number of radiation tracks crossing a specified area.

f, refers to the mean inter-fraction interval, in days. For example, if five treatments per week are given $f = 7\text{days}/(5–1) = 7/4 = 1.75$ days.

g, the ratio of a specified normal tissue dose divided by the tumour dose.

h, the incomplete repair parameter for closely spaced treatments.

KERMA, refers to the kinetic energy released per unit mass, in units of $J\ kg^{-1}$.

K, the BED equivalent of cellular repopulation, expressed as Gy $days^{-1}$.

LET, the linear energy transfer parameter, defined as the energy release per unit length of track in the track plane, expressed in units of keV μm^{-1}. (Further definitions are given in chapter 1.)

LET_U, the value of LET at the turnover point of the LET–RBE relationship.

LET_C, the value of LET of the low-LET control radiation quality.

LET_x, any specified value of LET for the test high-LET radiation.

N, the number of dose fractions in a treatment course (or schedule).

RBE, defined as the ratio of dose for a low-LET (control) radiation divided by the dose of the high-LET test radiation in order to achieve the same specified bioeffect.

RBE_{max}, the limiting value of RBE at very low dose (approaching zero dose) for any specified high-LET radiation when compared with a low-LET radiation.

RBE_{min}, the asymptotic limiting value of RBE at very high dose for any specified high-LET radiation when compared with a low-LET radiation.

RBE_C, an intermediate value of RBE where the following conditions apply: $R_{max}/R_{min}^2 = (\alpha/\beta)_H/(\alpha/\beta)_L$.

Radiation quality, refers to the LET of a radiation at a specified energy.

SF, the surviving fraction of cells in an experiment.

S, a formulation for combining the geometrical sparing (g factor) with the uncertainties of knowledge regarding the most appropriate RBE value in normal tissues and tumour.

T_K, the lag time, in days, that may occur before cellular repopulation is manifest.

Z, the nuclear charge.

z, the tumour dose if the normal tissue dose is specified as d.

Chapter 1

Particle physics for biological interactions

Basic descriptions of the particle beam parameters, dosimetry and the different forms of linear energy transfer (LET) are provided, together with some of the physical uncertainties that are inevitably present in particle therapy. The potentially important concept of the average inter-track separation distance (s) is introduced. This will depend on beam geometry since s will increase with depth in divergent beams, and also near-instantaneous values of s will increase with reduction of dose rate. The interaction of the above factors with radiobiology is quantified by the relative biological effect (RBE), which influences the actual dose given to a patient. A review of the influence of the reference (or control) radiation on RBE studies is provided. This concludes that only beams which ionise mostly via the Compton scattering process should be used, namely 137-caesium (^{137}Cs) or cobalt-60 (^{60}Co) isotopes, or megavoltage photons, or electrons; otherwise, with orthovoltage or lower-voltage x-rays, the RBEs obtained will be lower than what is appropriate for clinical use. The important potential issue of the reduction of RBE with increasing depth placement of spread-out Bragg peaks in the case of passively scattered (divergent) beams, but not in scanned (non-divergent) pencil beams, which may be related to differences in s and simultaneous reductions in the dose rate, is considered and suggestions made for further studies and applications.

1.1 Physical beam parameters, essential dosimetry and reference (or control) radiation requirements for RBE studies

This chapter, intended more for the benefit of biologists rather than physicists, includes a short qualitative description of the physics base of photon and particle therapy, including linear energy transfer (LET) and its variants, and finally the choice of the control or reference radiation for relative biological effect (RBE) studies. It is assumed that the reader will be familiar with the Bragg peak and how these peaks are spread out to cover a defined clinical target volume. By increasing the beam energy, the peak will occur at greater depth values. A comprehensive

doi:10.1088/978-0-7503-6209-2ch1

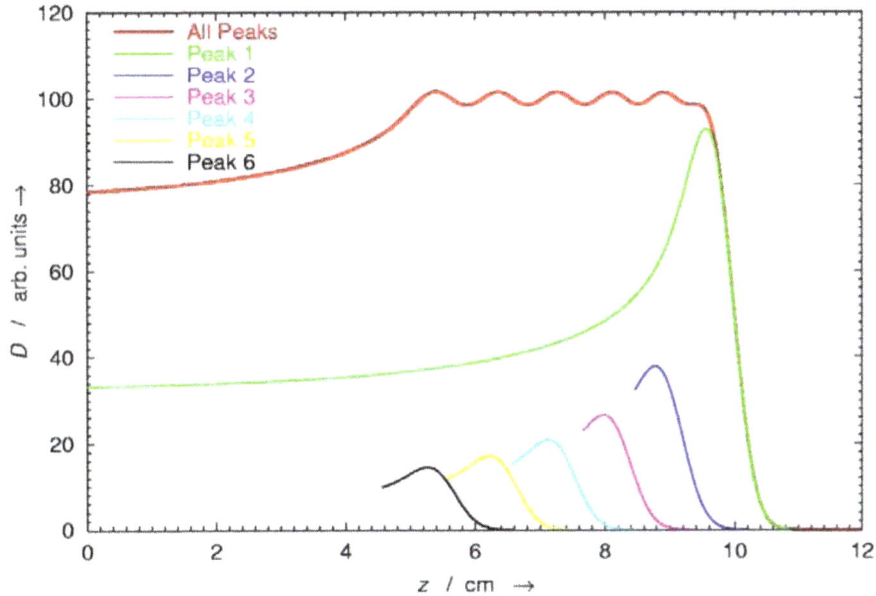

Figure 1.1. Absorbed dose D is shown as a function of depth z in water from a spread-out Bragg peak (SOBP, uppermost curve) and its constituent pristine Bragg peaks (for the lower curves, for clarity, all but the deepest pristine Bragg peak are only partly drawn). In many cases the clinical target volume is larger than the width of a pristine Bragg peak. Appropriate modulation of the proton energy range by using different energies from the highest (Peak 1), which provides dose to the greatest depth, and then with progressively reduced energies to provide peaks at each of the lower depths, the lowest energy providing Peak 6. The fluence (here proportional to the height of each peak) is also varied in order to provide the intended uniform dose to the target, although in this example there is some undulation of the 'All Peaks' summated dose from each separate energy contribution because of the low number of peaks used for illustrative purposes. Reproduced from Newhauser & Zhang (2015). © IOP Publishing Ltd. CC BY 3.0.

account of 'the physics of proton therapy', by Newhauser & Zhang (2015), is appropriate only for physicists, but their figure 15 is reproduced here as figure 1.1, and shows the dose (D) for multiple Bragg peaks obtained by using different proton energies resulting in peaks at different depths (indicated by z on the abscissa) to form a plateau of relatively uniform dose when they are all summated. It should be noted that the flat section of the green line is composed of low-LET radiation, with the high LET being within the Bragg peak and with the maximum LET at its end. The reader is encouraged to cross-refer to this diagram while reading this chapter.

Spread-out Bragg peaks (SOBPs) include a range of carefully selected energies which result in a plateau of relatively uniform dose, but will inevitably have greater LET towards its distal end as the Bragg peaks in that region are not as 'diluted' in terms of LET by lower-LET parts of the beam as occurs at the proximal part of the SOBP. The use of SOBPs is essential to cover the physical dimensions of malignant or benign tumours and their associated margins where cellular extensions can be found.

First, it is necessary to understand the basic concepts that underpin radiation dosimetry and the important differences between photon and positively charged particle therapies. For those less familiar with radiotherapy physics or who wish to revise the key aspects, a brief summary is provided, concentrating on important definitions that lead up to the concept of LET and its various forms. For more complete descriptions, the reader should consult standard textbooks.

Radiation fluence refers to the number of radiation beamlets (or individual tracks, *N*) within a beam which crosses a unit surface area, that is, N/A, where A is the area covered by the whole beam, and so the units are in cm^{-2}.

It should be noted that the fluence rate may vary considerably with technique, and will influence the near-instantaneous inter-track distances, as well as contribute to dose-rate changes.

KERMA signifies the kinetic energy released per unit mass of a specified mass of medium, by release of secondary particles such as delta rays and all ionisation products. However, some of the energy released (in J kg^{-1}) will be sufficient to pass beyond the volume of the mass of interest and be absorbed elsewhere. Consequently, it was necessary for the physicist L. H. Gray to define the **absorbed dose** as the energy absorbed by a mass of interest, again in J kg^{-1}, which should include not only the primary ionisation events but also all secondary particles such as delta rays, neutrons, recoiled neutrons/protons and fragmented ions that make a contribution.

Most dose calculations are performed for unit density water, so mass and volume have the same number. For denser structures, such as bone or lower-density air cavities, the absorbed dose is larger and smaller, respectively, and is often assumed to be mainly dependent on electron density in the case of megavoltage x-rays (photons) in the most commonly used clinical range (4–8 MeV); lower-energy x-rays (especially below 100 keV, which may form part of the x-ray spectrum from x-ray generators, which may have higher peak energies such as 200–300 keV) cause ionisation by the photoelectric effect in proportion to the atomic charge cubed (i.e. Z^3). In contrast, uncharged fast neutrons preferentially interact with neutron-deficient nuclei such as hydrogen, producing recoil protons, so that richly hydrogenated compounds, such as lipid-rich tissues (such as myelin in brain white matter and fat) have a greater KERMA than water.

To arrive at the absorbed dose, use is made of energy transfer coefficients and radiation absorption parameters. It is important to note that the loss of dose with depth for a divergent radiation, for example x-rays emanating from a high-Z metal target, are mostly due to inverse square law (ISL) effects as well as due to tissue absorption. For highly collimated beams, such as pencil beams, ISL effects are much reduced.

Particle beams can delivered in two ways:

1) Scanned pencil beams, where divergence is minimal until the very end of the range.
2) Passively scattered beams (often using a double system of scattering filters), with resultant divergence and ISL effects. The divergence of the beam with tissue depth reduces the instantaneous fluence.

There is some further divergence effect in all cases, caused by Coulombic force scattering of similarly positively charged particles (when stripped of their electrons), but this depends on their energy (and so velocity) and mass (each of which reduce the scattering when large), so that such late divergence occurs with scanned pencil beams when the velocity slows down sufficiently.

In particle therapy the intended absorbed dose is normally prescribed as an equivalent dose. This can cause confusion to practitioners, since the equivalent dose has been expressed in different ways, for example the cobalt equivalent Gy, or Gy equivalent (or eq-Gy), or Gy-RBE or RBE-Gy, where the particle dose has been reduced by the working RBE value in order to achieve the same intended effect as from, say, megavoltage x-rays or photons. Further confusion is caused by the standard expression for equivalent Gy, for example as

$$\text{Gy} - \text{RBE absorbed dose} = \text{particle absorbed dose} \times \text{RBE},$$

but it is important to realise and understand the rearrangement, which is used in practice, as

$$\text{particle absorbed dose} = \text{Gy} - \text{RBE absorbed dose} \div \text{RBE}.$$

The physician chooses the most appropriate equivalent Gy (or RBE-Gy) dose of photons (or x-rays); this is then divided by the RBE to provide the physical absorbed dose of particles given to the patient.

In routine clinical megavoltage x-ray (photon) therapy, the ionisation is relatively uniform along the radiation track. The depth dose curve for a monoenergetic and non-divergent beam shows a fairly constant fractional loss of absorbed dose per unit distance traversed from its initial maximum (d_{max}) dose so that at deeper distances (denoted by x) the dose d_x can be approximated as $d_x = d_{\text{max}}\ \mathrm{e}^{-\mu x}$, where μ is the attenuation coefficient. The same is not true along a charged-particle beam since slowing of the particle increases the energy loss (E) per unit distance (x), denoted by $\mathrm{d}E/\mathrm{d}x$. This is because of the increasing probability that opposite Coulombic charges will interact, causing more ionisation and so increased KERMA and locally absorbed dose, the extreme case being at the distal part of the Bragg peak itself. Since the ionisation probability changes with depth it is useful to consider a further parameter, the LET, which reflects the closeness of local ionisations along a beam track. LET is not only relevant to charged particles but also to low-energy photons/x-rays since whenever photon energy falls to the keV range, their secondary particles have lower energy and a higher LET.

Linear energy transfer, or LET, is defined as the energy lost per unit length of medium by a charged particle, where the unit of length is small (1 μm), which covers the approximate thickness of a chromosome. LET is expressed, for example, as 1 keV μm^{-1} (equivalent to 1.602 J m^{-1}). There are several variants of LET; the most appropriate for use in RBE estimation remains debatable, but the choice is as follows:

1. L_Δ, where Δ refers to the maximum limit of energy (e.g. L_{100} would consider only energies below 100 keV μm^{-1}), also LET as total energy loss (L_∞).

This latter parameter reflects 'stopping power' in the medium, and so includes its density, with units expressed as MeV cm^2 g^{-1}, or J m^2 kg^{-1}.

2. If there are different energies in a beam, as might be the case with fast neutrons or SOBP charged particles, a LET spectrum can be used, calculated as either a 'track average' or as 'absorbed dose average' (or energy average) LET.
3. In micro-dosimetry, the unsatisfactory aspects of 'average LET' are often overcome by graphical presentations of LET plotted against dose fraction per log LET interval.
4. The lineal energy (y), which takes account of stochastic energy deposition (whereas LET does not). This is defined as $y = \varepsilon / d_{av}$, where ε is the energy imparted in a volume, with d_{av} being the mean track chord length in the volume.
5. The final variant, with attractive properties for biomolecular considerations, is to account for delta rays ejected from tracks. These delta rays are radially distributed and responsible for most bioeffects and ionisations collected by detectors. With considerable acumen, Katz *et al* (1971) proposed the use of $Z^{*2}.\beta^{-2}$, where $Z^* =$ the effective nuclear charge of an atomic nucleus of atomic charge Z and β is the relativistic velocity (v/c), in order to estimate the effective radius of ionisation, and which should correlate with bioeffectiveness. It must be realised that as fully stripped ions slow down they pick up electrons while causing ionisation (so Z^* becomes less than Z), the parameter will change with depth. This is discussed further in chapter 8.

The loss of energy E with distance in a medium is well described by the Bethe–Bloch equation:

$$-\frac{dE}{dx} = \frac{4\pi}{m_e c^2} \cdot \frac{nz^2}{\beta^2} \cdot \left(\frac{e^2}{4\pi\varepsilon_0}\right)^2 \cdot \left[\ln\left(\frac{2m_e c^2 \beta^2}{I \cdot (1 - \beta^2)}\right) - \beta^2\right].$$

This equation can be simplified as

$$-dE/dx(\text{Energy/cm}) = K\ (\text{charge}^2/\text{velocity}^2),$$

where K replaces the constant physical parameters.

It can easily be seen that for a proton (charge = 1) or carbon (charge = 6, if all electrons are stripped away), the energy loss will depend on the Z number but will increase sharply as velocity falls. This occurs as particles slow down through a medium. After such slowing, they interact with orbital electrons in nearby molecules and cause ionisation. The Bragg peak represents a sharp rise in dE/dx with loss of velocity or energy at increasing depth. The initial energy or velocity will govern the complete range (or depth) of energy deposition, so beams with higher incident energies at the level of the skin will have Bragg peaks at greater depths.

1.1.1 Straggling and fragmentation

These terms are used to describe the variation in path length caused by differences in energy and velocity reduction through a medium or tissue, due largely to differences in interactions along the beam path because of variations in electron density/tissue composition and other stochastic events. It normally denotes a blurring-like effect on the beam towards its distal edge, but there is also some degree of lateral straggling for particles that are more easily scattered. Thus, the beam edge is not so sharp with protons, which are lighter than helium or carbon ions. For even heavier ions such as carbon, there is a distinct fragmentation tail caused by nuclear interactions and emitted gamma rays, which result in a tail of dose beyond the end of the Bragg peaks. For lighter particles such as protons, fragmented ions do not occur but, as with heavier particles, the tissue interactions can cause emission of gamma rays and some neutrons.

1.1.2 Separation of charged particles with increasing tissue depth

The Coulombic forces due to the nuclear charge will cause charged particles to separate from each other gradually in proportion to their tissue depth and also in inverse proportion to their mass and velocity. This will occur in a beam traversing a vacuum. This is often referred to as 'Coulombic scattering', but which in matter will also include much wider-angle scattering due to repulsive-charge interactions with atomic nuclei (as in the classical example of Rutherford scattering). So, protons (charge = 1, mass unit = 1) will separate less than electrons (charge = 1, mass = ~1/2000 of mass unit); compared to protons, heavier ions (also containing neutrons, so having mass greater than their Z number) show lesser deviation despite their increased charge, even if fully 'stripped' of electrons before their acceleration, although some particles will gain electrons during their transit through matter.

There appears to be no formal term which describes the average or median inter-track separation distances, which may contribute to biological effect changes over and above the LET, as discussed below. It is easy to crudely estimate the mean inter-track separation distances (s) by the following basic approach (see figure 1.2).

The overall area A is divided by the number of tracks to provide (A/N) the average area surrounding each track; if this is assumed to be a small square area (represented by s^2), then $A/N = s^2$. If, on average, the track occupies the centre of each square, then the average track separation will be s, which is $\sqrt{(A/N)}$, and which can also be expressed as $\sqrt{\frac{1}{F}}$, where F is the fluence (defined above). This might be an important parameter to use in the analysis of cell-survival studies and treatment outcomes, as it could modify the effect of LET and dose. For example, even if the LET parameter is calculated to be the same at, say, the mid-Bragg peak for the same particle type but accelerated to two quite different energies resulting in Bragg peaks at two different depths (where the particle energies will then be the same), any reduction in bioeffectiveness could be due to greater separation of tracks in the case of the particles that were accelerated to the higher energy. Such a process would depend on increasing track separation due to Coulombic scattering, and even more

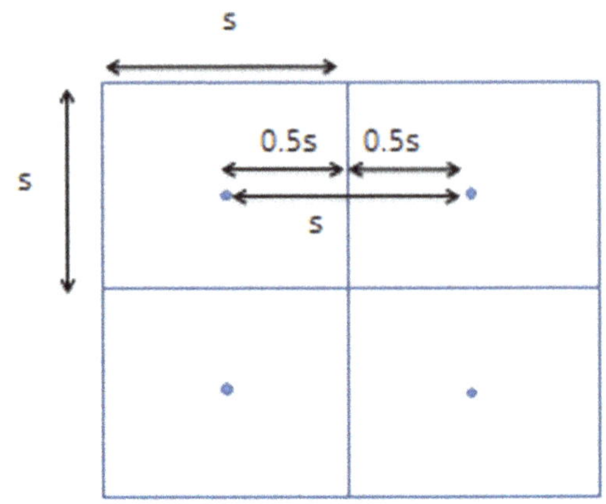

Figure 1.2. Four particle tracks are represented in cross section by central points within a square of side s; the inter-track distance is then s. For N tracks, the overall area (A) is Ns^2.

so by the deliberate use of scattering filters, causing ISL geometric dispersion of the beam at increasing depths.

This can be further expressed in a very simple way.

Consider tracks of radius a, with volume $\pi a^2.x$ when considered as a cylinder extending to depth x. The inter-track distance is s, so that the fractional volume occupied by a single track compared with its surrounding volume of s^2x is

$$\frac{\pi a^2 x}{s^2 x} = \frac{\pi a^2 N}{A} = \pi a^2.\ F$$

(since $s^2 = 1/F = A/N$).

For the same fluence, as the overall area (A) of a beam reduces, the closeness of tracks per unit area (and volume) increases. But if A increases, the fluence falls and the closeness of tracks decreases. For different ions, the specific Katz track radius may be used.

Such an effect can actually be visualised using GEANT4 and FLUKA in-silico simulations, shown to the present author by Drs David Colling (Imperial College) and Francesca Fiorini (Oxford), respectively. Although the LET may be similar for each track at each depth, their increased separation may be sufficient to diminish the bioeffect since more cell nuclear material or even whole cells may be unirradiated. Some evidence for a reduced bioeffectiveness with depth only in the case of passively scattered beams is given below.

1.1.3 Particle accelerators

Synchrotrons and cyclotrons are the commonest accelerators used for charged-particle medical beams. These terms can confuse since modern cyclotrons are in fact synchro-cyclotrons, but the more basic nomenclature remains useful. Printing space does not permit a full description of these. For a summary of how these accelerators operate, the reader should refer to short accounts such as Peach *et al* (2011), designed for hospital readers, with more complete accounts by Wilson (2001) in his excellent textbook, which contains ample worked examples concerning beam control, and so on. Cyclotrons have a circular cavity arrangement to accelerate protons to their peak energy, when they are then extracted. To produce lower energies that result in Bragg peaks at depths less than the maximum range, the beam must be degraded within metal or plastic strips of differing thicknesses (which become highly radioactive and must be situated sufficiently remote from the patient because of induced radiation including neutrons). Cyclotrons deliver high dose rates (0.5–1 Gy s^{-1}); for example, 12 Gy in 24 s is not unusual.

In contrast, synchrotrons, which are used to accelerate protons or particles heavier than helium, occupy a much larger floor space and operate by a single radiofrequency accelerator combined with magnetic focussing and defocussing in bending the beam around a geometrical arrangement of magnets, which lead the beam back to the original point for further acceleration. The magnetic field strength must be carefully increased to match the particle energies at each 'cycle'. When the desired energy is obtained, the 'particle bunch' is extracted and then delivered.

Considerable research has been devoted to laser-induced particle production. Here an intense laser beam is used to strike a target (which may be water or other hydrogenated materials for proton production) or thin metal foils for heavier ion production. The instantaneous dose rates are extremely high; the resultant beam, delivered in femtosecond bursts, and the repetition rate of the laser beam essentially governs its output.

Whatever the technique used for acceleration, there are two options for controlling beam size. First, the pencil beams delivered from the accelerator can be passively scattered by a filter(s) to cover a wider area, but with a small neutron contamination, depending on the efficiency and composition of the filter. The alternative is to use the pencil beam and magnetically deflect the beam to the positions required (active scanning), which avoids neutron production and provides better dose conformity to the intended targets.

In each case the energies delivered from these accelerators have a spread in terms of energy and in spatial properties. Some useful terms to denote these are as follows:

Luminosity refers to the total energy emitted, often expressed per unit time.

Emittance measures the average spread of particle coordinates with respect to their position in three-dimensional space and their momentum, with dimensions of length (e.g., metres) or length times angle (metres times radians). In a low-emittance particle beam, the particles are confined to a small distance and have nearly the same momentum. The probability of particle interactions will be greater, resulting in higher luminosity.

Also, further beam parameters include energy spread (in standard deviations), pulse repetition rate (f), bunches per macropulse (Mb) and effective bunch rate ($f.Mb$).

1.1.4 Proton range uncertainties

The energy spread of protons, their interactions in non-homogenous tissue, as well as physiological movement of tissues, all contribute to range uncertainties caused by variations in Bragg peak positions. These uncertainties will vary, depending on anatomical site, from millimetres to several centimetres (in the case of physiological movements such as breathing). Patient positioning variations, gain or loss of weight during treatment, with resultant changes in subcutaneous fat depths, and tumour shrinkage can all critically affect particle range, dose and LET distribution, with implications for tumour control and toxicities. Imaging of the SOBP position is improving; for example, proton nuclear activation of positron-emitting isotopes within the body results in a PET scanning signal detection to an accuracy of around 2 mm.

A clinical example of some of these considerations, as well as RBE allocation uncertainties, is given in figure 2 in Jones (2015, available on Open Access). This example illustrates the interdependence of dose, LET and RBE on the potential clinical outcomes. The proton 'dose' shown was calculated using an RBE conversion factor of 1.1. (the equivalent x-ray dose is divided by 1.1). The required 76 Gy dose to the target volume is achieved in both cases, but the proton plan spares the heart, a considerable volume of lung, and breast tissue, so reducing the later risk of breathlessness on exertion, sudden cardiac death and of radiation-induced breast cancer. The small ringed area anterior to the high-dose volume shows the position of the spinal cord, and the dose received to this structure appears to be the same for both treatment plans. Despite these attractive features, what if the RBE of 1.1 used in the dose prescription is higher than that of the tumour and lower than that of the spinal cord? Then, there would be enhanced risks of both tumour recurrence and spinal damage (resulting in paralysis of the lower limbs) when compared with the x-ray-based treatment. Also, the effect of increasing particle range, as might happen in a patient with weight loss (so reducing the subcutaneous fat and allowing the beam to travel further) might lead to a higher LET and dose in the spinal cord, increasing the risk of paralysis, while also lowering LET and dose to the tumour, so reducing the probability of tumour control. Weight gain may cause the opposite effects. The simplest allowance for changes in tissue distances would be to allow millimetre exchanges, assuming uniform tissue density. In this way, each millimetre lost or gained will shift the high-dose boundary in either direction by the same amount. The ballistic advantages, changes in dose distribution and these more uncertain aspects of proton beam therapy (PBT) should be mentioned in informed-consent procedures to patients, with explanation of how these risks can be minimised.

To reduce range instabilities, meticulous daily assessment of patient dimensions, accurate tumour localisation and patient immobilisation, etc, including confirmatory measurements made by non-ionising techniques such as ultrasonography, are necessary requirements. Improved dose-computing techniques and four-dimensional planning (the three dimensions of space and the fourth of time is included), including adaptive techniques to changes in normal tissues and tumour positions/dimensions with time, are even more important in PBT than conventional radiotherapy. Further details of these techniques, including proton radiography, are available elsewhere.

There has always been concern that the highest LET and RBE will occur towards the end of the particle range, even if the Bragg peaks are 'spread out' by the use of range filters or by the spot-scanning method. This is because of the greater proportion of high-LET radiation in the distal part of the beam; more proximal sections have a lower average LET due to a greater proportion of low LET in the non-plateau section of the SOBPs. The distal end will have the highest LET, which might lead to unintended clinical effects. This concern did lead to the intelligent use of 'patch field' techniques, which align lateral beam edges (rather than distal edges) against sensitive anatomical structures, when using passive beam scattering. In contrast, lateral beam-edge uncertainties are not so well understood. Beams diverge with depth due to Coulomb scattering, as well as geometric divergence with passively scattered beams. Lateral scatter must carry implications for higher LET values, since deviated particles will form Bragg peaks in a more lateral direction. Also, the track separations increase and are less linear, so a more micro-volumetric assessment of energy transfer (i.e. MVET) is indicated, as well as the number of particles per unit volume, related to the inter-track distances explained above. There is already evidence that with spot-scanned, intensity-modulated proton therapy high LET values can be found outside the tumour-bearing target volumes. This is perhaps explained by a greater proportion of partially overlapping beam edges, along with the additional weighting applied to some beamlets and the smaller inter-track distances.

In the case of carbon ions, the dose profile of each single field (composed of multiple Bragg peaks as in figure 1.1) was designed to compensate for the inevitable increase in LET along its path (Kanai *et al* 1997): deeper regions, where the LET is highest, receive less dose; shallower regions are allowed a higher dose because of the lower prevalent LET. Such an elegant arrangement has not been used for proton beams, but should be an urgent consideration especially when single or few field directions are used and if important functional normal tissue is exposed at these distal beam regions. Confirmation of a marked increase in side effects probably caused by enhanced RBE has been found for lung fibrosis in patients treated by single SOBP proton fields (Underwood & Paganetti 2016) and within the central nervous system (Eulitz *et al* 2023). The weighting of proton dose towards the distal end of the beam should be reduced to compensate for such an effect, although the extent will need to be determined by the dose per fraction used, using LET-RBE models as described in chapters 8 and 9.

1.2 Physics interacting with biology

1.2.1 Relative biological effect

The study of the relative biological effectiveness (RBE) of different radiation qualities is important, since the RBE concept is used in hadrontherapy dose prescription. RBE is defined as

$\text{RBE} = \frac{\text{Dose of control (low LET) radiation}}{\text{Dose of reference (higher LET) hadron radiation}}$ for the same bioeffect using each class (or quality) of radiation.

For RBE to exceed unity, the numerator must be greater than the denominator; for this to occur, the numerator must have the lower LET. If this is not the case, the RBE values will be less than 1.

RBE is dependent on the LET of the radiation, with initial increase in RBE with LET, followed by a reduction at higher LET values due to overkill or cell killing inefficiency, the turnover point LET (or LET_U) being dependent on the nuclear charge (z) of the ion, its velocity and possibly mass, but not apparently the cell type. Combinations of kinematic properties have been assessed by Jones and Hill (i.e. DATE) for many ions. It appears that each ion, from hydrogen to iron, has a unique value of LET_U.

RBE is also inversely related to dose for reasons related to differences in cellular radiosensitivities and the slope of the effectiveness curves between the reference (or control) low-LET radiation and the higher-LET state. This is illustrated in figure 1.3, based on the linear quadratic model of radiation effect (E), where $E = \alpha d + \beta d^2$, d being the dose, α and β the biological coefficients, and with subscripts L and H for the low- and high-LET states; more details regarding the radiobiology are given in chapter 2 and subsequently. The RBE falls from 1.27 to 1.2 with increasing dose due

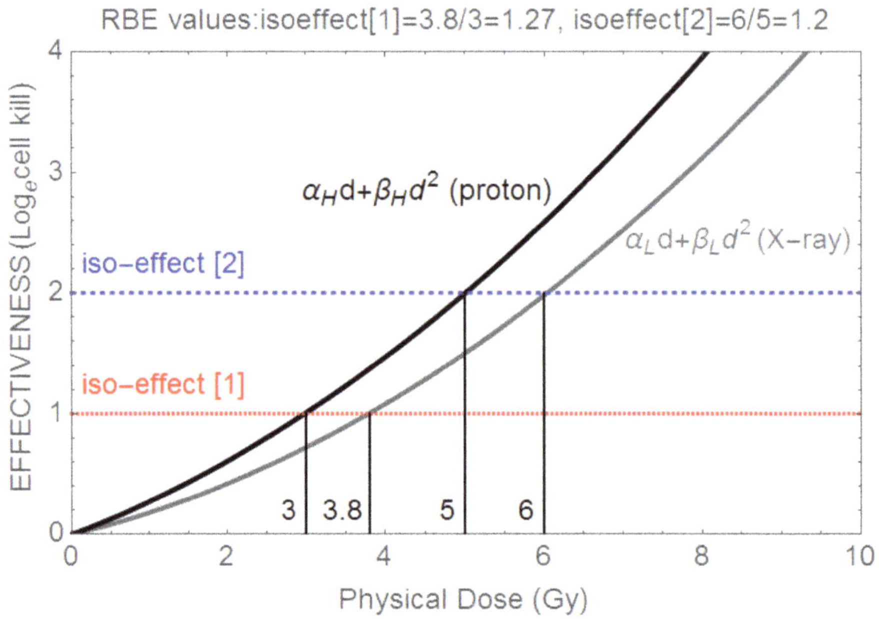

Figure 1.3. Demonstration of the RBE principle for two dose-effectiveness curves produced by x-rays (photons) and protons (assuming $\alpha_L = 0.15$ Gy^{-1}, $\alpha_H = 0.24$ Gy^{-1}, $\beta_L = 0.03$ Gy^{-2} and $\beta_H = 0.032$ Gy^{-2}) and where two different iso-effect levels [1] and [2] are considered and their corresponding RBEs are shown. The numbers 3, 3.8, 5 and 6 refer to the physical doses where each iso-effect line meets each curve, respectively: d_H followed by d_L for iso-effect [1] and d_H and d_L for iso-effect [2]. RBE is given by d_L/d_H in each case, as shown above the figure frame.

to the geometry of the curves and will reduce further with increasing dose. Such a change is an inherent feature of the linear quadratic (or LQ) model providing that the LET-induced increment in α exceeds that in β (as further discussed in chapters 8 and 9).

The RBE concept was included in the dose-prescription system for fast neutron therapy and continues to be important in proton and ion beam therapy; it is also potentially relevant in nuclear medicine and some forms of brachytherapy, but has not yet been used in their clinical applications. It is also useful when considering ultra-high dose rates or FLASH radiotherapy where the dose-rate intensity increases such that the near-instantaneous micro-volumetric LET increases at the same time as increasing oxygen depletion rates, with resultant changes in radiosensitivity parameters α and β so that the ratio of α/β increases substantially (discussed in chapters 2, 8 and 14) with emerging radioresistance.

In experiments to determine RBE, the choice of the control (or reference) radiation has varied considerably: examples include low-voltage x-rays (100–200 keV peak) and orthovoltage (200–350 keV peak), which inevitably contain lower energies than the peak value, along with variable degrees of filtration to remove the lowermost keV x-rays within the x-ray spectrum. Other examples include caesium-137 (^{137}Cs) or cobalt-60 (^{60}Co) gamma rays, megavoltage electrons, and more rarely megavoltage x-rays in the clinical range 4–10 MeV. The lower the energy of any beam, the greater is the LET: this applies to x-rays and gamma rays, protons, all ions and electrons, because lower energies result in more localised energy release and absorption, a higher LET, and results in more clustered DNA damage. This will increase RBE up to a saturation level beyond which RBE falls at even higher LET values. Conversely, the higher the energy of a particle or photon beam, then the local LET (and RBE) is reduced, because the ionisations are less clustered.

Since the reference radiation (sometimes called the control radiation) supplies the numerator dose for the RBE estimation, this must exceed the hadron radiation dose for the same bioeffect in order for the RBE to be greater than 1. Should the control RBE irradiator have an LET that is greater than the test hadron LET, then the RBE will be less than 1. Choosing a control irradiator that has a higher LET than that of the photons/x-rays used in hospital clinics will give a lower estimate of RBE than would be the case in the hospital setting for the same cellular system.

1.2.2 Choice of the control (or reference) radiation source

It follows that the choice of the reference radiation will have an important effect on the RBE ratio found. For example Hall & Gaccia (2011) quote typical LET values (keV μm^{-1}) of 2 for 250 keV (but the filtration is unspecified), 0.2 for 60-Co, 4.7 for 10 MeV protons and 0.5 for 150 MeV protons, while megavoltage photons are not mentioned. More comprehensive data, though even these are incomplete, can be found in Report 16 by the ICRU (1970). These suggest, by extrapolation, that megavoltage photons in the clinical range of 4–8 MeV would have a LET value of around 0.2 keV μm^{-1}. A useful collation of data in Andrews (1978) shows a mean LET of 0.5 keV μm^{-1} for 3 MeV photons and 60-Co irradiation, but stopping powers (or LET_∞) of 0.18 for 2 MeV electrons as well as being the theoretical minimum for any charged particle, and hence an important limit or baseline for relative biological effect studies. The average Compton electrons produced from 60-Co gamma rays have a LET_∞ of 0.26 keV μm^{-1}, so a slightly lower value around 0.2 keV μm^{-1} would be expected from clinical range megavoltage photons.

Further information is contained in some publications, such as Spadinger and Palcic (1992), where an LET range of 5.5–6 keV μm^{-1} is quoted for 25 keV x-rays and 1.7 keV μm^{-1} for 122 KeV x-rays (the average value obtained with 250 KeV x-rays with 0.35 mm copper and 0.4 mm tin filtration), with a value of 0.2 keV μm^{-1} for 11 MeV electrons, which are likely to closely resemble megavoltage photons in the clinical range.

From the above data, it seems reasonable to use a control radiation of either electrons of photons, according to the experiment being done, with a LET value of around 0.2 keV μm^{-1} as would be achieved with a clinical photon or electron beam. The added value of having a megavoltage photon beam would be for comparative combined ballistic and radiobiological studies in humanoid phantoms between charged particles and clinically relevant photon energies.

Some important examples of the unsuitability of orthovoltage and lower-voltage x-ray beams as the control/reference radiation are as follows:

1. For the collated proton RBE data of Paganetti *et al* (2002), orthovoltage radiations, 14 low-voltage or orthovoltage x-ray irradiations had an RBE less than 1 and only one such experiment showed an RBE just over 1. The probability of this being due to chance or experimental error is low: use of the sign test provides the probability of there being no difference as being $p = 0.00061$, a highly significant result.
2. The literature contains a report by Amols *et al* (1986), who measured cell-survival data in DLD-1 human tumour cells. Their results clearly demonstrate a statistically significant RBE difference between orthovoltage and megavoltage radiation ($p = 0.001$). A small difference is also measured in RBE between megavoltage photons and megavoltage electrons, but the difference is not statistically significant ($p = 0.25$). All biological, dosimetric and microdosimetric data were obtained under nearly identical geometric conditions, but this was only using one cell line.

The past literature contains many contributions which concentrate on the influence of lower photon energies in the low kilovoltage range on RBE, but these are mainly in the context of radiation protection, because this class of x-rays is used so much in routine diagnostic medicine. Such work has confirmed that RBE varies inversely with photon and particle energy (see, for example, the review by Hill (2004)).

RBE should be taken into account in clinical radiotherapy using positively charged particle beams, where RBE effects can be significant even in the case of protons. Papers by Belli *et al* (2000), Britten *et al* (2013) and Marshall *et al* (2016) are examples of such work, containing well-documented experimental detail. There is presently a potential shift of opinion to include more flexible (or variable) RBE values than the constant values previously assumed in proton therapy, in order not to (a) underdose certain radiosensitive tumour classes and (b) overdose late-reacting normal tissues of clinical importance. This is discussed in chapters 7, 9 and 10.

The urgent need to clarify RBEs in critical experimental normal tissues exposed to proton and other ion beams will require careful choice of control radiation if the purpose of such studies is to provide information that will be useful for ultimately clinical purposes. Some potential forms of control radiations can easily be eliminated, as is the case for orthovoltage x-rays because of their low expense and convenience, and should be avoided, since they will lead to lower estimates of RBE. 60-Co units also have some significant disadvantages. These include the lower dose rates with time, since it is advisable to use the same exposure times (within differences of only 1–2 min at most) for the control and test irradiations, due to ongoing repair of sub-lethal radiation damage. Longer treatments will have slightly lower bioeffectiveness, and this will influence the estimated RBE ratio. Also, the need to compensate for radioactive decay on a weekly or monthly basis may sometimes be forgotten or wrongly applied; the LET can be lower than for megavoltage photons, and drift of dose rate with time, and modification of source treatment distances to compensate for radiation decay, with accompanying changes in depth dose distributions. There are also problems associated with radiation protection of staff, shielding requirements, and source replacements are required with time, are expensive, and have their own difficulties.

Some laboratories do have a 137-Cs irradiator, which is more compact and delivers monoenergetic photons close to 0.5 MeV, which should have a LET close to that of cobalt beams. Again, radioactive decay has to be compensated for and dose-rate effects may accrue with time, although this can be overcome by using shorter source-to-target distances. Such a unit can be fitted into the size occupied by a large double refrigerator without additional shielding.

Megavoltage electrons are a reasonable choice for the control radiation in RBE studies. However, electron dosimetry, although much improved in recent years, has limitations due to its high scatter, especially for small field sizes, as well as the energy-dependent relationship of electron buildup with depth, which must be taken into account in any laboratory experiment. Electron fields are essentially SOBPs, often with lower RBEs than one in megavoltage electron plateau regions, but there remains uncertainty as to their higher RBE values with falloff of dose and energy towards their end of range. It must not be forgotten that Auger electrons (from low-energy radioactive emissions) can have very high RBEs. However, a broad electron beam operating at, say, 8–10 MeV would give a satisfactorily uniform dose for radiobiological experiments, but could not be used for beam ballistics combined with radiobiology comparisons.

There is interest in some particle therapy centres across Europe, including international laboratories like CERN, in addressing the clinically important RBE issue. For there to be comparable results, it is very important that the reference radiation be standardised. The best standard to choose, despite the additional expense, would undoubtedly be megavoltage x-rays from a linear accelerator operating at typical energies used in the clinic. It is already the case that national radiation standards laboratories such as the National Physical Laboratory

(NPL; Teddington, UK) contain a standard hospital linear accelerator for dosimetry comparisons and maintenance of standards. Likewise, laboratories which aim to contribute useful RBE data should use a control megavoltage linear accelerator with optional use of 4–10 MeV photons or electrons for their studies. A single 137-Cs source could also be useful.

Interestingly, since hospital linear accelerators are normally replaced every 10 years, it is relatively easy to obtain one which can be refurbished for experimental use. These would have a gantry for variable beam angles and collimation down to small field sizes.

Further considerations arise for dose rates, as the reference radiation should ideally operate at the same dose rate as the test radiation, since potentially large differences in cell survival can follow more protracted treatments due to DNA repair occurring during the radiation exposure. Even for very rapid dose rates, such as from laser-generated protons, matching of dose rate should be attempted in the reference radiation, although this is expected to be of most greatest significance in hypoxic cells. Ultra-high dose rates are considered further in chapters 2, 9 and 14.

1.2.3 Can RBE reduce with the depth of the SOBP placement in the case of passively scattered but not pencil scanned beams?

1.2.3.1 A hypothesis for passively scattered beams in contrast with pencil scanned beams

In general, and for whatever particle energy, RBE increases with depth due to the progressive increase in LET, especially within the Bragg peaks. However, there is evidence that if the same LET and dose is given at the same SOBP positions when these are situated at markedly different depths (which is achieved by using a different incident energies), then the RBE is reduced in the case of SOBPs placed at the deepest position in the case of passively scattered beams, but the RBE remains constant regardless of SOBP placement depth in scanned beams. These intriguing experiments, in the case of scattered beams, were led by V. Megnin-Chanet (Institute Curie), and were designed to study proton RBE at various depths using the Orsay proton beams (Calugaru *et al* 2011). Using two different incident energies of 76 and 201 MeV, with mid-SOBPs at 20.5 and 160 mm, respectively, and also near the distal ends of the SOBPs at 26.9 and 185 mm, respectively, with identical LET characteristics towards their distal ends. The main physical differences appeared to be the beam widths: 3 and 12 cm diameters, respectively, indicating greater lateral dispersion at the increased SOBP placement depth due to passive beam scattering. They observed a reduction of the RBE in two human cell lines from around the highest RBEs of 1.3–1.33 at 3 cm depth down to 1.0 (at 12 cm depth). Although the dose rates did differ with increasing depth, if DNA repair kinetics are considered the changes in minutes required to deliver the dose ranges used cannot account for the substantial change in RBE (the dose-rate effect at the low-to-medium dose-rate range is discussed further in chapter 2).

In contrast, Britten *et al* (2013) found no such RBE change in two cell lines with incident energies of 87 and 200 MeV at Bloomington, but where scanned pencil beams were used. These beams, without metallic filter-related scatter, consist of essentially parallel tracks and so deliver shorter inter-track separation distances (s) over most of their range, even when magnetic deflection is used to cover lateral parts of a target. There is little geometric dispersion with these pencil beams until the very end of their range, so s is relatively well preserved with depth. Some Coulombic scattering does diverge the beams, mostly near to the extreme range when energy and velocity are reduced.

The experimental depth changes and contrasting RBE findings of these two experimental studies are important and are illustrated schematically in figure 1.4, with a further summary in figures 1.5 (a, b). Alternative explanations for the findings of the Paris and Bloomington experiments might include chance, or a cellular batch effect, or the cell types used. These latter hypotheses are unlikely as each institute used two different cell lines with different radiobiological properties. The most likely explanation is the maintenance of a high fluence rate in each pencil beam compared with a marked reduction in fluence rate in the scattered beams when the SOBP placement is at least partly responsible and associated with a reduced dose rate (see chapter 11 for further interpretations). These fluence rates will be proportional to the inter-track distances (s).

Since all the other physical parameters such as LET and energy distributions will be very similar for SOBPs placed at superficial or deep locations, the most obvious physical explanation of this phenomenon, although speculative, is that increasing

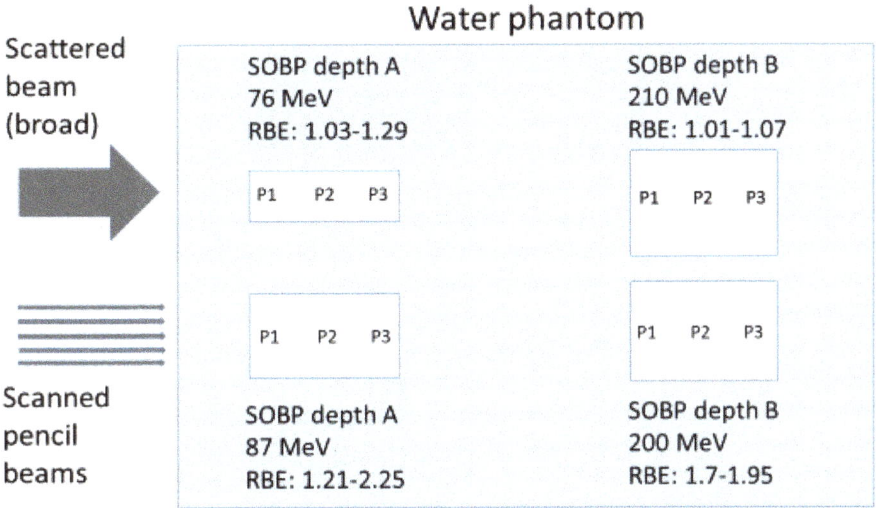

Figure 1.4. Schematic diagram of the experimental setup design and ranges of RBE found in (a) HeLa and SQ20B cells in a broad scattered proton beam using two similar SOBPs placed at different depths by using energies of 76 and 201 MeV (Calugaru *et al* 2011), and (b) in V-79 and Hep-2 cells (Britten *et al* 2013) in a pencil scanned beam using two SOBPs based on energies of 87 and 200 MeV, respectively. P1, P2 and P3 refer to the same distances along each of the SOBPs regardless of their depth placement and where the experimental RBE studies were done.

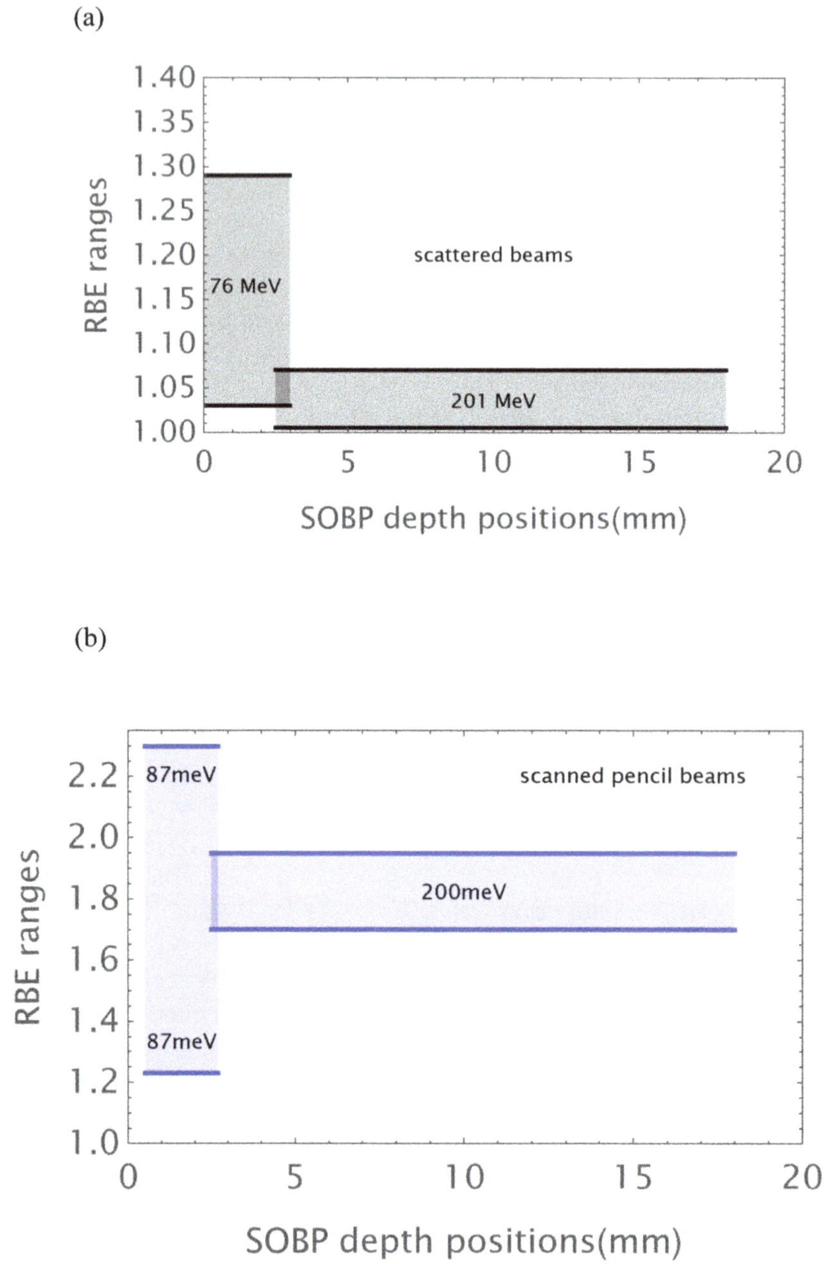

Figure 1.5. Depth ranges of the entire SOBP placement for the specified incident beam energies and experimental RBE ranges for (a) Calugaru *et al* (2011), and (b) Britten *et al* (2013) experiments given in the text.

track separation caused by the broad beam divergence in passively scattered beams is responsible. There may also be an associated loss of RBE with depth owing to increasing gamma-ray contributions, but these are small and would be at least partly offset by neutron production in matter, and this should be much the same in both experimental setups in each of the two publications. The scattering from metallic foils is designed to achieve a broad beam, but with inevitable reduction in dose rate and radiation fluence. Of course, there will be an increase in RBE along the SOBP in all of these experimental situations regardless of the SOBP placement depth, but it is important to realise that there are separate *relative* differences in the RBE due to the SOBP placement position in scattered beams.

If it is assumed that the RBE is proportional to the inter-track distance which decreases with depth (x) in passively scattered beams, all other factors being equal (e.g. dose, energy, LET), and if the rate of change of this effect depends on the operative RBE, then

$$d(\Delta RBE)/dx = -K.\ \Delta RBE,$$

where ΔRBE represents the RBE value in excess of 1.

Integration then provides, for RBE values >1, $1 + \mathrm{RBE}_x = 1 + \mathrm{RBE}_0\, e^{-cx}$, where RBE_x is the RBE value in excess of 1 at a specified depth of x cm, RBE_0 is the RBE value in excess of 1 at the smallest depth, and c is a constant assumed to be controlled by track separation. This simplified view is justified for initial testing purposes where the depth x of the SOBP is controlled by varying the incident particle energy.

For the Megnin-Chanet experiments, and using their pooled data for two different human cell lines, the above function provides a value of $c = 0.009$ and 0.013, respectively, for the mid-SOBP and distal SOBP positions used for the comparisons, and so it is possible to plot the reduction in RBE with increasing depth, as shown in figure 1.6. Further experiments are required at multiple depths to confirm this hypothesis and achieve a more robust value for parameter c.

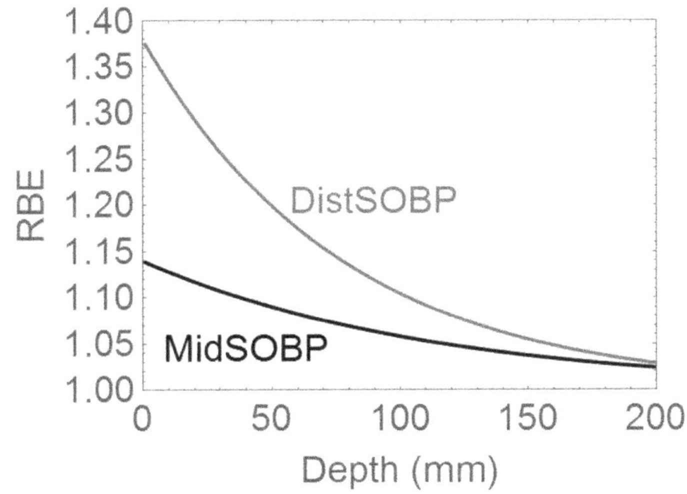

Figure 1.6. Putative relationship between RBE with depth of similar experimental reference points at the mid-SOBP and distal SOBP obtained by increasing particle energy to achieve progressively deeper SOBP placement positions, from data averaged for two human cell lines (HeLa and a head and neck squamous cell cancer line) for caesium and cobalt referenced RBE values obtained using the above equations.

The other approach might be to consider the inter-track distances (s). Using similar triangles, the radius of a divergent overall beam field is proportional to the distance (x) that it traverses. For two different depth positions, 1 and 2, indicated by the respective subscripts, the overall beam radii r_1 and r_2 are proportional to their respective depths (x_1 and x_2) due to the similar triangle rule; the areas A_1 and A_2 are given by πr_1^2 and πr_2^2. The inter-track distance, when squared, is $s^2 = A/N$, and since N remains constant, then the ratio of inter-track distances (s_1/s_2) at two different depths will be the same as x_1/x_2. Using one of the data examples in Calugaru *et al* (2011), from x = 2.69–18.5 cm, the inter-track distance ratio (S/R) will change from the shallowest depth, where s_1 is normalised to 1, down to 2.69/18.5 = 0.145 (in the absence of precise knowledge of N or F). When this process is applied to the data, and by using a similar exponential function as in the above example, then the relationship between RBE and inter-track separation ratio (S/R) can be expressed as $1+0.0055\ e^{(4.14\ S/R)}$, and this function is plotted in figure 1.7.

Also, further work has studied the reduction of dose rate, and inevitable increased instantaneous inter-track distances, at increasing entire SOBP depth placement with higher energies in scattered beams (a consequence of the considerably larger field size with depth, as given in the Calugaru *et al* (2011) report). Further modelling on these radiobiological factors provides a rationale to explain the large differences in RBE found in their experiments, although it can be difficult to follow without a full understanding of the experimental setups. It is crucial to appreciate that, although the RBE always increases along a SOBP, placement of the SOBP at a much greater depth results in a marked reduction in the RBE within it. This work is presented separately in chapter 11.

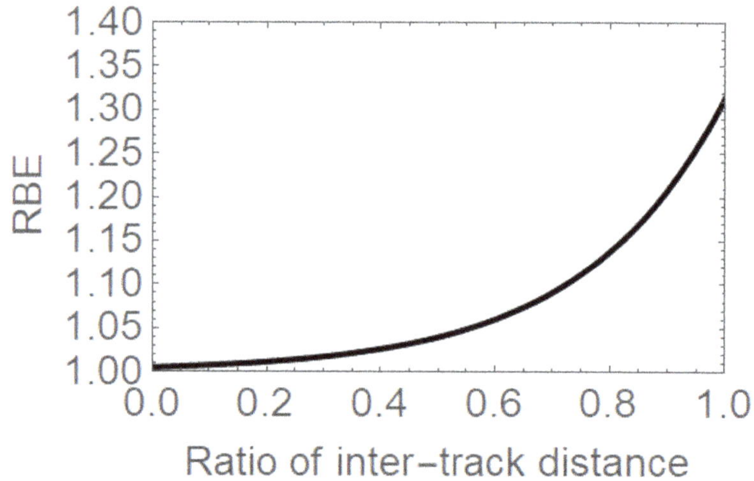

Figure 1.7. Plot of RBE with inter-track distance ratio (SR), normalised to s = 1, where the RBE is 1.33, but with an RBE close to 1 when the SR is around 0.1 for scattered proton beams, as in Calugaru *et al* (2011).

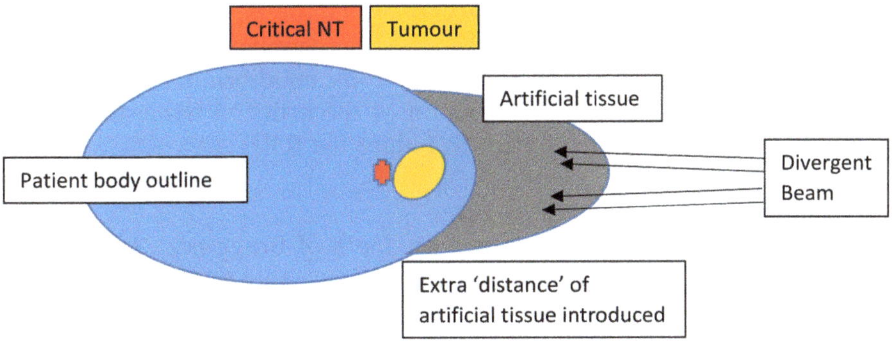

Fi.gure 1.8. Diagram of possible addition of a synthetic medium to change the effective target depth in order to reduce RBE further in passively scattered beams.

Such exploratory data needs to be extended, with RBE estimations at many depths in a panel of cell lines, in order to fully verify and extend this hypothesis using further micro-dosimetry considerations.

Although speculative, if such a reduction in RBE with depth of SOBP position can occur in some cell lines with divergent beams, it may be possible to investigate reducing potential RBE problems in normal tissue adjacent to a tumour by electively increasing the path length (and energy) of the radiation and adding tissue-equivalent material outside the skin (as shown in figure 1.8), aiming for the RBE to be close to 1 at the critical distance. The length of additional material would require careful calculation to produce the SOBP at the required tissue depth, but with loss of RBE this could be advantageous where the local biological characteristics confer a high normal tissue RBE in a critical structure and which exceeds any critical normal tissue dose sparing advantage. The alternative way of reducing the normal tissue RBE is to increase the dose per fraction of the particle therapy (these aspects are discussed in later chapters).

It is vital that further research should be conducted on this topic. A more recent study on total-body irradiation of mice showed no survival difference between scanned and scattered beams, but this was a study of acute rather than late toxicity (which are governed by different mathematical relationships with respect to radiation dose, as will be discussed in chapter 2). However, scanned beams significantly increased lymphocyte micro-nucleus frequency (an index of radiation effectiveness), erythrocyte glutathione peroxidase activity and heart oxidised glutathione levels (which are radioprotectors) compared to scattered beams (Chaouni *et al* 2020).

It is paradoxical that so much effort is devoted to meticulous dosimetry along the beams, yet relatively little resources have been dedicated to radiobiological considerations. The lack of divergence in pencil beam scanning, with no significant reduction of RBE with SOBP depth, is also of concern, since high RBE values beyond the 1.1 value used in the standard prescription process can be exceeded wherever the SOBP is placed. This is an obvious explanation for 'unexpected' normal tissue toxicity occurring with use of scanned pencil beams, which are presently preferred by particle accelerator manufacturers. Further discussion and modelling on this important topic can be found in chapters 7, 9 and 10.

The possible detriment would be loss of electronic equilibrium buildup in skin and subcutaneous tissue due to the introduction of the artificial tissue that allows the beam to diverge to the required extent to reduce the RBE.

1.2.3.2 A corollary: ultra-high dose rates

The converse effect to loss of dose rate with depth of Bragg peak placement is the possibility (or inevitability) that intensification of dose rate to ultra-high or FLASH dose rates will change radiosensitivity in the opposite direction; that is, RBE will increase in proportion to the increments in α and β parameters. The product of fluence × LET is relevant here since it is expressed in units of energy transfer per unit volume on a micro-volumetric scale, the metric then being MVET, as explained in Jones (2022).

Just as increasing LET causes increasing radiosensitivity, so should increasing MVET do so, although the specified LET remains constant. Simultaneously, oxygen depletion accompanies dose-rate intensification, which can reduce radiosensitivity, sometimes severely so in very low oxygen tension states. The net effect of these two processes will be to modestly increase α but markedly reduce β, since the β parameter is the most sensitive to oxygen tension. Consequently, the cellular α/β ratio will increase, as was found in the fitting of a lung fibrosis experimental data set. It was found that the increase in α/β increase could be approximated by a cube root or near cube root function of the ratio of the dose rates of the reference or standard dose rate of around 0.5–3 Gy hr^{-1} and the FLASH dose rate.

In the previous section it was explained that the mean inter-track distance, s, is approximated by the inverse square root of the fluence, F, or $s = \sqrt{\frac{1}{F}}$, and this extends to the inter-track separation in a volume of interest as $s' = \sqrt[3]{\frac{1}{F}}$, which leads to a relationship of $s' = \sqrt[3]{\frac{R}{R_{\text{ref}}}}$, where R is the relevant dose rate and R_{ref} the conventional dose rate.

This new hypothesis is discussed, with some graphical examples for charged particles, in chapters 2, 9, 11 and 14, since it allows estimations of biological effectiveness changes if dose rates change between the conventional and FLASH dose range, as well as being relevant to the reduction in RBE with SOBP depth.

References

Andrews J R 1978 High LET radiobiology and radiotherapy *The Radiobiology of Human Cancer Radiotherapy* (Baltimore, MD: University Park Press) pp 241–4

Amols H I, Lagueux B and Cagna D 1986 Radiobiological effectiveness (RBE) of megavoltage *x*-ray and electron beams in radiotherapy *Radiat. Res.* **105** 58–67

Belli M, Bettega D, Calzolari P, Cera F, Cherubini R *et al* 2000 Inactivation of human normal and tumour cells irradiated with low energy protons *Int. J. Radiat. Biol.* **76** 831–9

Britten R A, Nazaryan V, Davis L K, Klein S B, Nichiporov D, Mendonca M S *et al* 2013 Variations in the RBE for cell killing along the depth-dose profile of a modulated proton therapy beam *Radiat. Res.* **179** 21–8

Calugaru V, Nauraye C, Noël G, Giocanti N, Favaudon V and Mégnin-Chanet F 2011 Radiobiological characterization of two therapeutic proton beams with different initial energy spectra used at the Institut Curie Proton Therapy Center in Orsay *Int. J. Radiat. Oncol. Biol. Phys.* **81** 1136–43

Chaouni S, Leduc A, Pouzoulet F, De Marzi L, Megnin-Chanet F *et al* 2020 Biological effects of scattered versus scanned proton beams on normal tissues in total body irradiated mice: Survival, genotoxicity, oxidative stress and inflammation *Antioxidants (Basel)* **9** 1170

Eulitz J, Troost E, Klünder L, Raschke F, Hahn C *et al* 2023 Increased relative biological effectiveness and periventricular radiosensitivity in proton therapy of glioma patients *Radiother. Oncol.* **178** 109422

Hall E J and Giaccia A 2011 Radiobiology for the radiologist ed E Hall, E J Hall and A J Giaccia *Radioprotection in Radiobiology for the Radiologist* 7th edn (Philadelphia, PA: Lippincott Williams and Wilkins) chs 6 and 7, pp 253–70

Hill M A 2004 The variation in biological effectiveness of *x*-rays and gamma rays with energy *Radiat. Prot. Dosimetry* **112** 471–81

ICRU 1970 *Linear Energy Transfer (ICRU Report 16)* (Bethesda, MD: International Commission on Radiation Units & Measurements)

Jones B 2015 Towards achieving the full clinical potential of proton therapy by inclusion of LET and RBE models *Cancers (Basel)* **7** 460–80

Jones B 2022 The influence of hypoxia on LET and RBE relationships with implications for ultra-high dose rates and FLASH modelling *Phys. Med. Biol.* **67**

Kanai T, Furusawa Y, Fukutsu K, Itsukaichi H and Eguchi-Kasai K O H 1997 Irradiation of mixed beam and design of spread-out Bragg peak for heavy-ion radiotherapy *Radiat. Res.* **147** 78–85

Katz R, Ackerson B, Homoyooufar M and Sharma S C 1971 Inactivation of cells by heavy ion bombardment *Radiat. Res.* **47** 402–25

Marshall T I, Chaudhary P, Michaelidesová A, Vachelová J, Davídková M, Vondráček V, Schettino G and Prise K M 2016 Investigating the implications of a variable RBE on proton dose fractionation across a clinical pencil beam scanned spread-out Bragg peak *Int. J. Radiat. Oncol. Biol. Phys.* **95** 70–7

Newhauser W D and Zhang R 2015 The physics of proton therapy *Phys. Med. Biol.* **60** R155–209

Paganetti H, Niemierko A, Ancukiewicz M, Gerweck L E, Goitein M, Loeffler J S and Suit H D 2002 Relative biological effectiveness (RBE) values for proton beam therapy *Int. J. Radiat. Oncol. Biol. Phys.* **53** 407–21

Peach K, Wilson P and Jones B 2011 Accelerator science in medical physics *Br. J Radiol.* **84** S1–S10

Spadinger I and Palcic B 1992 The relative biological effectiveness of 60Co gamma-rays, 55 kVp *x*-rays, 250 kVp x-rays, and 11 MeV electrons at low doses *Int. J. Radiat. Biol.* **61** 345–53

Wilson E J N 2001 *An Introduction to Particle Accelerators* (Oxford: Oxford University Press)

Underwood T S A and Paganetti H 2016 Variable proton relative biological effectiveness: how do we move forward? *Int. J. Radiat. Oncol. Biol. Phys.* **95** 56–8

Chapter 2

The essential radiobiology background

A summary of radiobiological modelling is given, based on the linear quadratic (LQ) model of radiation effect and the transformation of survival curve theory into the biological effective dose (BED) concept, which is useful in the clinic in many practical applications. Descriptions and formulations for conventional photon-based therapy are extended to particle therapy across a wide range of topics, including very-low- to high-dose ranges, repopulation effects and the dose-rate effect (including both enzymatic repair processes and ultra-high dose rates). The BED equations for the particle therapies include the RBE_{max} and RBE_{min} concepts, which refer to the respective α and β parameters of the LQ model and which dominate the overall RBE at low and high doses, respectively. Their use leads to a variable rather than a constant RBE with dose. Parameters for use in these equations are provided.

2.1 Introduction

The information given in this chapter is intended as a summary of the analytical methods that have been developed for expressing radiation effects in explicit equations. Some existing basic knowledge is assumed. There are two sections: the first describes the models and their background; the second considers the choice of some key parameters. As a reminder, the time course of radiation effects is important and is summarised in figure 2.1.

2.2 Background and models

2.2.1 The linear quadratic model

Douglas Lea, a pupil of Rutherford, fitted the average yield of severe (or lethal) chromosomal aberrations per cell (E), in the form of $E = \alpha d + \beta d^2$ (Lea 1962). For many years, this finding was largely ignored because of the increasing use of target theory models that had little biological basis. The linear quadratic (LQ) model later became important for two reasons.

doi:10.1088/978-0-7503-6209-2ch2

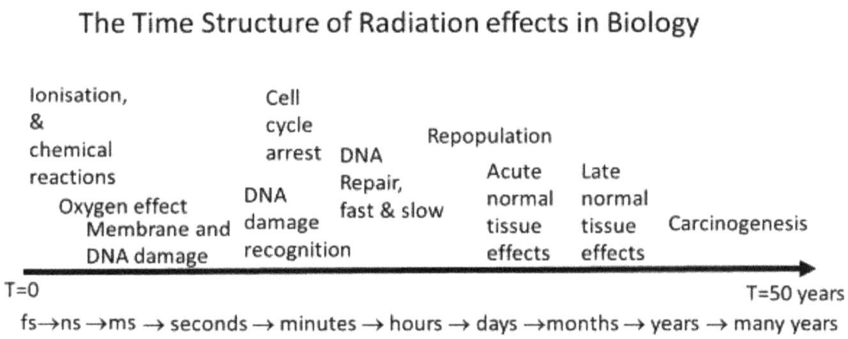

Figure 2.1. The essential time structure of radiation effects from near-instantaneous effects to those which require many years before their expression.

First, several mathematically complex theoretical approaches, separately based on micro-dosimetry, molecular damage (and its repairability/non-repairability) and chromosomal aberration yields, all approximate to the LQ formulation, as in Rossi & Zaider (1992), Curtis (1986), Chadwick & Leenhouts (1973) and Campbell & Warenius (1989).

Second, animal and human fractionation data were fitted by transformations of the LQ model. Douglas & Fowler (1976) used fractionation effect (or FE) plots. These use a simple algebraic transformation of the LQ model as $1/D = \alpha/E + (\beta/E)d$, where D is the product of each 'fractional' dose d multiplied by the number of fractions n and where the fractionated form of the LQ model is $E = n(\alpha d + \beta d^2)$ or $D(\alpha + \beta d)$. The reciprocal of total dose when plotted against dose per fraction produced reasonably good linear fits of isoeffective fractionation data, where the same biological end point was obtained using different dose-fractionation schedules in experimental tissue experiments. These plots were used to obtain the α/β ratio, a useful single parameter, by dividing the intercept (α/E) by the slope (β/E) of the FE plot.

Thames *et al* (1982), using multiple isoeffective data sets, later showed the very important and clear dissociation between classes of tissues with different α/β ratios by plotting only dose per fraction against total dose: acute-reacting tissue (rapidly growing tumours or normal tissues including many normal epithelial tissues) had high α/β ratios (7–15 Gy), but late-reacting tissue (slowly growing tumours or low turnover biosystems including all stable normal tissues) had low α/β ratios (2–3 Gy). In comparison to the previously used non-biologically based 'power-law' models, which failed at low and high dose limits, and were initially and incorrectly thought to apply to all tissues and tumours, the LQ approach was more flexible, and produced better data fits as well as modelled predictions that could be applied over a wide range of doses.

Critics of the LQ model appear to be fixed on its simplicity as represented in many textbook diagrams, where the DNA double helix is used to demonstrate single-hit and double-hit lesions; such a concept is naïve, in that the LQ end point must be the yield (or probability) of lethal events per cell or even across a whole tissue, so that α and β must represent the ultimate coefficients of lethality, or clinical effects, rather than some of their initial DNA damage precursors. Criticism has rightly been raised as to how such a simple formulation can represent the entire pathway of injury from a cellular to the tissue level, where many biological processes (inflammatory mediators, cytokines and cellular sub-compartmental kinetics, fibrosis, vascular damage and tissue hypoxia, and nutrient depletion) may all influence the end result. However, even complex industrial processes, as well as cellular processes, are governed by key rate-limiting steps which can simplify any analysis of outcomes. It can only be concluded that tissue α/β ratios are a useful summary of multiple processes, which contribute to the effect being considered.

The present book considers high-LET effects from protons (and other ions) as well as standard low-LET effects. It is useful to consider the dimensions of LET (energy released per micrometre of track). Micrometres are a more appropriate measurement for chromosomal damage, resulting from multiple smaller DNA changes, but where these accumulate in a critical three-dimensional (3D) space to produce lethal chromosomal breaks. The chromosomal diameter is around 700 nm, and each non-replicating chromosome is covered by heterochromatin protein, which can also be chemically disrupted by the clustered radiation in high-LET beams, releasing native damaged DNA to the oxidative micro-environment of the cell, and disrupting any ongoing background repair mechanisms. Consequently, as LET increases, the complexity of local DNA disruption renders the repair enzymes ineffective, and accumulation of such local damage can ultimately result in a lethal chromosomal break.

A good example of the LQ model's clinical utility is given in figure 2.2, where the model has been used to delineate an isoeffective dose curve for spinal cord myelitis (which can cause paralysis), based on the low risk associated with a dose of 50 Gy in 25 fractions, with data points given by many empirically derived clinical fractionation schedules used in the clinic by the present author, and considered to be very safe (grey points), whereas the doses used to treat common cancers are indicated by the red points. The curve provides an effective upper limit which should not be exceeded in the spinal cord tissue if uniformly irradiated in cross section. Details of how to construct such a curve, using the biological effective dose (BED) concept, are given in later sections.

Summary of LQ model:

Contrary to many statements in textbooks, and common misconceptions, α and β are *not* specific coefficients for single-strand (SSB) and double-strand (DSB) DNA breaks, the yield of which are dose dependent, and they are in most instances efficiently repaired by cellular enzymatic mechanisms. A large number of SSBs and DSBs are required to exist in reasonably close proximity, and avoid repair in order to produce a lethal event, normally accompanied by the appearance of a lethal chromosomal aberration, which will cause cell death due to asymmetric segregation of genetic information usually at the next mitosis. Consequently, SSBs and DSBs are necessary

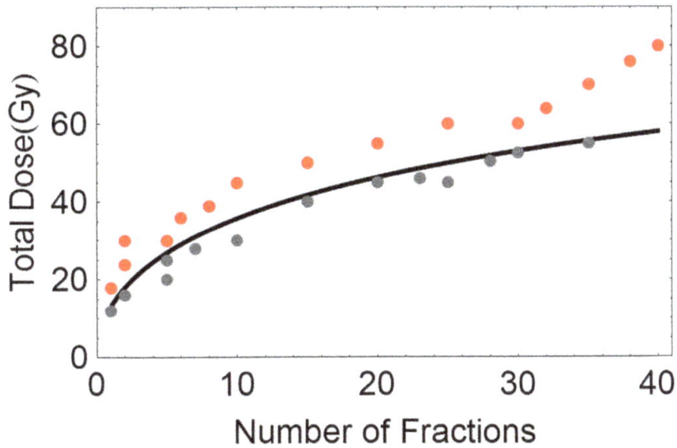

Figure 2.2. LQ-model-based plot of the relationship between total dose and number of fractions which result in the same low risk (isoeffect) of spinal cord paralysis, obtained using an α/β ratio of 2 Gy. The grey points are considered to be safe and are based on many standard fractionation schedules used by the author in the UK for radical and palliative radiotherapy. The red points are the radical doses often used to treat squamous cell cancers (plotted using an α/β ratio of 10 Gy) and which exceed the isoeffect curve. Clinical radiotherapy may utilise the grey dose-fractionation points to palliate cancer close to the spinal cord, but when the red point curative doses are given, great care is taken to ensure that the spinal cord doses must be lower and so fall near to or further beneath the spinal cord isoeffect curve.

precursors, but not sufficient requirements, for lethality: additional spatial and temporal considerations may or may not lead to lethality. Consequently, in cell survival experiments, α and β must reflect the probability of lethality with increasing dose and are best defined as follows:

α is the coefficient of lethal events per cell per unit dose (in units of Gy^{-1}).

β is the coefficient of lethal events per cell per unit dose squared (in units of Gy^{-2}).

In this way, α and β probably reflect the number of lethal chromosomal events with dose and dose squared, respectively.

It follows that the probability of cell survival (where there are no lethal events), referred to as the survival fraction (SF), is obtained using Poisson statistics, where

$SF = e^{-(\text{expected number of lethal events})} = e^{-\alpha d - bd^2}$ or $SF = e^{-n(\alpha d - bd^2)}$ for n fractions of dose d.

Summary of events:

DNA-level events: Base changes, SSBs, DSBs, short patches, long patches.

Cellular response systems: Repair is achieved by multiple mechanisms; but misrepair or inability to completely repair can result in lethality according to local complexity/clustering.

These lesions if sufficiently concentrated in a particular location on a chromosome or chromatid will lead to structural instability of the chromosome.

Chromosomal and chromatid-level events are caused by asymmetrical breakage at stressed sections (thus multiple or heavily clustered radiation damage will cause more mechanical stress).

Cellular responses: Time-dependent recognition and repair of DNA damage according to the half-times of enzymatic repair, and attempted rejoining of small breaks resulting minimally in some loss of heterozygosity and mutagenesis; asymmetric chromosomal breaks result in lethality.

The numbers of lethal events per cell are expressed as α and β per unit dose and dose squared, respectively.

The LQ can alternatively be expressed as follows:

$\alpha = \Sigma$ (localised unrepaired DNA damage $\Rightarrow$ lethal chromosomal injury events per cell)/dose.

$\beta = \Sigma$ (localised unrepaired DNA damage $\Rightarrow$ lethal chromosomal injury events per cell)/dose^2.

The greater the degree of local clustering of ionisation (as with high LET), then α and β are expected to increase.

The predominant mode of cell killing at low dose is via α-mediated damage, especially direct damage (less sensitive to oxygenation status), invoking a repair mechanism called non-homologous end-joining (NHEJ) operating on strand breaks throughout the cell cycle, and is highly susceptible to increased LET (Takahashi *et al* 2014); the damage is cumulative with dose and not dependent on further dose commitments, so the damage caused will not depend on the dose rate at low to conventional dose rates, although can be modified by oxygen depletion at ultra-high dose rates.

The other mode of cell killing, which dominates at high doses, is via β-mediated damage, especially indirect damage (more sensitive to oxygenation status or sensitising drugs). Inter-track cooperation may occur, and a superior repair mechanism, recombination repair (RR), operates by recombination and chromatid exchanges from non-damaged DNA regions; this form of cell killing is less susceptible to increased LET, and exhibits a pronounced dose-rate effect in the conventional to low dose-rate range, because of the requirement for two separate dose-related events which lead to the squared term. Time protraction permits repair of the first hits before second nearby hits can lead to more significant DNA lesions, which contribute to lethality.

Note that experimental lethality coefficients α and β, as determined in cell survival experiments or from *in vivo* tissue work, will also include other cell-killing processes such as follows:

- Apoptotic cell death (which saturates at low dose) so is a fixed proportion at clinically used doses above 1.5 Gy.
- Autophagy.
- Bystander effects (again occurs mainly at low doses).

These three mechanisms are explained further in radiobiology textbooks.

2.2.2 Model variants

Clinicians especially should be aware of two classes of models that can assist with RBE determination, and therefore fractionation issues:

A. *Bottom-up models*. Examples include the developing GEANT4-DNA project, and detailed micro-dosimetry studies, such as the local-effect model (Kase *et al* 2008) based on LET values, together with assumed or measured (the so-called low-level) sub-cellular and cellular parameters, which allow

RBE to be predicted, although the model remains to be perfected. This and other variants can be used to guide the choice of dose and so aid treatment planning by application on a voxel-to-voxel basis, etc. These are discussed further in chapters 8 and 9.

B. *Top-down models.* These use high-level parameters (at the clinical level) such as the BED model which contains tissue or tumour α/β ratios, or models which separately use the α and β parameters and will be discussed below and in many later chapters. They link our present knowledge of clinical radiobiology with fractionation phenomena and can be applied usually with ease using relatively simple mathematics for low- and high-LET radiations. They are essentially phenomenological, but with a real biological basis and can be regarded as semi-empirical. These can be an effective check in clinical applications, and clinicians and physicists should ideally be able to perform such calculations with reasonable competence and understand their implications and limitations.

Obtaining a model that contains the multi-scaled nature of the events must remain a future goal, although may not be fully obtainable because it is not possible to define the event probabilities down to individual cells or indeed to know all the contributing parameters, with the dynamic heterogeneity of individual cellular radiosensitivities which vary with position in the cell reproductive cycle, the biochemical redox state, the nuclear and cell volumes, repair proficiency, etc. At present, averaged parameter values during treatment are assumed in most cases, although cellular repopulation is accommodated as a variable.

This type of challenge exists in many parts of science, including physics, where the separate quantum and gravitational models have yet to be unified in a single framework, despite each model being highly accurate in their own domains. However, there are some realistic assessments of the scaling of RBE from the low-LET α/β ratio in some micro-dosimetry-related models, as in Japan and Germany (Elsässer & Scholz 2007, Kase *et al* 2008), for example to predict brain RBE using the preferred α/β of 2 Gy, and further simpler options are given in chapters 8 and 9.

2.2.3 Biological effective dose

Barendsen (1982), Dale (1985, 1989) and Fowler (1989) all contributed to the application of the BED concept to clinical and experimental data sets. In earlier publications the term 'extrapolated response dose' was used, but this is synonymous with the BED.

For standard megavoltage low-LET radiation the following approach is taken. From the surviving fraction (SF) of cells after radiation exposure, included in a Poissonian probability function for the probability of no lethal damage (i.e. survival) when the expected number per cell is E, consequently

$$\mathrm{SF} = e^{-(E)} = e^{-\alpha d - bd^2}, \tag{2.1}$$

and for n fractions it follows that

$$\mathrm{SF}^n = e^{-n(\alpha d + bd^2)}. \tag{2.2}$$

By taking the natural logarithm and multiplying by -1, and replacing $-\ln(\mathrm{SF}^n)$ by E (sometimes called the 'log cell kill'), a much simpler expression is obtained:

$$E = n(\alpha d + \beta d^2). \tag{2.3}$$

Next, consider the lowest possible dose as a limit; then, the βd^2 term can be ignored.

It follows that E approaches $n\alpha d$ as $d \to 0$, and so $E/\alpha = nd$ at near-zero dose. The nd product is the total dose (D) required for a given effect using a large number of very small dose fractions, and represents a ceiling of dose. At very low doses, this is the BED, expressed in units of Gy. In this way, BED can be defined as the total dose required for a specific bioeffect, if the dose is delivered in a very large number of fractions of low dose.

Then division of equation (2.3) throughout by α, with some rearrangement, leads to the important BED expression:

$$\mathrm{BED} = nd\left(1 + \frac{d}{\alpha/\beta}\right). \tag{2.4}$$

This applies to low-LET radiation, noting here that the first term in parenthesis is 1 (higher values than 1 exist in high-LET conditions).

For any specified BED, the equivalent dose in 2 Gy fractions (the EQD-2) is simply

$$\mathrm{EQD}^2 = \mathrm{BED}/(1 + 2/(\alpha/\beta)). \tag{2.5}$$

It must be noted that BED, expressed as $\mathrm{Gy}_{[x]}$, should be further qualified by x, which is the specific α/β ratio used.

2.2.4 Repopulation allowances

BED modifications are required to account for ongoing tumour cell repopulation during treatment. Since tumour cells grow exponentially in good growth conditions, it is now standard to express this process as a reduction of BED by using a BED-dose equivalent of repopulation, obtained in the following way.

Repopulation effects may be incorporated in the LQ model. The SF following radiotherapy is given by equation (2.1) above, but the surviving clonogenic cells will repopulate independently of the radiotherapy, so that the SF must be increased by a factor which accounts for the exponential cellular repopulation during treatment given over a time t, so the equation becomes

$$S = e^{-n(\alpha d + \beta d^2)}.\, e^{\frac{\ln 2.t}{T_{\mathrm{eff}}}} = e^{-n\left(\alpha d + \beta d^2\right) + \frac{\ln 2.t}{T_{\mathrm{eff}}}}, \tag{2.6}$$

where T_{eff} expresses the effective doubling time of the repopulating cells, which may vary during treatment.

By taking natural logs of each side of the equation, the logarithmic SF, expressed as the negative natural logarithm (or radiation log cell kill, E_t) at time t, is given by

$$- \ln S = E_t = n(\alpha d + \beta d) - 0.693\frac{t}{T_{\text{eff}}}. \tag{2.7}$$

The sign of the repopulation factor is now negative, and the cell kill part of the equation is positive for consistency.

There has been much debate regarding the form of the repopulation factor and the nomenclature of the doubling time. It is reasonable at this stage to distinguish between the actual clonogen cellular doubling time, T_C, the potential doubling time, T_{pot}, and the effective doubling time denoted by T_{eff}. The T_{eff} is a rather flexible parameter in that it may initially correspond to the pre-treatment tumour volume doubling time, T_D, but in some tumours may shorten during treatment and approach the value of the pre-treatment T_{pot}.

For normal tissues no allowance for repopulation should normally be necessary for repopulation during treatment in the case of late-responding tissues. Inclusion of normal tissue repopulation, or 'recovery', following treatment may be required when considering re-treatment after an interval of many months or years. This is discussed further in chapter 12. There is currently no general agreement on how to include a variable repopulation factor for acute tissue effects, where α/β ratios will be larger and appear to increase during the treatment from average values of 4, 12 and 35 Gy in the first 2, 2–4 and 4–6 weeks of treatment, respectively, as far as the skin is concerned (Hopewell *et al* 2003). These last considerations should be of importance in acute-reacting tissue BEDs. Most BED applications are for late normal tissues where the α/β ratios remain stable during treatment. More work needs to be done on tumour BED values in the context of more flexible α/β ratios. Some caveats have also been provided by Dale and colleagues about the use of EQD-2 in repopulation estimations, with methods for their correction (Dale *et al* 2023).

2.2.5 Biological effective dose and repopulation

To allow for the effect of repopulation during treatment, the standard BED equation requires a negative repopulation factor that here assumes a constant rate of BED compensation during treatment:

$$\text{BED} = \text{D}\left[1 + \frac{d}{(\alpha/\beta)}\right] - KT, \tag{2.8}$$

where K (in units of Gy day^{-1}) is the daily BED equivalent of repopulation and T is the overall treatment duration. Typical values of K used for squamous cell cancers are 0.5–1.0 Gy_{10} day^{-1}. These are considered to be average values throughout treatment. It is emphasised that K values are in units of physical dose, and do not normally represent the physical dose per day required to offset repopulation. This important difference can lead to errors in calculating compensatory schedules for unintentional treatment interruptions, as shown by Dale *et al* (2002), and the situation is more complex for high-LET treatments (see chapter 12). For slower growing tumours, e.g. breast and prostate, there is little evidence for repopulation until durations of 7 weeks or more have elapsed when the K value may be close to 0.2–0.3 Gy day^{-1} (Thames *et al* 2010). In the case of very anaplastic or poorly differentiated tumours with total lack of growth control mechanisms, it is possible that repopulation will be continuous without a lag time. The term K includes several parameters: it is obtained by dividing the conventional repopulation correction factor by the α parameter (just as BED is obtained by dividing the log cell kill E by α), so that

$$K = \frac{0.693.\ t}{\alpha.\ T_{\mathrm{eff}}}. \tag{2.9}$$

Since α increases with increasing LET, so will the K value reduce, and the dose to compensate for unintended treatment interruptions will change compared to the dose required for megavoltage photons. These subtleties are further discussed in chapter 12.

2.2.5.1 Alternative patterns of repopulation

The above formulation assumes *continuous* repopulation (i.e. the repopulation rate is continuous, at the same rate during the entire treatment time). For tumours where steady-state repopulation begins after an apparent time lag of T_K days, the repopulation term is modified to be $K(T-T_K)$. The BED is then

$$\mathrm{BED} = nd(1 + d/(\alpha/\beta)) - K(T - TK). \tag{2.10}$$

This pattern of repopulation can be described as being *discontinuous*. For head and neck cancers, T_K is between 21 and 28 days. This approach is only valid if $T > T_K$. It would be incorrect to assume that all tumours behave like most differentiated squamous cell cancers. For ultra-short fractionation schedules with overall times shorter than 21 days, the repopulation correction factor (RCF) can either be omitted, as there is relatively little repopulation, or it is possible to assume that a longer T_{eff} is operational, for example, assuming that the T_{eff} is 5–10 times larger, especially if the tumour is poorly differentiated. An alternative formulation, based on a *progressive* or *delayed* reduction in the cell-loss factor during treatment can also be used. This model is based on a continuously changing repopulation rate, governed initially by the volume doubling time. Later during treatment, when φ values are small, T_{eff} approximates to the pre-treatment T_{pot} value. This model predicts a slowly increasing extra dose required to counteract repopulation as treatment time is increased, which simulates accelerated repopulation, and there is the attractive feature of no sudden discontinuities. A wider discussion and alternative approaches are given by Jones & Dale (2007) and in Dale (2019), Dale & Jones (2022) and Dale *et al* (2024).

2.2.6 BED expression of high-LET radiation

For higher-LET radiations, it is necessary to include the separate increments in α and β due to increasing LET, noting that the former normally exceeds the latter, as in Jones *et al* (2006) and Carabe-Fernandez *et al* (2007). Some authors ignore the smaller β increments for low-dose treatments (see chapters 8 and 9), but the β contribution to effectiveness become progressively more important with higher dose per fraction (often referred to as hypofractioned radiotherapy).

First, it is necessary to apply basic limit theory to the basic LQ model in the form of the following isoeffective equation (where the same bioeffect is produced by two forms of radiation in each case, designated by subscripts L and H for low LET and high LET, respectively) as

$$n_L(\alpha_L d_L + \beta_L d_L{}^2) = nH(\alpha_H d + \beta_H d_H{}^2), \tag{2.11}$$

To simplify further, assume that $n_L = n_H$, so that

$$\alpha_L d_L + \beta_L d_L{}^2 = \alpha_H d + \beta_H d_H{}^2. \tag{2.12}$$

Since RBE is defined as the ratio of the control or reference low-LET dose to the high-LET test radiation dose for the same bioeffect, i.e. RBE $= d_L/d_H$, then as d approaches zero dose, by neglecting β terms in equation (2.14), RBE is given by α_H/α_L, which is referred to as the RBE_{max}. Also for high dose, by neglecting the α terms in equation (2.14), RBE (or d_L/d_H) will approach a value of $\sqrt{}(\beta_H/\beta_L)$, which is called RBE_{min}.

It follows that

$$\text{RBE}_{\text{min}}{}^2 = \beta_H/\beta_L \tag{2.13}$$

and that

$$\beta_H = \text{RBE}_{\text{min}}{}^2.\ \beta_L. \tag{2.14}$$

To obtain the high-LET BED_H the entire isoeffect linear quadratic equation (2.14) must be divided throughout by α_L, the low-LET α parameter, as was done in the original BED derivation. This procedure ensures that the high-LET BED and the low-LET BED are compatible and expressed in the same units.

To simplify further, the right-hand side of the isoeffect is only considered from here on and in its fractionated form. Then the high-LET BED will be given by dividing $E = n_H(\alpha_H d + \beta_H d^2)$ by α_L, to obtain

$$\text{BED} = \frac{E}{\alpha_L} = D_H\left(\frac{\alpha_H}{\alpha_L} + \frac{\beta_H}{\alpha_L}d_H\right). \tag{2.15}$$

From the above equation, where D_H is used to express the total dose given by $n_H.d_H$, and then using RBE_{max} (to replace both α parameters) and RBE_{min} to replace β_H by the expression in equation (2.15), then

$$\text{BED} = D_H\left(\text{RBE}_{\text{max}} + \frac{\text{RBE}_{\text{min}}{}^2\, d_H}{\left(\frac{\alpha}{\beta}\right)_L}\right). \tag{2.16}$$

It is then possible to pursue isoeffect calculations using the equality

$$\text{BED} = D_L\left(1 + \frac{d_L}{\left(\frac{\alpha}{\beta}\right)_L}\right) = D_H\left(\text{RBE}_{\max} + \frac{\text{RBE}_{\min}{}^2\, d_H}{\left(\frac{\alpha}{\beta}\right)_L}\right). \tag{2.17}$$

And since $D_L = n_L.d_L$, and $D_H = n_H.d_H$, then if two schedules with the same number of fractions are compared, it follows that

$$d_L\left(1 + \frac{d_L}{\left(\frac{\alpha}{\beta}\right)_L}\right) = d_H\left(\text{RBE}_{\max} + \frac{\text{RBE}_{\min}{}^2\, d_H}{\left(\frac{\alpha}{\beta}\right)_L}\right). \tag{2.18}$$

One can then obtain the value of d_H, from the positive root of the above equation which, with $(\alpha/\beta)_\text{L}$ replaced by k, is

$$d_H = \frac{-k.\ \text{RBE}_{\max} + \sqrt{k^2.\text{RBE}_{\max}{}^2 + 4d_L{}^2\text{RBE}_{\min}{}^2 + 4\text{d}_L.\ k.\ \text{RBE}_{\min}{}^2}}{2\text{RBE}_{\min}{}^2}. \tag{2.19}$$

The RBE will then be d_L/d_H.

As an example, if the megavoltage photon dose per fraction is 2 Gy, and the $\text{RBE}_{\max}$ is 1.6 with $\text{RBE}_{\min} = 1.05$, d_H is found to be 1.54 Gy when $\alpha/\beta = 3$ Gy. The operative RBE will be $2/1.54 = 1.3$. If the photon dose is changed to 6 Gy, then the equivalent d_H is 5.15 Gy and the RBE reduces to 1.16.

For dose inhomogeneity it is sometimes convenient to use a factor x, where $x = 1.07$ would indicate a 7% dose increment or $x = 0.93$ a 7% on dose reduction, so that

$$\text{BED} = D_L x_L\left(1 + \frac{d_L.\ x_L}{\left(\frac{\alpha}{\beta}\right)_L}\right) = D_H x_H\left(\text{RBE}_{\max} + \frac{\text{RBE}_{\min}{}^2\, d_H.\ x_H}{\left(\frac{\alpha}{\beta}\right)_L}\right). \tag{2.20}$$

a range of BED values can, in principle, be expressed as an equivalent uniform BED just as in the case of equivalent uniform dose (Niemierko 1997), but in such cases there is loss of information on the extreme values which can influence outcomes; in addition, position is lost. It is arguably better to use a BED display superimposed on 3D anatomy or to use representative points where possible.

2.2.7 Dose rate, total fraction treatment time and incomplete repair between treatment fields

Protraction of radiation exposure from the conventional dose rates of around 1–3 Gy min^{-1} to lower rates of around 0.5 Gy hr^{-1} is known to reduce cell kill in most instances (changes due to dose-rate intensification beyond the conventional are considered in chapter 14). Delivery of large single fractions often require a long time, due to setting up several treatment fields, with gantry rotations (which are slower because of the heavier particle therapy gantries) and treatment alignment checks.

This can take as long as 2 hr or more in some instances, which allows considerable repair of sub-lethal damage (operating through the β radiosensitivity parameter), which usually has a half-time of repair of around 10–15 min *in vitro*, with additional longer values in some biosystems, as discussed below.

For explanatory purposes, dose-rate effects are firstly expressed for low-LET conditions, for dose rate R, treatment duration T and where μ is the sub-lethal damage repair rate coefficient (linked only with the dose-rate-sensitive β parameter). The standard LQ equation becomes $E = \alpha RT + \beta R^2T^2.f(\mu T)$. In each case RT can be replaced by either d for a single fraction or nd for multiple fractions. Again, by dividing throughout by α, then

$$\mathrm{BED} = R.\,T\left(1 + \frac{R.\,f(\mu T)}{\left(\frac{\alpha}{\beta}\right)_L}\right). \tag{2.21}$$

The $f(\mu T)$ term used is fully expressed as

$$(2/\mu T)(1 - (1 - \exp[-\mu T])/(\mu T)), \tag{2.22}$$

which can be simplified to $2(\mu \mathrm{T})$ for $T > 10$ hr.

For biphasic repair where there are two operative repair systems each with different time constants μ_1 and μ_2, respectively, in proportions x and $(1 - x)$, each with incomplete repair functions f_1 and f_2, the BED equation becomes

$$\mathrm{BED} = xR.\,T(1 + (\mathrm{R.\,T}/\left(\frac{\alpha}{\beta}\right).f_1) + (1 - x)R.\,T(1 + (\mathrm{R.\,T}/\left(\frac{\alpha}{\beta}\right)f_2). \tag{2.23}$$

2.2.7.1 Consideration of sub-fractional doses

Sub-fractional doses refer to where a given fraction of radiotherapy is split into two or more periods of time when radiation is given ('beam on'), which is usually accompanied by duration of time when no beam exposure occurs ('beam off'). In such cases, which may be given in a large single fraction, as in radiosurgery applications, it is often convenient to consider a dose D in a single fraction (or repeated doses D to give the required total dose) but with n numbers of sub-fractions of dose d. This should not be confused with the standard use of n as being the number of fractions of dose d leading to a total dose of D in standard fractionated radiotherapy as used above.

If a single-fraction treatment is given with n sub-fractions of dose d, each given in a sub-fraction time t_f, but to a total beam-on duration of t, and with all beam-off time being added to a total treatment time of T, then to include repair between fractions and the dose-rate effect during each individual fraction, the BED can be approximated, as in Jones & Hopewell (2019), to be

$$\mathrm{BED} = nd\ (1 + \left(\frac{nd}{k} - \frac{d}{k}\right) f\,(\mu T) + \frac{d}{k} f\,(\,\mu t)). \tag{2.24}$$

The original publication used t_f instead of t in the above equation, and subsequent verification shows this to be a better approximation especially for higher doses and longer exposure times.

This equation is applicable for large single fractions of dose $D(=nd)$, when the sub-fractions d refer to exposures to different isocentres, or if treatment is interrupted by gantry movement to deliver different radiation fields. An additional repopulation correction factor may be required for the separate case of multiple fractionated treatments given over a much longer duration.

This approach was extended to biphasic repair in the case of a single fraction with sub-fractions as

$$\begin{aligned}\mathrm{BED} = x.\ nd(1 &+ \left(\frac{nd}{k} - \frac{d}{k} f\,(\mu_1 T) + \frac{d}{k} f\,(\mu_1 t)\right) \\ &+ (1-x).\ nd(1 + \left(\frac{nd}{k} - \frac{d}{k} f\,(\mu_2 T) + \frac{d}{k} f\,(\mu_2 t)\right).\end{aligned} \tag{2.25}$$

For high LET, the same equations can be used with the $\mathrm{RBE}_{\min}$ terms linked to the $f\,(\mu T)$ or f_1 and f_2 functions, with $\mathrm{RBE}_{\max}$ replacing 1 in the relative effect part. So, for a single repair process:

$$\mathrm{BED} = nd(\mathrm{RBE}_{\max} + \left(\frac{nd}{k} - \frac{d}{k}\right) f\,\mu T\mathrm{RBE}^2_{\min} + \frac{d}{k} f\,\mu t\mathrm{RBE}^2_{\min}), \tag{2.26}$$

and for the biphasic repair processes:

$$\begin{aligned}\mathrm{BED} = x.\ nd(\mathrm{RBE}_{\max} &+ \left(\frac{nd}{k} - \frac{d}{k} f\,(\mu_1 T)\mathrm{RBE}^2_{\min} + \frac{d}{k} f\,(\mu_1 t)\mathrm{RBE}^2_{\min}\right) + \\ (1-x).\ nd(\mathrm{RBE}_{\max} &+ \left(\frac{nd}{k} - \frac{d}{k} f\,(\mu_2 T)\mathrm{RBE}^2_{\min} + \frac{d}{k} f\,(\mu_2 t)\mathrm{RBE}^2_{\min}\right).\end{aligned} \tag{2.27}$$

From the data analysed by Pop *et al* (2000) and used by Hopewell *et al* (2012), the value of x is 0.495 with μ_1 as 3.647 hr^{-1} and μ_2 as 0.321 hr^{-1} (these, respectively, represent exponential half-times of repair of 0.19 and 2.16 hr, respectively, with a spinal cord α/β of 2.47 Gy). For short durations of time of up to 2.5 hr, the original form of the equation gave results 3% above the minimum BEDs and around 4% below the average BEDs estimated in vertibular Schwannoma treatments to 13 Gy, when compared with more complex summation formulations representing incomplete repair of very closely spaced fractions and continuous repair during the radiation exposure published by Canney & Millar (1997). The above simplified approach appears to be useful for the assessment of radiosurgery techniques (Jones & Hopewell 2019, Tuleasca *et al* 2019), although there are many pitfalls in BED estimation which has resulted in confusion with published amendments to some articles, for example as published by Hopewell *et al* (2023).

The total treatment time T is given by the sum of beam-on and beam-off times until the treatment is completed, i.e. $n\, t_f + g(n - 1)$. Use of this expression allows n to be replaced by a function of time in the BED estimate and assessment of the effect of splitting the delivered dose into separate sub-fractions, as shown in figures 2.3(a) and (b) for two different examples of dose per fraction at standard 2 Gy and hypofractionated 7.5 Gy doses for photons (x-rays) and protons. The use of $\alpha/\beta = 2.47$ instead of the standard 2 Gy gives reasonably accurate BED values for doses less than around 10 Gy. Users may wish to use $\alpha/\beta = 2$ Gy.

There is greater separation of the curves in figure 2.3 because of the larger fraction size, but there should be no complacency about the lesser separations for smaller fraction sizes in a fractionated treatment course, since it will be the total BED that will influence outcomes. To obtain the total BED, the BED for a single fraction is multiplied by the number of fractions. For example, in the above graphics the 2 Gy per fraction with two sub-fractions, each delivered in 1 min and with a beam-off time of 10 min, results in a BED of around 4.48 $\text{Gy}_{[2]}$, which if given for 30 fractions gives a BED of approximately 134.4 $\text{Gy}_{[2]}$, whereas the 7.5 Gy dose per fraction yields a BED of 26.9 $\text{Gy}_{[2]}$, which if given four times provides a BED of 134.5 Gy, which are comparable. These BEDs are above standard central nervous system (CNS) tolerance (60 Gy in 30 fractions provides a BED of 108.58 $\text{Gy}_{[2.47]}$), the excess BED being due to the RBE effect. These proton doses have not been reduced for any RBE effect, so will require reduction. This can be found by solving the quadratic in d for 30 fractions:

$108.58 = 30\, d(1.4 + 1.05^2 . \frac{d}{2.47})$, so that the corrected dose per fraction should be 1.68 Gy of protons.

Similarly, a dose reduction will be required for the five-fraction hypofractionated schedule, found from the solution of $108.58 = 5\, d\left(1.4 + 1.05^2 . \frac{d}{2.47}\right)$, which provides a proton dose per fraction of 5.58 Gy instead of 7.5 Gy.

This shows that the precise time durations of treatments when including beam-off times can change the total BED in conventional and hypofractionated treatments. For this reason, detailed exposure and beam ‘downtime’ durations should be recorded for future analysis as well as for estimating significant changes in BED due to longer fractional delivery times (e.g. because of gantry rotations during each treatment fraction in proton therapy).

The above examples use RBE values appropriate for a mid-SOBP, but if distal SOBP RBE values are used the BEDs will be higher, though there should be no complacency about assuming that there will be less repair since the RBE_{min} part of the equations (on which repair operates) will have increased and which allows greater repair capacity for sub-lethal damage. Figures 2.4(a) and (b) show a comparison between mid-SOBP and distal SOBP regions, where it can be seen that there is a considerable reduction in BED with time even in the higher-LET and RBE region of the distal SOBP, although the BED values are higher.

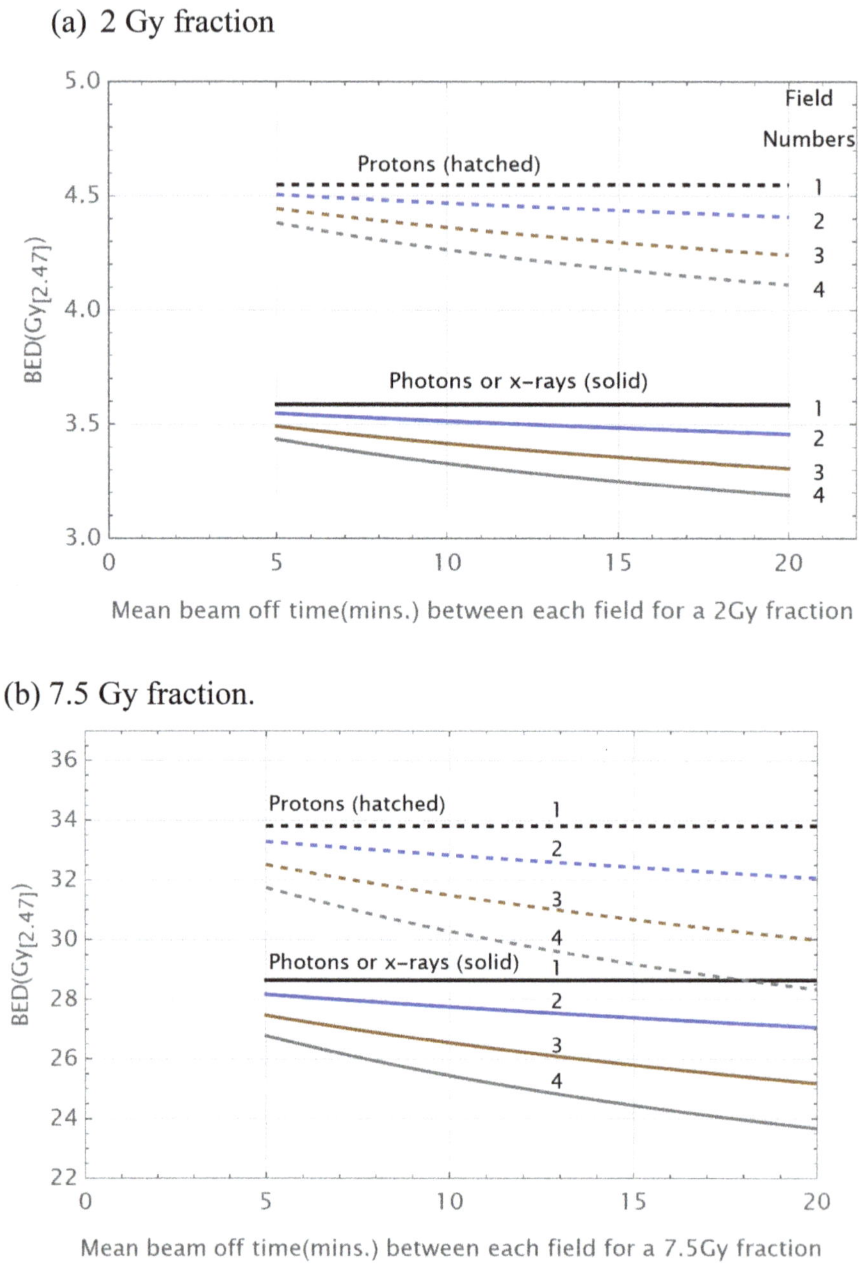

Figure 2.3. (a) and (b): Relationships between number of sub-fractions and BED per fraction with variation in the time of each sub-fraction (or field) delivery for the CNS, using biphasic repair equations, repair half-times of 12 min and 2.3 hr, with $\alpha/\beta = 2.47$ Gy. Plotted using equation (2.27) for protons with assumed $RBE_{max} = 1.4$ and $RBE_{min} = 1.05$, and where n is the number of fields used per fraction and which is varied in order to represent the use of different field numbers (as indicated on the graphs). The physical dose is 2 Gy in (a) and 7.5 Gy in (b) for both photons and protons with a treatment delivery dose rate of 1 Gy min^{-1}.

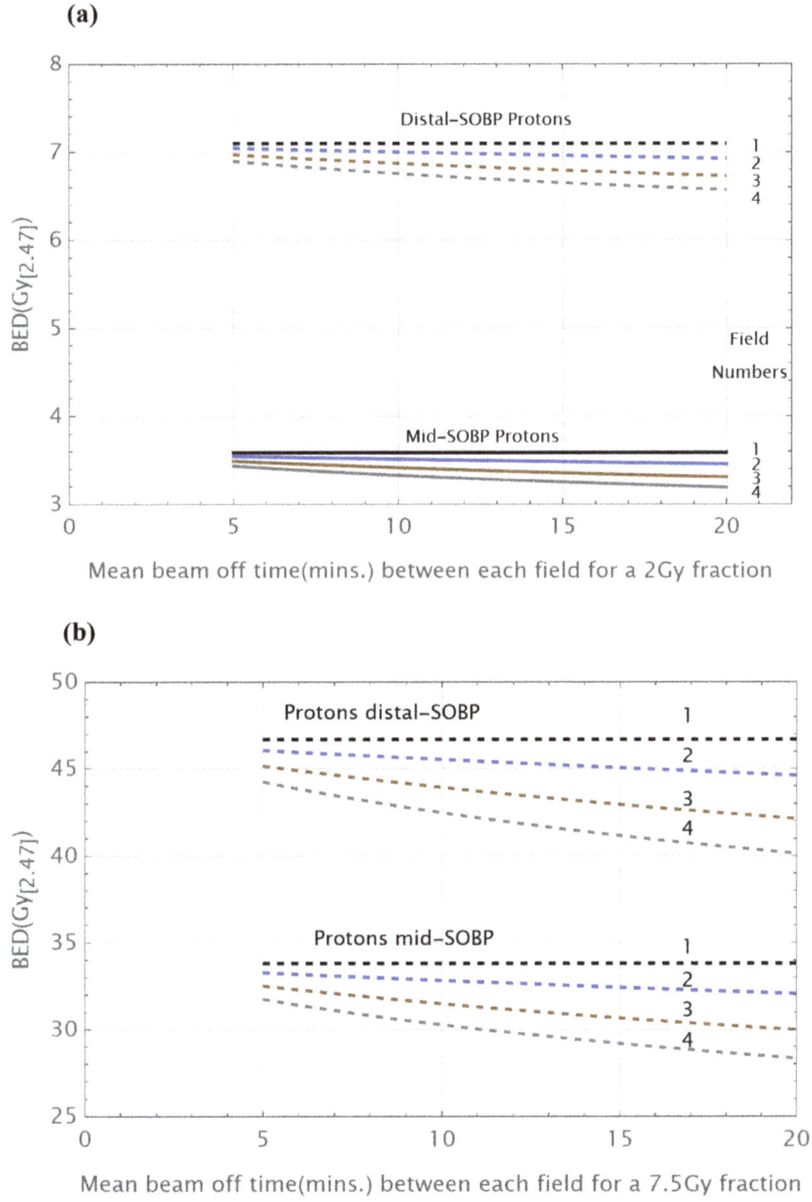

Figure 2.4. Relationships between number of sub-fractions and BED per fraction with variation in the time of each sub-fraction (or field) delivery for protons (details as in figure 2.3). The mid-SOBP has assumed $RBE_{max} = 1.4$ and $RBE_{min} = 1.05$, but $RBE_{max} = 2.5$ and $RBE_{min} = 1.15$ and where n is the number of fields used per fraction (as indicated on the graphs). The physical dose is 2 Gy in (a) and 7.5 Gy in (b).

For a single proton treatment delivered without interruptions in beam delivery, isoeffective doses can be obtained with a single fraction of megavoltage photons or gamma rays which have times longer than a few minutes, the durations of treatment should be used. A single instantaneous dose per fraction of 12.5 Gy (gamma rays)

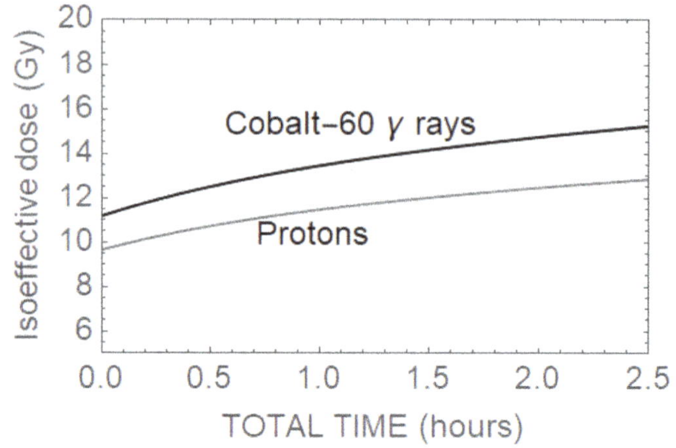

Figure 2.5. Plot of isoeffective doses and total treatment time to match the same effect (or BED) as a single dose of 12.5 Gy given by megavoltage protons or cobalt gamma rays given in 0.5 hr. Note that this applies only in the case of the specified parameters used for a variable RBE.

delivered instantaneously has a BED of around 75.76 $Gy_{[2.47]}$, but when the time is extended to 0.5 hr this value becomes 61.66 Gy. The isoeffective dose is 10.71 Gy for a proton beam with an assumed $RBE_{max} = 1.75$ and $RBE_{min} = 1.09$ (note that this would be 11.36 Gy if a 'standard' 1.1 RBE correction for the 12.5 Gy dose). For further extensions of time, isoeffective doses may be individually solved for this BED value, as shown in figure 2.5. It should be noted that the total doses required to maintain an isoeffect for $\alpha/\beta = 2.47$ Gy (as might be the case in very slow-growing tumours) increases with treatment time to match the required BED. If this is not done then tumour control could be reduced, although the fall in BED should be protective on normal tissues. The doses should be recalculated using more specific tumour α/β ratio values. Where normal tissue toxicity is of great concern, an elective decision to deliver a treatment fraction or individual fractions over a slightly longer time may be appropriate.

Readers may wish to consider using BEDs from their own dose protocols, which could be a BED given, say, over a designated time, such as a half-hour or 1 hr using photons, and then finding the solution for the equivalent dose of protons at relevant LET and RBE values using the equations given above and also in chapters 8 and 9. In principle, these refinements could be added to treatment planning systems. The textbook by Wigg (2008) contains comprehensive summaries of dose-rate radiobiology and practical applications, as does the shorter review by Dale & Jones (1998); Fowler (2012) provides a more recent review of DNA repair half-times. Suffice it to say that tumour repair half-time rates may be shorter than in some normal tissues, but with some reduced repair capacity if there is an absence of a repair pathway, especially the recombination repair (RR) mechanism. Further work needs to be done on this important topic.

2.2.8 Closely spaced fractions

Unlike the dose-rate effect where $f(\mu T)$ terms cause reduced effects with increasing time, closely spaced fractions incur higher effects by imposing a multiplicative factor $(1 + h)$ to replace the in place of the $f(\mu T)$ term: readers should note that sometimes a term h is used where $h > 1$, which can cause confusion.

The standard BED is then

$$\mathrm{BED} = nd\left(1 + \frac{d(1 + h)}{\alpha/\beta}\right). \tag{2.28}$$

To find h values based on the mean inter-fraction interval (f), formulations and tables are available in Dale (1985) and Jones *et al* (2001). As with the dose-rate effect, the overall influence of a higher LET causing larger increments in α will diminish the magnitude of closer fraction spacing to some extent, but this aspect needs careful assessment since breakdown of normal tissue tolerances have occurred with closely spaced fractions in the past, in late-reacting normal tissues such as the spinal cord.

The high-LET BED equation for incomplete repair becomes

$$\mathrm{BED} = nd\left(\mathrm{RBE}_{\max} + \frac{d(1 + h).\ \mathrm{RBE}_{\min}^{2}}{\alpha/\beta}\right). \tag{2.29}$$

2.2.9 Hypoxia

For hypoxia studies, the separate oxygen enhancement ratios for the α_{L} and β_{L} terms can be incorporated as OER_{α} (defined as the ratio $\frac{\alpha_{\mathrm{oxic}}}{\alpha_{\mathrm{hypoxic}}}$) and OER_{β} (the ratio $\frac{\sqrt{\beta_{\mathrm{oxic}}}}{\sqrt{\beta_{\mathrm{hypoxic}}}}$), as multipliers of the dose, so that

$$\mathrm{BED} = nd.\left(\mathrm{OER}_{\alpha} + \frac{d.\ \mathrm{OER}_{\beta}}{\alpha/\beta}\right). \tag{2.30}$$

The same replacements can in principle be used within the high-LET BED equation, as

$$\mathrm{BED} = nd.\left(\mathrm{RBE}_{\max}.\ \mathrm{OER}_{\alpha} + \frac{d.\ \mathrm{OER}_{\beta}.\ \mathrm{RBE}_{\min}^{2}}{\alpha/\beta}\right). \tag{2.31}$$

Care must be taken to use the appropriate OER, which will itself diminish with LET. This aspect has been explored by several authors (Furusawa *et al* 2000, Wenzl & Wilkens 2011, Bopp *et al* 2016).

The effect of hypoxia in high-LET radiation can be seen in graphical presentations of the work of Furusawa *et al* (2000). Not only are the OER_{α} values lowered by hypoxia, but also the LET_{U} turnover points for RBE occur at much higher values of LET. One example from Jones (2022) is shown here as figures 2.6(a) and (b) for carbon and neon ions on human HSG cells.

The phenomenon of extreme radioresistance occurring with ultra-high dose rates (FLASH exposures) in moderately hypoxic cells is thought to be caused by high

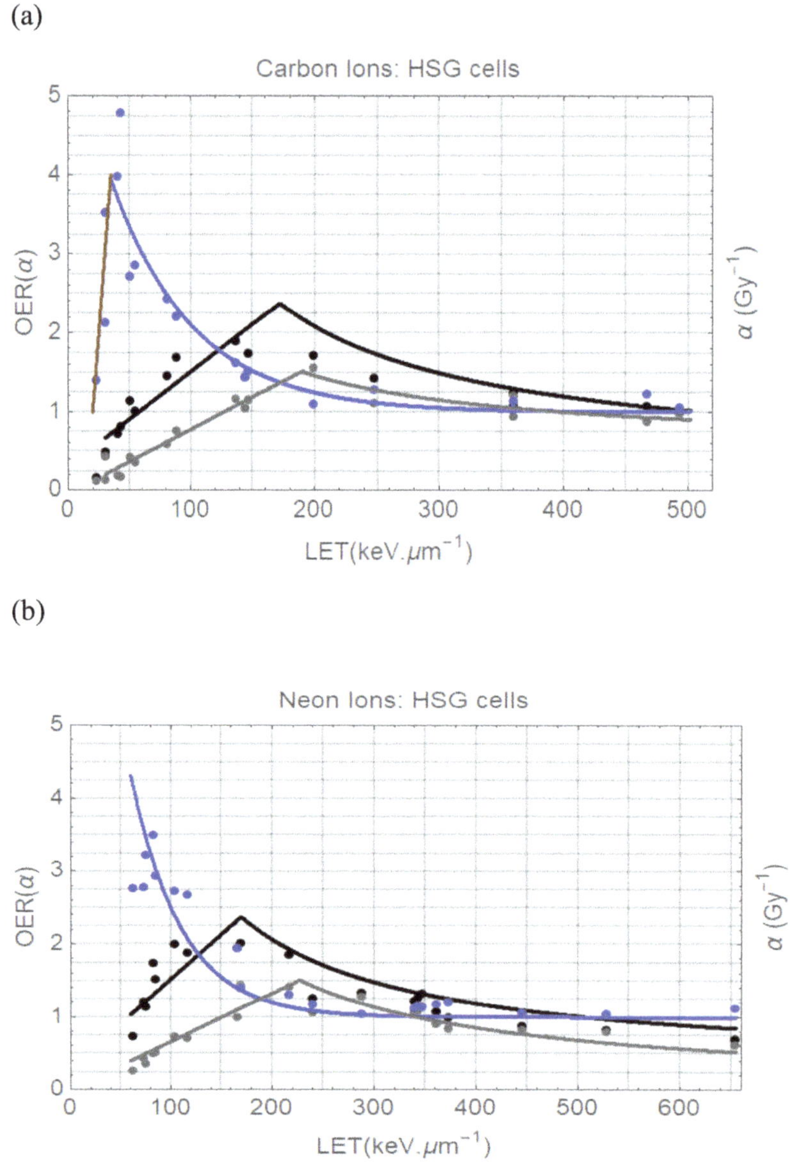

Figure 2.6. (a) and (b): Relationships between LET and both OER(α), which is the ratio of the α radiosensitivities in oxic and hypoxic conditions, and the ï ¡ radiosensitivity parameter in HSG cells irradiated with carbon and neon ions in oxic (black data points, fitted line and curve) and hypoxic (grey data points and fitted curve) conditions. The blue data points and curve (and in (a) the brown line) show the change in OER(α) with LET. (Data from Furusawa *et al* (2000), no standard errors provided.)

oxygen depletion rates as a consequence of rapid ionisation and free-radical interactions which cause severe hypoxia. Intriguingly, the intensification of dose rate may also increase RBE_{max} whilst more severely reducing RBE_{min} (as in Jones 2022) due to increased α and sharply reduced β values. These effects will be considered in further detail in chapters 9 and 14.

2.2.10 Very low doses

Deviations from the LQ model in fast-growing cells with a high G2 cell cycle phase content exist, and have been described as a phenomenon of 'low-dose hypersensitivity', thought to be related to induced repair, in other words induction of repair enzyme systems with increasing dose. Such cells will have high α/β ratios. These have been modelled empirically by Joiner *et al* (2001), as in Marples *et al* (2004), but more mechanistically using the Michaelis–Menten enzyme kinetics approach and induction of additional enzyme capacity in Jones & Morgan (2007). This is relevant to high-LET radiations as the extreme initial slope represents a state of enhanced radiosensitivity, represented by an increase in the α coefficient, and so represents the equivalent of a high-LET situation where there is an increased yield of non-repairable damage, and which does not exhibit a slightly higher SF at doses up to 1.5 Gy before resuming the normal LQ survival curve shape. For intermediate LET values one can assume intermediate patterns of this phenomenon. In most practical applications the doses will exceed the dose range (0–1.5 Gy at the most) in which this phenomenon operates.

These formulations can be transformed to higher-LET situations by replacing α with either α_H or $\alpha_L.R_{max}$, and β by either β_H or $\beta_L.R_{min}{}^2$. The low-LET formulations are

$$\mathrm{SF[overall]} = f.\ e^{-\frac{\alpha d}{\rho_{\mathrm{res}}}-\frac{\beta d^2}{\rho_{\mathrm{res}}}} + (1-f).\ e^{-\alpha d-\beta d^2}, \tag{2.32}$$

where

$$\rho_{res} = x + \rho(1-x) \tag{2.33}$$

and

$$\frac{v}{V_{\max}} = \frac{\alpha d + \beta d^2}{K_M + \alpha d + \beta d^2} = \rho, \tag{2.34}$$

where f is the fraction of cells in the G2 phase, and x is the fraction of DNA repair that is active at zero dose. The saturation of repair rate (ρ) is described by $v/V_{\max}$, where v is the rate at dose d.

The change in effective K_M from a minimum to maximum value is described by

$$K_{M\mathrm{eff}} = K_{M\max} + e^{-jd}(K_{M\min} - K_{M\max}). \tag{2.35}$$

Values of $f = 20\%$, $K_{init} = 10$, $K_{min} = 0.01$ and $j = 6$ were used to fit data in the above source reference.

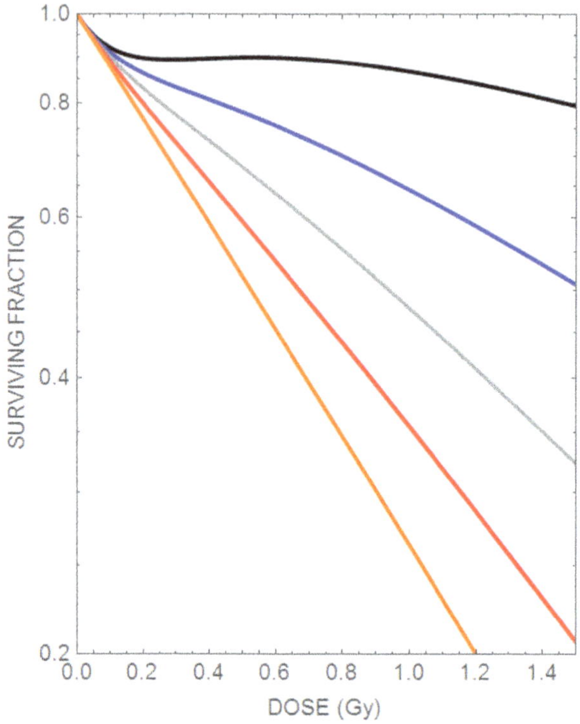

Figure 2.7. Theoretical plot of the effect of increasing the radiosensitivity (assumed here due to LET) causing progressive loss of low-dose hyper-radiosensitivity. The black curve has $\alpha = 0.1$ Gy^{-1}, blue $\alpha = 0.4$ Gy^{-1}, grey $\alpha = 0.7$ Gy^{-1}, and red $\alpha = 1.0$ Gy^{-1}. The orange line represents α_U, the maximum possible radiosensitivity for the cell line (here $\alpha_U = 1.3$ Gy^{-1}).

The more pragmatic equation developed by Joiner *et al* (2001), shows the effective change in α with dose as

$$\mathrm{SF} = \exp\left[-\alpha_r d\left(1 + \left(\frac{\alpha_s}{\alpha_r} - 1\right)\right).\ \exp\left(-\frac{d}{d_C}\right) - \beta d^2\right]. \tag{2.36}$$

This is of considerable interest since as α_r (the 'normal' LQ parameter) becomes larger and approaches α_s (the more sensitive parameter, which describes the initial steep slope of the phenomenon), then the plotted function will shift towards the steep initial slope (as shown in figure 2.7). This may have relevance to high-LET radiations since the α_s probably reflects the high-LET condition (or the α_U, the ultimate value of α at high LET, discussed in later chapters 8 and 9, since there is effectively no repair at such low dose, just as there is reduced or absent repair at high dose with high-LET radiations depending on the LET value). Consequently, α_r can be replaced by α_H (or by α_r.RBEmax) up to a limit of α_U, at any high LET. So, at the LET–RBE turnover positions representing maximum efficiency:

$$\mathrm{SF} = \exp\left[-\alpha_H d\left(1 + \left(\frac{\alpha_U}{\alpha_H} - 1\right)\right).\ \exp\left(-\frac{d}{d_C}\right) - \beta_H d^2\right]. \tag{2.37}$$

Failure to account for low-dose hypersensitivity (LDH) can influence the interpretation of RBE. For example, the study by Mara *et al* (2020) in Austria compared several models for RBE estimation in cell lines with different α/β. Cells with high α/β values (which correlates with faster growth rates) did show LDH, and the experimental dose range included low-dose values in the LDH range, resulting in altered α values which contribute to RBE. The rank order of models changed completely for the cells with low α/β values, where the LDH phenomenon did not occur (and where the models used in chapters 8 and 9 provided the best estimates of the measured RBE). This shows that experiments should be more carefully designed to avoid inclusion of doses within the LDH range.

2.2.11 Higher doses per fraction

There continues to be discussion about deviations from the LQ model at higher doses, even if these may be artefacts due to experimental conditions. In different cell systems and growth conditions, deviations have been observed at doses above the 6–10 Gy range. This effect can occur at least partly because of the statistical issues that arise for lower SFs in colony-forming assays where the number of colonies growing are smaller in number. Nevertheless, there are also some theoretical reasons why some apparent straightening of the cell survival curve might occur with increasing dose.

Three approaches are presented here.

1. The first assumes that second or third lethal chromosomal breaks on the same chromosome result in 'wasted dose', being incapable of causing additional lethality, with resulting high-dose inefficiency of the survival curve.
2. The second is a pragmatic model which assumes a final slope beyond a fixed dose. Alternative approaches include that of Park *et al* (2008), who suggested methods for a gradual transition of the dose–response from the LQ to increasing linearity at higher doses. It is claimed that such approaches may be better suited for assessing high-dose radiotherapy, but others (e.g. Fowler 2008, 2010) suggest that caution needs to be exercised in their application.
3. The third is based on the effect of time protraction to deliver a higher dose, allowing more sub-lethal damage repair during the radiation exposure. Careful assessment of the time taken to deliver higher doses should be made in the interpretation of data sets and whether the change in time is sufficient to allow significant changes in cell survival.

To return to the two models presented here: they are shown graphically with a comparison to the standard LQ model in figure 2.8.

The yield of lethal injury is conventionally represented by the number of lethal chromosome breaks per cell, broadly represented by $\alpha d + \beta d^2$, as initially

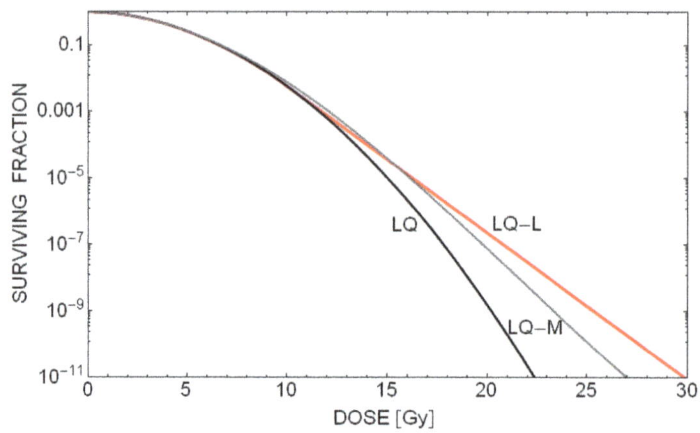

Figure 2.8. Three theoretical survival curves taken to high doses capable of causing tumour sterilisation. The curves appear to deviate around 10 Gy. The standard LQ model shows progressive curvature, the LQ-M (chromosomal) model 1 gradually straightens and the LQ-L (or LQ-linear) model 2 follows a constant slope after a dose of 10 Gy has been achieved.

Table 2.1. Derivation of chromosomal number considerations in apparent straightening of the cell survival curve with increasing dose.

- The nuclear chromosome number is M.
- Total number of lethal chromosome breaks per cell, $E = \alpha d + \beta d^2$.
- Expected average number of lethal breaks per chromosome at dose $d = (\alpha d + \beta d^2)/M$.
- Probability of no breaks on an individual chromosome $= \exp[-(\alpha d + \beta d^2)/M]$.
- Probability of any number of lethal breaks on an individual chromosome $= 1 - \exp[-(\alpha d + \beta d^2)/M]$.
- The average number of lethally damaged chromosomes per cell becomes $M(1 - \exp[-(\alpha d + \beta d^2)/M]) = E_M$.
- So the surviving fraction becomes $\text{SF} = \exp[-E_M]$.

determined by Douglas Lea in 1942 (Lea and Catcheside 1942). Since some of these breaks will be second or third breaks on the same chromosomes (this being likely since some chromosomes are larger than others), such an effect would require modification of the yield of 'effective' lethal chromosomal events, defined as lethal breaks restricted to only one chromosome (second, third, etc., breaks on the same chromosome representing no further lethality risk). This makes a difference when Poisson statistics are considered, and such an interpretation is given in table 2.1.

The model provides a relatively simple formulation but requires radiosenstivity and chromosomal number input. Straightening of the LQ curve occurs at reasonable doses in the 6–10 Gy range depending on the radiosensitivities and scaling used. This model may be appropriate for normal tissue with a normal chromosome content of $M = 46$. Rapidly dividing cells have the added complexity of chromatids, and tumour cells may possess greater than 46 chromosomes per cell. Another complexity is that chromosomal volumes are variable, so some chromosomes will be more susceptible than others to random radiation damage. The chances of lethal breaks and multiple such breaks on the smallest chromosomes can probably be ignored, so one might compromise on there being an effective smaller input number of M to the model. A number of around 36–40 is suggested. Some unpublished work showed that a greater number of cell survival curves were better fitted by this model than the standard LQ model, but the difference was not statistically significant. However, the model is attractive for normal tissue modelling purposes and may be biologically more realistic than the assumption of an arbitrary dose beyond which a straight line is assumed, to be considered next.

Since the chromosomes are of variable volume, random lethal break distributions will favour the larger ones, so there is likely to be an 'effective value' which is less than the 46 chromosomes of a cell. This is not known at the present time but is potentially obtainable by experiment. A disadvantage of this model is that it is not possible to use the BED concept with accuracy: this is because series expansion of the exponential term does not converge well on the pure function, and there is increasing dependence on knowledge of α and β terms rather than α/β. Consequently, graphical methods are necessary to determine the reduction of effect or the equivalent dose to produce the same effect, and then apply BED equations. The method in its present form may be a useful research tool since by fitting appropriate data sets the effective value of M could be obtained.

Jones & Dale (2015) presented an alternative simple approach, inclusive of a BED approach, which assumes that the transition from pure-LQ cell kill to purely logarithmic (i.e. straight-line) cell kill is abrupt rather than gradual and occurs at a specific fractional dose (c) after which the same slope is maintained. In terms of the number (L) of lethal lesions created.

At low fraction doses (less than c) equation (2.1) holds, i.e. $E = \alpha d + \beta d^2$ and up to a limit of $E = \alpha c + \beta c^2$, but at a dose of c the gradient given by the first differential coefficient of the linear quadratic equation $(\alpha + 2\beta c)$ at dose c, so that for doses which exceed c (i.e. d–c):

$$E = \alpha c + \beta c^2 + (\alpha + 2\beta c)(d - c), \tag{2.38}$$

which provides a constant slope for $d > c$.

Following exactly the same procedures as were applied in the basic BED derivation (see equations (2.1)–(2.5)), the BED for N fraction treatments involving fraction doses greater than c is given by

$$\mathrm{BED}_N = N\left(c + \frac{c^2}{(\alpha/\beta)} + \left(1 + \frac{2c}{(\alpha/\beta)}\right)(d - c)\right), \tag{2.39}$$

which simplifies to

$$\mathrm{BED}_N = Nd\left(1 + \frac{c}{(\alpha/\beta)}\left(2 - \frac{c}{d}\right)\right). \tag{2.40}$$

For purposes of illustration, we assume that the crossover from LQ cell kill to linear (logarithmic) cell kill occurs at 10 Gy, i.e. $c = 10$. Then, again following the steps used earlier, for a single-fraction treatment to be isoeffective to a conventional 30 × 2 Gy treatment (BED = 72 Gy_{10}):

$$\text{Then,}\ 1 \times d \times \left(1 + \frac{10}{10}\left(2 - \frac{10}{d}\right)\right) = 72,$$

i.e. the single-fraction isoeffective tumour dose (d) is 27.3 Gy (see the 22.3 Gy derived above for the 'pure-LQ' case).

In the case of a late-reacting normal tissue with $\alpha/\beta = 3$ Gy (for 60 Gy in 30 fractions, BED = 100 Gy_3), then solve

$$1 \times d \times \left(1 + \frac{10}{3}\left(2 - \frac{10}{d}\right)\right) = 100,$$

which provides a single-fraction dose of 17.4 Gy (see the 15.9 Gy derived for the 'pure-LQ' case).

The effect of changing the dose at which the transition occurs is shown in figure 2.9.

High-LET formulations for each method.

1. Chromosomal M model: use the BED formulation containing RBE_{max} and RBE_{max} instead of the standard BEDs:

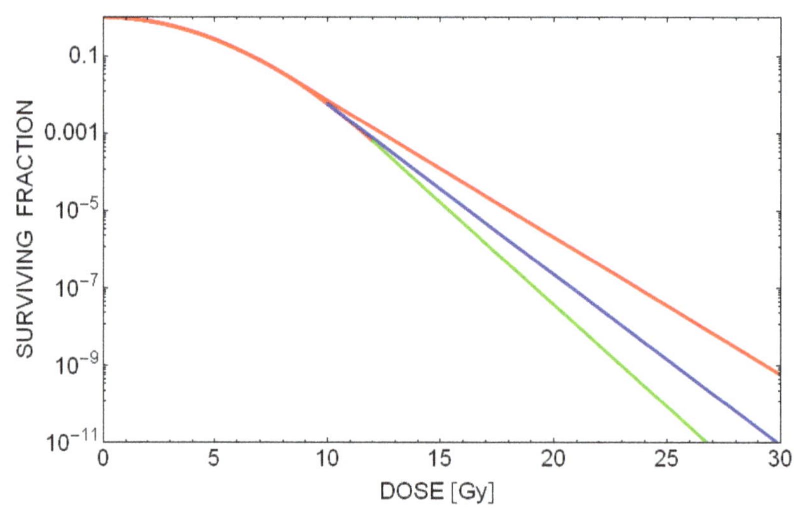

Figure 2.9. Changing the transition points on the LQ survival curve at 8 Gy (red), 10 Gy (blue) and 12 Gy (green).

$$E_M = M(1 - \text{Exp}[-(a_H d + \beta_H d^2)/M])\ or$$
$$E_M = M(1 - Exp[-(\alpha_L.\ R_{\max} D + \beta_L.\ \text{RBE}_{\min}{}^2 d^2)/M]),$$

where M is the 'effective number of chromosomes'.

2. For the straightening of the LQ curve after a dose c, it can be shown by similar rearrangements as in the standard model case that

$$\text{BED}_N = Nd\left(\text{RBE}_{\max} + \frac{\text{RBE}^2_{\min} c}{(\alpha/\beta)}\left(2 - \frac{c}{d}\right)\right) \tag{2.41}$$

It is important to understand that standard BED equations (those assuming that the LQ model holds for indefinitely large fraction doses) will always underestimate the isoeffective doses required for treatments involving high fraction doses. However, caution must be taken in applying this alternative and untested BED approach, but it might be useful for those who wish to analyse their data and attempt to isolate what is the best dose for c in particular situations such as normal tissue type, or tumour class.

In practice, because the dose–response curves 'straighten out' (compared with the increasing curvature predicted by the LQ model), the isoeffect doses calculated using the above methodology provide lower tolerance or isoeffective dose estimates compared with the standard LQ approach. To that extent the standard BED calculations tend to 'fail-safe'; both the required tumour and normal tissue doses will be underestimated, but the degree of underestimation is probably greater in the latter case. This is because the late-reacting normal tissue dose–response curve has greater curvature (and lower α/β ratio) than has the tumour. In the case of slow-growing tumours with α/β ratios that are close to that of the late-reacting normal tissue, there should be less difference. However, the LQ model will continue to underestimate the effect and will fail-safe with respect to normal tissue late-reacting effects. This must be understood by the physicians and physicists involved in the treatment planning process. These methods may of course be useful in obtaining correlations with clinical data sets.

The inclusion of normal tissue and tumour repopulation effects, and further more detailed considerations on fractionation, as well as the increasingly important topic of re-treatment of recurrent tumours are discussed further in chapter 12.

The third potential mechanism can be illustrated by plotting cell survival curves for different exposure times, as shown in figures 2.10(a) and (b), where treatment exposure time extension leads to reduced survival and apparent 'straightening' of the survival curve. The degree of change in survival is much greater in the case of low α/β ratios.

2.3 The α/β ratio and its choice for modelling particle therapies

Models can only be sufficiently informative for clinical decision making if their input parameters are reasonably accurate and if the model is used in a fail-safe way,

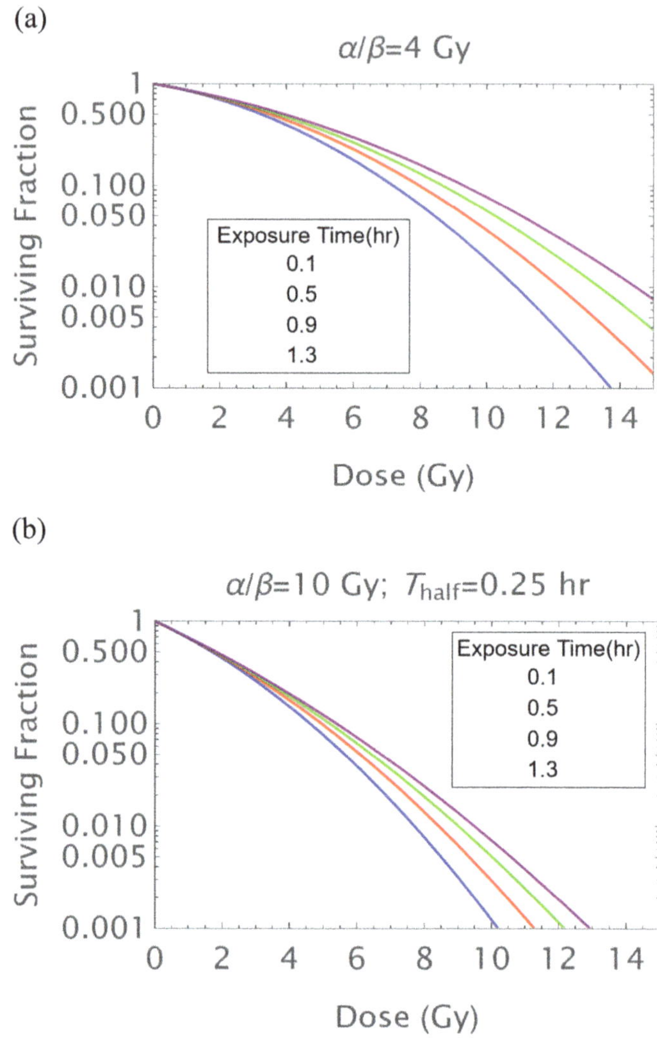

Figure 2.10. (a) and (b): The assumed α/β ratios and repair half-times are shown on each graph, where variations in surviving fraction with exposure time are plotted between 0.1 and 1.3 hr.

sometimes varying these parameters to consider worst-case scenarios. The radiobiology literature contains many examples of such parameters, especially the key α/β ratio of important normal tissues and certain tumour types, although in the latter case with considerable variation. Unfortunately, good predictive assays are not available, although it is clear that correlations between concepts like repair capacity will correlate with radiosensitivity and that α and β may reflect some of the limiting repair processes such as NHEJ and RR, respectively. Much work is needed to establish firm links between molecular-based assays and the modelling parameters.

2.3.1 The α/β ratio

The α/β ratio is the ratio of the two radiosensitivity parameters in the LQ model of radiation effect and is expressed in units of Gy. The ratio is a relatively robust parameter, especially in the case of late-reacting normal tissues with little change between species; inversely related to the fraction sensitivity during radiotherapy; well-characterised for certain classes of tissue and tumours in experimental cell lines, animals and humans; and inversely proportional to cell turnover.

The α/β ratio probably reflects many cellular processes, such as DNA repair and changes in radiosensitivity due to cell cycle position, and in the case of tumours the extent of hypoxia, although a single α/β value can only represent the average contributions of these processes during therapy. It is an especially useful parameter within BED equations.

The function of the α/β ratio is to act as a coefficient which controls the fractionation sensitivity. When fraction size is changed, the resulting total dose needs to be modified in order to provide a constant BED (and the same bioeffect). It is important to understand that different tissues and tumours can possess quite different α/β ratios, so that they respond differently to different changes in dose fractionation. The use of α/β ratios in hadrontherapy is more complex, as discussed below. Although it is used as a constant term, it can increase in proportion to cell cycling activity, or with increasing LET and at ultra-high dose rates. Hypoxia also modifies α/β since oxygen influences α by a lesser amount than β.

2.3.2 Applications of BED equations

The BED equations have many uses, including the calculation of the following:

- Isoeffect (or equieffect) doses for different fractionation schedules (see chapter 6).
- Compensatory radiation doses after unintended under- or overdosage (See chapter 13).
- Modified dose-fractionation schedules after unintended treatment interruptions (see chapter 12).
- Re-treatment dose-fractionation schedules, by using time-related changes in tissue re-treatment tolerances (see chapter 12).
- Changes in tissue tolerances and tumour doses due to dose-rate effects, ranging from low dose rates to ultra-high or FLASH dose rates (see chapters 9, 11 and 14).

BED equations can be adapted for the purposes of charged-particle therapy (CPT) using protons and ions, as well as for drug-related effects (cytotoxic chemotherapy or other biotherapies) and for the influence of changes in radiation tolerance due to factors such as age/surgery by allocating a BED equivalent for these factors, as shown below.

BED equations are derived from the basic LQ model of radiation effect, by dividing the number of lethal events per cell by the α parameter. Although the BED equation consists of a simple mathematical (quadratic) form, clinical BED calculations require considerable care, especially in the choice of α/β ratio used: this applies to both conventional x-ray-based megavoltage radiations and CPT using hadrons.

There are some important rules concerning BED equations:

1. BEDs can be added for different components of an overall treatment given by different types of radiation (e.g. for a treatment combining x-rays and electrons, the overall BED = electron BED + x-ray BED, or for a treatment comprising x-rays and an ion-beam boost, then the overall BED = x-ray BED + ion-beam BED).
2. Additional risk factors such as chemotherapy, age or other medical conditions can be included as overall BED = radiation BED + risk factor BED. The latter is determined from clinical studies which contain multiple radiation dose levels with and without the risk factor, where an isoeffect can be identified and allowing simultaneous equations to be used, as shown by Jones *et al* (2006).
3. Calculations which involve a specified bioeffect in a given tissue or tumour type should be done only using the same α/β ratio; it follows that different α/β ratios cannot be used to describe the same bioeffect.
4. It is assumed that the α/β ratio reflects an average value during treatment. During a course of radiotherapy lasting 4–8 weeks, the ratio is probably stable in the case of slow-growing tumours and slow-cell-turnover tissues. However, in the case of tissues or fast-growing tumours and normal tissues that exhibit real or apparent acceleration of their proliferation rates during treatment, the α/β ratio may itself increase; this has been shown to be the case for acute-reacting normal epithelial tissues, where α/β increases from 5 to 35 Gy from the first few weeks to the sixth week in human and animal skin (Hopewell *et al* 2003).

2.3.3 Special considerations for particle therapy

The reader should be cautious about some published high-LET BED values, since they have incorporated a constant RBE value. The literature can be confusing, as this work can still be regarded as being in a developmental stage despite many of the underlying principles being understood around 40 years ago, but before the more widespread utilisation of the LQ model and BED concept. Subsequent improvements have now produced a more coherent framework for isoeffect applications. Two suggested methods for BED isoeffect calculations in modern hadrontherapy are provided below: these use both low- and high-LET α/β ratios in specific situations, but principally the low-LET α/β in association with RBE conversion factors. It must be stressed that 'dose' in these calculations refers to the physical dose and not the cobalt equivalent or any other form of RBE-weighted dose, unless otherwise stated.

The relationship between $(\alpha/\beta)_L$ and $(\alpha/\beta)_H$ is linked in the following way by the maximum and minimum RBE parameters:

$$\frac{\text{RBE}_{\text{max}}}{\text{RBE}_{\text{min}}{}^2} = \frac{\left(\frac{\alpha}{\beta}\right)_H}{\left(\frac{\alpha}{\beta}\right)_L}. \tag{2.42}$$

It also follows that $$\left(\frac{\alpha}{\beta}\right)_H = \frac{\text{RBE}_{\text{max}}}{\text{RBE}_{\text{min}}{}^2}. \quad \left(\frac{\alpha}{\beta}\right)_L. \tag{2.43}$$

This provides a general method for estimating the α/β for high-LET radiations where these are not known. This equation can be further simplified by use of a combined RBE converting factor (R_C) as

$$\left(\frac{\alpha}{\beta}\right)_H = R_C \cdot \left(\frac{\alpha}{\beta}\right)_L, \tag{2.44}$$

where

$$R_C = \frac{\text{RBE}_{\text{max}}}{\text{RBE}_{\text{min}}{}^2}. \tag{2.45}$$

Consequently, a single number, R_C, can be used to convert low-LET α/β to the high-LET state.

The increase in RBE, when dose per fraction is reduced, is mainly due to the increase in repair of sub-lethal damage that occurs in the low-LET radiation case. Then, in principle, RBE_{max} and RBE_{min} may also be governed in part by the low-LET α/β ratio, such that a greater change in RBE with dose per fraction occurs in tissues with lower low-LET α/β ratios (due to their ability to repair low-LET radiation sub-lethal damage more effectively than tissues with higher α/β values). Recent analysis of fast neutron data sets in the UK has shown (for cells and tissues which are not seriously repair deficient) that the RBE_{max} and RBE_{min} are, respectively, inversely and directly related to the low-LET α/β ratio. RBE_{max} appears to be a reciprocal function of the low-LET α/β ratio, but RBE_{min} is linearly related to the square root of the low-LET α/β ratio. In other words, RBE is not only a combination of change in LET and dose (physical), but also is influenced by changes in cell cycling/repair (biological) as reflected in the α/β ratio.

It follows from the definitions of RBE_{max} and RBE_{min} and equation (2.39) that

$$\text{RBE}_{\text{max}} = \text{RBE}^2_{\text{min}} \cdot \frac{\alpha_H}{\beta_H}\left(\frac{1}{(\alpha/\beta)_L}\right) \tag{2.46}$$

and

$$\text{RBE}_{\text{min}} = \sqrt{\frac{\text{RBE}_{\text{max}}. \, (\alpha/\beta)_L}{(\alpha/\beta)_H}}. \tag{2.47}$$

It can clearly be seen that RBE_{max} is inversely proportional to the low-LET α/β and that RBE_{min} is directly proportional to its square root (all other terms being kept constant).

In biological data, the general relationships between RBE_{max}, RBE_{min} and $(\alpha/\beta)_L$ take the following form, where A and C represent the minimum values of RBE_{max} and RBE_{min}, respectively, and B and K are coefficients:

$$RBE_{max} = A + \frac{B}{\left(\frac{\alpha}{\beta}\right)_L}, \tag{2.48}$$

$$RBE_{min} = C + K\sqrt{\left(\frac{\alpha}{\beta}\right)_L}. \tag{2.49}$$

Such relationships can only apply for specific LET-determined situations, and the above equations were derived from fast neutron data (Jones *et al* 2011), consequently from an LET spectrum, although the RBE values obtained are close to those found towards the end of the range of proton SOBPs (Britten *et al* 2013), not surprisingly perhaps, since fast neutrons ionise mainly by formation of recoil protons. For many years neutron RBEs were used to provide RBEs for carbon-ion therapy in Japan (Kanai *et al* 1997). Thus the values of A, B, C and K are available for one fast neutron data set but remain to be determined for protons and heavier ions. Studies of how the basic physics-related RBE changes (A and C) with LET, the further parameters (B and K) and how they change between cells and tissues might offer a simple pragmatic approach to data fitting, but the constants would apply only to specific LET values. However, it would be preferable to derive RBE limits directly from LET, as will be shown in later chapters.

The local-effect model (Elsässer & Scholz 2007), developed and used in Germany, predicts RBE from LET and for cabon ions uses the low-LET α/β ratio along with a conversion factor based on beam micro-dosimetry (LET) and mean cellular nuclear volume. It essentially provides an RBE that is related to the low-LET α/β ratio, which varies with dose per fraction within its accepted range based on *in vitro* cell survival data. It has been applied successfully in clinical treatments of carbon ions at Darmstadt and Heidelberg using 3 Gy per fraction equivalent dose at the tumour target. The RBE is said to be underestimated by around 10%–20%, which ensures that the tumour cell kill will be higher than expected from the stated equivalent dose. It remains to be seen if the model will hold when larger fraction sizes beyond those used to obtain *in vitro* data are used.

In the micro-dosimetric kinetic model (MKM), developed in the USA and now used in Japan (Hawkins 2003, 2009, Inaniwa *et al* 2013), the predicted RBE also has a similar inverse dependency on the low-LET α/β, and could be similarly susceptible in hypofractionated conditions. Because of a longstanding controversy about whether β values change with increasing LET (see Jones 2010), this model did not include allowance for changes in β until more recently, as an improved version (Chen *et al* 2017). To verify models over a wider range of fractionation may require animal models rather than *in vitro* experiments since the amount of cell killing required to produce late tissue effects exceeds the *in vitro* range by several orders of magnitude. The alternative is to analyse human clinical data in greater detail with respect to LET, particle dose (BED) and tissue tolerances.

It is important to note that the α/β ratio must increase non-linearly with LET. This can cause confusion in modelling. Any attempt to convert between low- and high-LET α/β should be done for the two components of the LQ model separately, that is for RBE_{max} (for α) and RBE_{min} (for β).

2.3.3.1 Alternative approach for isoeffect calculations in the case of two high LET schedules

Rather than convert dose information between low- and high-LET conditions, there will be situations where only the high-LET radiosensitivity parameters are known. Then one can use the following approach without reference to low LET. Thus for two isoeffective schedules of high LET we have for N_1 factions and N_2 fractions of dose d_1 and d_2:

$$N_{1H}(\alpha_H d_{1H} + \beta_H d_1^2{}_H) = N2H(\alpha_H d2H + \beta_H d_2^2{}_H). \tag{2.50}$$

It is then permissible to divide throughout by α_H and obtain

$$D_{1H}\left(1 + \frac{d_{1H}}{\left(\frac{\alpha}{\beta}\right)_H}\right) = D_{2H}\left(1 + \frac{d_{2H}}{\left(\frac{\alpha}{\beta}\right)_H}\right). \tag{2.51}$$

Here the α/β is that of the high-LET parameters (these are less well established in the literature at the present time), but in this case the two RBE parameters RBE_{max} and RBE_{min} are no longer necessary. It would also be possible to use the single R_C conversion factor in the situation of comparing two identical high-LET radiations, so that equation (2.15) would become

$$D_{1H}\left(1 + \frac{d_{1H}}{R_C\left(\frac{\alpha}{\beta}\right)_L}\right) = D_{2H}\left(1 + \frac{d_{2H}}{R_C\left(\frac{\alpha}{\beta}\right)_L}\right), \tag{2.52}$$

which could also be used in this form along with the time factor corrections, as given below.

For unintended treatment interruptions, the most appropriate time and repopulation correction factors can be added for the case of tumour isoeffects. This is not necessary for late-reacting tissues. The equations are then

$$D_{1H}\left(1 + \frac{d_{1H}}{\left(\frac{\alpha}{\beta}\right)_H}\right) - K_H T_{1H} = D_{2H}\left(1 + \frac{d_{2H}}{\left(\frac{\alpha}{\beta}\right)_H}\right) - K_H T_{2H}, \tag{2.53}$$

where T_1 and T_2 are the respective overall treatment times for schedule 1 and 2, and K_H is defined as

$$K_H = \frac{0.693}{\alpha_{H}.\omega}. \tag{2.54}$$

Compared with the K values for low LET (K_L), there is little knowledge of K_H values in the literature. K_H can however be found from K_L by dividing by RBE_{max} (which is α_H/α_L), that is

$$K_H = \frac{K_L}{\text{RBE}_{\text{max}}}. \tag{2.55}$$

For $(\alpha/\beta)_{\text{H}}$ there is little in the way of large-scale clinical data for protons and heavier ions, although it is well established that α values increase with LET to a far greater extent than β values, which results in $(\alpha/\beta)_H$ being much larger than $(\alpha/\beta)_L$, as shown in large *in vitro* data sets. It is also possible to infer α/β values from sample clinical data. For example, the Japanese National Institute of Radiological Sciences (NIRS, Chiba) carbon-ion phase 1/2 non-small cell lung cancer studies showed an isoeffective tumour control for 44 Gy-eq in one fraction and 60 Gy-eq in four fractions given in 1 week (Okada *et al* 2010): then, the $(\alpha/\beta)_H$ can be found in the following equation, where an RBE of 2.5 is assumed to convert to physical dose in the middle of the SOBP for carbon ions at NIRS (Chiba):

$$\frac{44}{2.5}\left(1 + \frac{44}{(2.5)\left(\frac{\alpha}{\beta}\right)_H}\right) = \frac{60}{2.5}\left(1 + \frac{60}{(4 \times 2.5)\left(\frac{\alpha}{\beta}\right)_H}\right), \text{ from which } \left(\frac{\alpha}{\beta}\right)_H = 25.9 \text{ Gy}.$$

It is then possible to reestimate this parameter from isoeffective tumour control in patients treated with either one, four, nine or 18 fractions to cobalt-equivalent Gy total doses of 44 (in 1 day), 60 (in 1 week), 72 (in 3 weeks) and 86 (in 6 weeks), respectively, and allowing for repopulation at an assumed equivalent rate of 0.1 Gy day^{-1} between 1 and 3 weeks and of 0.3 Gy day^{-1} at times over 28 days. These repopulation rates are in K_H units and are consequently lower than the K_L values usually seen. The total dose solutions are then 25.9, 22.2, 23.9, 15.3, 19.1 and 37.7 Gy when each schedule is compared with another. This provides a mean $(\alpha/\beta)_{\text{H}}$ of 24 Gy (median 23.1) with a standard error of the mean of 3.3 Gy. This would imply an R_C value of 2.4 (if the $(\alpha/\beta)_L$ is 10 Gy). Then, by using equation (2.39), RBE_{min} is not unreasonably around 1.3; it follows that RBE_{max} is around 4.

It can be appreciated from the previous paragraph that changes in total dose are required to compensate for altered dose per fraction even in the case of high-LET radiations which have high $(\alpha/\beta)_{\text{H}}$ values. It is only when high-LET and very-low-LET radiations are compared that the fractionation sensitivity of the high-LET case is considered to be almost zero in relative terms: this is reflected by the differences in their α/β ratios.

Some recommendations for future work include the following:

- RBE_{max} and RBE_{min} values need to be better established for high-LET radiations and linked to specific LET values.
- Specific high-LET repopulation dose equivalents are required for different classes of tumours.
- α/β values specific for high-LET radiations can be used in some circumstances without RBE when identical high-LET radiations are compared, but not for comparing low- and high-LET schedules, or for calculating a combined BED where low- and high-LET radiations are used. A library of clinical $(\alpha/\beta)_H$ values must be gathered for protons and ions and would need cooperative international research, although the process has commenced in Germany, at GSI, Darmstadt (Friedrich *et al* 2013), and should be extended from only *in vitro* data to *in vivo* conditions. It will take a long time to establish a comprehensive set of radiobiological parameters specific for hadrontherapy under the circumstances of using only a physical dose, the high-LET parameters and no RBE factors. This is a reasonable long-term goal which will need to also include the defining of tissue tolerances and expected tumour control rates using such an approach. In the meantime, the use of RBE to convert known tolerance and tumour prescription doses remains the norm. The only alternative is to use data from Japan where dose per fraction has been varied and where good isoeffective dose data are available.
- Users should beware of over-reliance on *in vitro* α and β values; these are acquired using ideal cell culture conditions and in only one treatment fraction, which can hardly reflect the conditions in a tumour or normal tissue, with all the changes which inevitably occur during fractionated treatment.

In situations where under- or overdose has occurred and in subsequent calculations of compensatory equivalent x-ray schedules the most reasonable estimates of the parameters should be used; clinicians may prefer to use the safest choices, such as a high RBE_{max} in tissues which are highly fraction sensitive for x-rays, such as the CNS. The general advice for such calculations in the case of x-rays has been published by Jones & Dale (2018), but the additional effect of RBE must be included if there is any attempt to use (low-LET) x-ray tissue tolerances or x-ray tumour control data. The alternative approach is to use only high-LET α/β ratios within BED equations where the tolerance and tumour control BED values for the high-LET radiation are known. These are subtle but important differences.

***2.3.3.1.1 The α/β* ratios**

The low-LET α/β ratios for various tumours can be found in publications by Wyatt *et al* (2003) and Wigg (2008). It is unfortunate that, because of a worldwide reduction in radiation research applied to pure radiobiology over the past 20 years, relatively little progress has been made to obtain determine even better parameters from clinical data sets. Despite such setbacks, this remains an important area for research.

From the clinical experience of the present author, who has implemented many forms of the LQ model in clinical situations, it is recommended that a range of α/β values should be modelled. The variation in α/β will normally be greater for tumours than for normal tissues, since the former contain greater genetic and phenotypic heterogeneity. Another issue is that α/β may vary with age and be smaller in younger individuals, consequently making them more fraction sensitive; alternatively, an equivalent BED for age can be used. The responsible clinician should ideally be given a choice of a range of solutions to any clinical problem, calculated using a reasonable range of α/β values. It should also be noted that, more recently, the α/β values for human tumours are considered to be lower than those previously established from animal experiments. As such, a value of 5–8 Gy may be more reasonable than 10 Gy for many human cancers. Fowler stated that the fractionation effects were far less substantial for tumour α/β values greater than 7–8 Gy when compared with normal tissues with values of between 2 and 4 Gy (Fowler 2012).

Some normal tissues probably exhibit dual-response characteristics where the combined effects of severe acute reactions can make a significant contribution to the late effects; these are termed consequential late reactions. They may be the weighted product of the acute- and late-reacting α/β ratios and so can be greater than 3 Gy. An example is rectal damage, often quoted as 4 Gy, but in practical (and conservative) terms assumed to be 3 Gy. There probably are differences in terms of duration of radiation exposure. For the extreme example, the acute exposure of a large single fraction, we should assume the lowest α/β value since irradiation takes place in the situation of (relatively) low proliferation. But in the case of a more protracted irradiation, the acute-reacting epithelial tissue may increase its own α/β ratio with time: this is known to be the case in animal and human skin. Another important issue is that overall treatment time and dose per fraction, taken together, may influence the severity of the acute reaction sufficiently to have an impact on the late reaction. This aspect of clinical radiobiology is relatively neglected in recent times and deserves further attention.

It cannot be overemphasised that α/β ratio values in tumours need to be expressed as a function of their histological differentiation status, or in other words related to the complexity of genetic disorder, or chaos, within the tumour cell; that is, a choice of a larger value within the accepted range should be considered for poorly differentiated tumours and lower values for the well-differentiated state. The α/β ratios of normal tissues with respect to their late-reacting complications are considered to be more stable so that 2 Gy for the CNS and 3 Gy for all other tissues are usually used.

Obtaining reliable ranges of K values and, where applicable, T_K values for specific tumour and normal tissue classes are also important research aims.

The following data were compiled by the present author and Dr Joe Martin as part of an introductory DPhil project (as well as figures 2.7 and 2.8). Considerable use has been made of data within *Applied Radiobiology: Continuous Irradiation and Brachytherapy* (Wigg 2008), p. 28, table 1.3, and other sources. Values as in Bentzen & Baumann (2002), p. 135, table 13.1.

Tissues and species	α/β	**Upper (95%) confidence limit**	**Lower (95%) confidence limit**
Head and neck	10.0	n/a	n/a
Prostate cancer	3.1	2.6	3.6
Prostate cancer	1.5	0.8	2.2
Prostate cancer	1.49	1.25	1.76
Melanoma	0.6	−1.1	2.5
Melanoma	0.17		

Tumour	α	**Standard deviate**	β	**Standard deviate**	α/β
Melanoma	0.27		0.042		6.43
	0.33		0.038		8.68
	0.13		0.113		1.15
	0.27		0.047		5.74
	0.21		0.1		2.10
	0.28		0.087		3.22
	0.35		0.070		5.00
	0.53		0.078		6.79
	0.61		0.101		6.04
	0.33		0.048		6.88
Mean	0.33	0.22	0.072	0.027	4.58
Pancreatic	0.51		0.048		10.63
	0.47		0.052		9.04
Mean	0.49	0.028	0.050	0.003	9.80
Breast	0.51		0.031		16.45
	0.47		0.091		5.16
Mean	0.49	0.14	0.061	0.042	8.03
Prostate	0.44	0.27	0.037	0.028	11.89
Cervical	0.43	0.19	0.036	0.024	11.94
Colon	0.23		0.048		4.79
Astrocyt gd.1	0.37		0.11		3.36
Astrocyt gd.3	0.26		0.034		7.65
Glioblastoma	0.28	0.049	0.045	0.022	6.22
Glioma (paed)	0.30	0.20	0.030	0.018	10.00
Squ. cell car.	0.36	0.22	0.042	0.023	8.57
Adenocar.	0.45	0.32	0.039	0.033	11.54

Embryonal	0.61	0.24	0.029	0.054	21.03
Lymph/myel.	0.56	0.25	0.085	0.102	6.59
Oat cell car.	0.58	0.27	0.087	0.122	6.67
Osteosarcoma	0.38	0.19	0.063	0.038	6.03
Neuroblast.	0.75	0.33	0.059	0.062	12.71
Medulloblast.	0.55		0.019		28.95
Wilm's tumour	0.55		0.023		23.91
Ewing's sarc.	0.42	0.17	0.127	0.19	3.31
Rhabdomyos.	0.25		0.029		8.62
Burkitts lymp.	0.87		0.009		96.67
Acute mye.	1.24	1.2	0.052	0.083	23.85
Leukaemia					
ALL	0.59	0.19	0.012	0.017	49.17
AML	0.96	0.60	0.021	0.012	45.71
Chronic ML	0.09		0.007		12.86
Leukaemic ce.	0.65		0.065		10.00
Promyelocyt.	0.59	0.056	0.028	0.039	21.07
APL	0.44		0.018		24.44
Erythroleuk.	0.53	0.36	0.031	0.042	17.10
Acute non-lymp. leuk.	1.45		0.13		11.15

***In Vivo* Human Tumours**		**Wigg (2008) p. 210**	
Tissues and species	α/β	Lower (95%) confidence limit	Upper (95%) confidence limit
Oral cavity	10.0	6.5	10.3
Vocal cord	9.9		
Bladder ca.	10		
Cervix ca.	13.9		
Skin ca.	8.4		
Liposarcoma	0.4	−1.4	54
Melanoma	0.6	−1.1	2.5
Melanoma	0.17		

Tumours	α/β	Lower (95%) confidence limit	Upper (95%) confidence Limit
Head and neck			
Larynx	14.5	4.9	24
Vocal cord	13		
Oropharynx	16		
Buccal mucosa	6.6	2.9	Infinite
Tonsil	7.2	3.6	Infinite
Nasopharynx	16	−11	43
Various	10.5	6.5	29
Skin	8.5	4.5	11.3

Other analytical techniques have been used for tumours such as glioblastoma, where the α/β has been estimated to be 9.2 Gy (Jones & Sanghera 2007), and there is greater acceptance that α/β wil vary between tumours according to their proliferative and repair capacity. These may correlate with histological grading features: the more well differentiated, the lower the ratio.

Where α/β is not known but tumour potential doubling time (and volume doubling time) information is available, one can resort to a simple inverse relationship, given by $\alpha/\beta = 48.8/T_{\text{pot}}$, as derived from the plot shown in figure 2.8. This formulation was derived from the equation $K = 0.693/(\alpha.T_{\text{eff}})$, since it can be divided throughout by β and rearranged to give $\alpha/\beta = C/T_{\text{pot}}$, where C is regarded as a replacement constant and which assumes T_{pot} is the operative T_{eff} in most radiotherapy schedules. This is consistent with standard radiobiology dogma that low-proliferative states have low α/β and vice versa. For measured tumour volume doubling times (T_D), one can assume a high cell-loss factor of 90% for carcinomas (50% for sarcomas), which allows the estimation of the potential doubling time. The cell-loss factor (φ) is known to be related to T_{pot} by the relationship $\varphi = (1 - \frac{T_{\text{pot}}}{T_D})\%$.

In the case of normal tissue, it is standard practice to use $\alpha/\beta = 3$ Gy for most late effects (fibrosis in lung, kidney, soft tissues and heart), but the lower value of 2 Gy in the CNS (spinal cord and brain). Peripheral nerves and the cauda equina (below the spinal cord, but consisting of nerves derived from it) may have a α/β between 2 and 3 Gy, although the more conservative 2 Gy is often used. Another important area is the optic chiasm, where a α/β of 2 Gy should be used, whereas the optic nerve may behave more like peripheral nerves (figure 2.11).

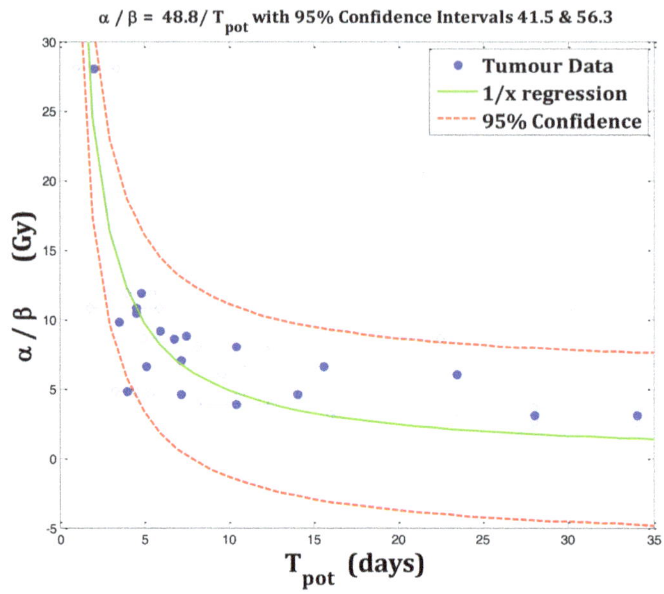

Figure 2.11. Plotted data from the literature of the cellular potential doubling time (T_{pot}) against the α/β ratio and fitted using a non-linear least-squares technique.

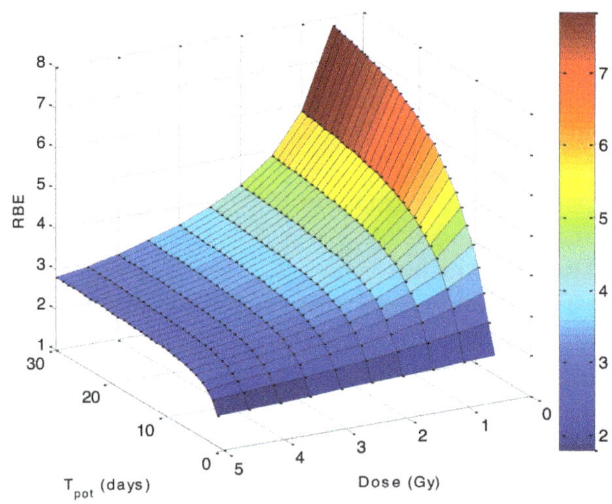

Figure 2.12. 3D plot of dose, T_{pot} and RBE for fast neutrons derived from data of Batterman for RBE relating to tumour recurrence times after treatment, using the inverse relationship with T_{pot} given above and an assumed cell-loss factor of 90%. This may represent the worst-case situation for a proton beam, but would need scaling to lower RBEs for the more usual clinical proton beam, but may be useful for heavier ion beams.

Using the above equations and assumption of the cell-loss factor linking T_{pot} and volume doubling times, it is possible to build up 3D plots of the relationship between volume doubling times, RBE in the case of fast neutrons (see figure 2.12), which ionise mostly by the means of recoil protons. This approach may reflect the operative RBE within the Bragg peak region for protons. Further information on neutrons and the implications for proton therapy can be obtained in chapter 5.

2.4 The design of experiments for RBE determination and other purposes

For many of the above reasons, the experimental design when using high-LET radiations to determine RBE, or to additionally investigate radiosensitisation by any molecular mechanism, must be carefully planned in order to obtain realistic and credible results with minimal distortions produced by the experimental circumstances. This is potentially an exhaustive topic because of the complexity of ion-beam radiotherapy and its chemical and biological interactions, and the considerable simultaneous influence of the reference radiation on RBE, which must be understood to a reasonable level.

The following list of precepts and caveats applies to the two classes of experiments: the reference (low-LET) radiation and the test (high-LET) radiation:

1. The same physical conditions must be respected in both reference and test experiments. These include the experimental setups, jigs and apparatus, and closely comparable if not identical dose rates should be used. The same laboratory environment should be used in both cases where possible. A similar time of day should be chosen for each category of experiments since diurnal rhythm effects can influence cell proliferation and survival. The temperature should be maintained at 37 °C in each case, and room-temperature cellular experiments must be avoided since enzymatic radiation repair is highly temperature dependent.
2. The physical beam properties must be reportable and include dose rates, beam intensities, beam-delivery mechanisms (e.g. passively scattered or pencil beam scanned beams), beam widths at the level of the experiment and a summary of dosimetry checks in and around the experimental area, beam dose profiles, etc. The analysis of biological data results can be influenced by many of these physical parameters.
3. Ideally, the same cellular 'batch' should be used for each class of experiments, since biological responses may vary considerably on different days when different harvested cells are used.
4. Avoid the use of low doses in the 0.5–1.2 Gy range for the reference radiation (and for equivalent survival levels) in the test irradiation, especially in rapidly dividing cells, due to the LDH phenomenon, which can distort the shape of the cell survival curves and so give inappropriate α, β and RBE values.
5. Avoid the use of higher doses where the cellular SF approaches a reasonable limit at less than 10^{-3} and beyond. This would depend on the cellular radiosensitivity values and the RBE. There are two reasons for this: the statistical uncertainty increases where low numbers of surviving colonies exist, and also the longer time taken to deliver the dose may influence the amount of sub-lethal damage repair during the exposures, especially those

of the reference radiation. If this is not done, the subsequent least-squares line-fitting process will tend to favour near-zero or negative β parameter values, where in fact they must remain positive. If low levels of SF in the 10^{-4} (and beyond) range is achieved it is best to exclude these results in the analysis. This has been a particular problem in carbon-ion RBE experiments.

6. The reference radiation should be carefully selected to be representative of megavoltage radiotherapy using photons or electrons. Low-voltage or orthovoltage x-rays, especially with unfiltered or poorly filtered beams, can reduce the RBE values obtained in experiments, sometimes below unity.
7. The same biochemical milieu is essential for each class of experiment. For oxygenation studies, the experimental apparatus should involve glass rather than plastic dishes and, where possible, metal rather than rubber tubing. All materials in the experimental apparatus should be of tissue-equivalent density or reasonably so. The effects of scattered radiation, potential neutron contamination, etc., should be identified by a competent physicist.
8. Generic conclusions should not be made on the basis of irradiations involving only one cell type, but use at least two and preferably more cell types with different radiobiological characteristics, principally with variation in their radiosensitivities. Ideally, a comprehensive panel of cells should be used. This has been a particular problem with the β parameter, which was for many years thought not to change with LET, as this is the finding in V-79 cells, which are not of human lineage. Cell lines with very high intrinsic radiosensitivities should not be used in standard experiments, but can be useful to show the effects of absent repair mechanisms if required.
9. There is arguably no satisfactory normal tissue cell line for *in vitro* experiments, although progress is being made with explanted tissues or spheroidal systems.
10. Be aware that coefficients of variation (CV), which is the standard deviation divided by the mean value, are high in biological experimentsm and since RBE is a ratio the CV values may be as large as 15%–30%. To reduce uncertainty, reasonable numbers of repeated experiments must be used at each dose level to reduce the standard errors. This may increase expense but will produce more reliable results.
11. Additional checks can be done for the cells used such as their proliferation rates and chromosome numbers, which tend to increase with laboratory passaging over many years and can influence radiosensitivity. The excess numbers of chromosomes include 'spare copies' and also will influence nuclear volume. Ideally, human-derived cells should be used, although hamster and other mammalian-derived cell systems can be used for proof of principle or piloting experiments.
12. Similar and further considerations apply to *in vivo* experiments, where experimentalists must have awareness of the many and substantial

differences that are found between animal and human tumours. Animal experimental tumour systems have the following:

(i) A higher metabolic rate (and so oxygen consumption), which is inversely proportional to a living organism's volume, and which effectively decreases oxygen diffusion distances from blood vessels, resulting in a greater hypoxic fraction in animal tumours compared with human tumours.

(ii) More rapid cellular proliferation rates, higher growth fractions (or cycling cells).

(iii) Tumour radiosensitivities tend to be reduced. For example, murine tumours usually require a dose which is around 3 times larger to achieve the same effect as in the human.

(iv) The optimum treatment duration for fractionated treatment is much shorter in animals, around 12 days, the duration at which accelerated repopulation begins, which is larger by a factor of over 2 or more in humans.

(v) Normal tissue tolerance levels tend to be around 10% higher in animals than in humans.

(vi) The dose restrictions mentioned above for *in vitro* experiments do not apply for *in vivo* experiments.

(vii) The use of 'top-up' doses where a large priming fraction is given followed by smaller doses per fraction is controversial, although economical. It must always be remembered that the use of large dose per fraction will reduce RBE.

(viii) Whereas it is difficult and expensive to reproduce highly fractionated experiments in animals, the increasing use of hypofractionation with more sophisticated forms of radiotherapy is increasing such that hypofractionated *in vivo* experiments are again becoming more relevant.

(ix) The time for which an experimental small animal can be kept alive is much shorter than the time taken for severe late tissue effects to appear in humans. This must be borne in mind since the yield of late effects may be underestimated.

It is consequently not surprising that many radiobiological 'therapeutic advances' found in animal experiments have not shown similar ranges of improvements in human clinical trials, due to the above factors and possibly others such as differences in molecular profiles and mutational characteristics.

References

Barendsen G W 1982 Dose fractionation, dose rate, and iso-effect relationships for normal tissue responses *Int. J. Rad. Oncol. Biol. Phys.* **8** 1981–97

Bentzen S M and Baumann M 2002 The linear quadratic model in clinical practice *Basic Clinical Radiobiology* ed G G Steele (London: Arnold)

Bopp C, Hirayama R, Inaniwa T *et al* 2016 Adaptation of the microdosimetric kinetic model to hypoxia *Phys. Med. Biol.* **61** 7586–99
Britten R A, Nazaryan V, Davis L K *et al* 2013 Variations in the RBE for cell killing along the depth-dose profile of a modulated proton therapy beam *Radiat. Res.* **79** 21–8
Campbell I R and Warenius H M 1989 Radiation-induced cell death by chromatin loss. A model to explain the shape of low-linear-energy-transfer cell survival curves *Br. J. Radiol.* **62** 338–43
Canney P A and Millar W T 1997 Biphasic cellular repair and implications for multiple field radiotherapy treatments *Br. J. Radiol.* **70** 817–22
Carabe-Fernandez A, Dale R G and Jones B 2007 The incorporation of the concept of minimum RBE (RBE_{min}) into the linear-quadratic model and the potential for improved radiobiological analysis of high-LET treatments *Int. J. Radiat. Biol.* **83** 27–39
Chen Y, Li J, Li C, Qiu R and Wu Z 2017 A modified microdosimetric kinetic model for relative biological effectiveness calculation *Phys. Med. Biol.* **63** 015008
Chadwick K H and Leenhouts H P 1973 A molecular theory of cell survival *Phys. Med. Biol.* **18** 78–87
Curtis S B 1986 Lethal and potentially lethal lesions induced by radiation—a unified repair model *Radiat. Res.* **106** 252–70
Erratum in: *Radiat. Res.* 1989 **119** 584
Dale R G 1985 The application of the linear quadratic theory to fractionated and protracted radiotherapy *Br. J. Radiol.* **58** 515–28
Dale R G 1989 Time-dependent tumour repopulation factors in the linear quadratic equations – implications for treatment strategies *Radiother. Oncol.* **15** 371–82
Dale R G 2019 Radiation repair models for clinical application *Br. J. Radiol.* **92** 20180070
Dale R G and Jones B 1998 The clinical radiobiology of brachytherapy *Br. J. Radiol.* **71** 465–83
Dale R G and Jones B 2022 Radiotherapy treatment interruptions during the COVID-19 pandemic: the UK experience and implications for radiobiology training *Radiat. Phys. Chem.* **200** 110214
Dale R G, Plataniotis G A and Jones B 2024 A generalised method for calculating repopulation-corrected tumour EQD2 values in a wide range of clinical situations, including interrupted treatments *Eur. J. Med. Phys.* **118** 103294
Douglas B G and Fowler J F 1976 The effect of multiple small doses of x-rays on skin reactions in the mouse and a basic interpretation *Radiat. Res.* **66** 401–26
Elsässer T and Scholz M 2007 Cluster effects within the local effect model *Radiat. Res.* **167** 319–29
Fowler J F 1989 The linear quadratic formula and progress in fractionated radiotherapy *Br. J. Radiol.* **62** 679–94
Fowler J F 2008 Linear quadratics is alive and well: in response to Park *et al* (IJROBP 2008: 70: 847–852) *Int. J. Radiat. Oncol. Biol. Phys.* **72** 957
Fowler J F 2010 21 years of biologically effective dose *Br. J. Radiol.* **83** 554–68
Fowler J F 2012 Personal communication
Friedrich T, Scholz U, Elsässer T, Durante M and Scholz M 2013 Systematic analysis of RBE and related quantities using a database of cell survival experiments with ion beam irradiation *J. Radiat. Res.* **54** 494–514
Furusawa F, Fukutsu K, Aoki M *et al* 2000 Inactivation of aerobic and hypoxic cells from three different cell lines by accelerated (3)He-, (12)C- and (20)Ne-ion beams *Radiat. Res.* **154** 485–96
Erratum in: *Radiat. Res.* **177** 2012 129–31

Hawkins R B 2003 A microdosimetric-kinetic model for the effect of non-Poisson distribution of lethal lesions on the variation of RBE with LET *Radiat. Res.* **160** 61

Hawkins R B 2009 The relationship between the sensitivity of cells to high-energy photons and the RBE of particle radiation used in radiotherapy *Radiat. Res.* **172** 761–76

Hopewell J W, Nyman J and Turesson I 2003 Time factor for acute tissue reactions following fractionated irradiation: a balance between repopulation and enhanced radiosensitivity *Int. J. Radiat. Biol.* **79** 513–24

Hopewell J W, Moore J, Villafuerte C J, Paddick I, Jones B, Hill M A and Tsang D S 2023 Improving the accuracy of biologically effective dose estimates, from a previously published study, after radiosurgery for acoustic neuromas *World Neurosurg.* **172** e130–143

Hopewell J W, Millar W T and Lindquist C 2012 Radiobiological principles: their application to γ knife therapy *Prog. Neurol. Surg* **25** 39–54

Inaniwa T, Suzuki M, Furukawa T *et al* 2013 Effects of dose-delivery time structure on biological effectiveness for therapeutic carbon-ion beams evaluated with microdosimetric kinetic model *Radiat. Res.* **180** 44–59

Joiner M C, Marples B, Lambin P, Short S C and Turesson I 2001 Low dose hypersensitivity: current status and possible mechanisms *Int. J. Radiat. Oncol. Biol. Phys.* **49** 379–89

Jones B, Dale R G, Deehan C, Hopkins K I and Morgan D 2001 The role of biologically effective dose (BED) in clinical oncology *Clin. Oncol.* **13** 71–81

Jones B, Dale R G and Gaya A 2006 Linear quadratic modelling of increased late normal tissue effects in special clinical situations *Int. J. Radiat. Oncol. Biol. Phys.* **64** 948–53

Jones B, Carabe-Fernandez A and Dale R G 2006 Calculation of high-LET radiotherapy dose required for compensation of overall treatment time extensions *Br. J. Radiol.* **79** 254–7

Jones B, Underwood T C, Carabe-Fernandez A and Dale R G 2011 Further analysis of fast neutron relative biological effects and implications for charged particle therapy *Br. J. Radiol.* **84** S11–8

Jones B and Hopewell J W 2019 Modelling the influence of treatment time on the biological effectiveness of single radiosurgery treatments: derivation of 'protective' dose modification factors *Br. J. Radiol.* **92** 20180111

Jones B 2010 The apparent increase in the β-parameter of the linear quadratic model with increased linear energy transfer during particle irradiation *Br. J. Radiol.* **83** 433–6

Jones B and Hopewell J W 2019 Spinal cord re-treatments using photon and proton based radiotherapy: LQ-derived tolerance doses *Phys. Med.* **64** 304–10

Jones B and Dale R G 2015 Radiobiology of high dose per fraction *Stereotactic Body Radiotherapy* ed A Gaya and A Mahadevan (Berlin: Springer) ch 5 pp 67–86

Jones B and Morgan D 2007 Radiotherapy fractionation *Radiobiological Modelling in Radiation Oncology* ed A Gaya and A Mahadevan (London: British Institute of Radiology) ch 4 pp 70–1

Jones B and Dale R G 2007 Repopulation effects *Radiobiological Modelling in Radiation Oncology* (London: British Institute of Radiology) pp 79–95

Jones B and Sanghera P 2007 Estimation of radiobiological parameters and equivalent radiation dose of cytotoxic chemotherapy in malignant glioma *Int. J. Radiat. Oncol. Biol. Phys.* **68** 441–8

Jones B and Dale R G 2018 Radiobiological compensation of treatment errors in radiotherapy *Brit. J. Radiol.* **81** 323–6

Kanai T, Furusawa Y, Fukutsu K *et al* 1997 Irradiation of mixed beam and design of spread-out Bragg peak for heavy-ion radiotherapy *Radiat. Res.* **147** 78–85

Kase Y, Kanai T, Matsufuji N *et al* 2008 Biophysical calculation of cell survival probabilities using amorphous track structure models for heavy-ion irradiation *Phys. Med. Biol.* **53** 37–59

Lea D E and Catcheside D G 1942 The mechanism of induction by radiation of chromosome aberrations in *Transcendentia J. Genet.* **44** 216–245

Lea D E 1962 *Action of Radiation on Living Cells* 2nd edn (Cambridge: Cambridge University Press)

Mara E, Clausen M, Khachonkham S *et al* 2020 Investigating the impact of alpha/beta and LET_d on relative biological effectiveness in scanned proton beams: an *in vitro* study based on human cell lines *Med. Phys.* **47** 3691–702

Marples B, Wouters B G, Collis S J, Chalmers A J and Joiner M C 2004 Low-dose hyper-radiosensitivity: a consequence of ineffective cell cycle arrest of radiation-damaged G2-phase cells *Radiat. Res.* **161** 247–55

Niemierko A 1997 Reporting and analyzing dose distributions: a concept of equivalent uniform dose *Med. Phys.* **24** 103–10

Okada T, Kamada T, Tsuji H *et al* 2010 Carbon ion radiotherapy: clinical experiences at National Institute of Radiological Science. (NIRS) *J. Radiat. Res. (Tokyo)* **51** 355–64

Park C, Papiez L, Zhang S, Story M and Timmerman R D 2008 Universal survival curve and single fraction equivalent dose: useful tools in understanding potency of ablative radiotherapy *Int. J. Radiat. Oncol. Biol. Phys.* **70** 847–52

Pop L A, Millar W T, van der Plas M and van der Kogel A J 2000 Radiation tolerance of rat spinal cord to pulsed dose rate (PDR-) brachytherapy: the impact of differences in temporal dose distribution *Radiother. Oncol.* **55** 301–15

Rossi H H and Zaider M 1992 Compound dual radiation action. I. General aspects *Radiat. Res.* **132** 178–83
Erratum in: *Radiat. Res.* 1993 **133** 274

Takahashi T, Kubo M, Ma H *et al* 2014 Non-homologous end-joining repair plays a more important role than homologous recombination repair in defining radiosensitivity after exposure to high-LET radiation *Radiat. Res.* **182** 338–44

Thames H D, Withers H R, Peters L J and Fletcher G H 1982 Changes in early and late radiation responses with altered dose fractionation: implications for dose-survival relationships *Int. J. Radiat. Oncol. Biol. Phys.* **8** 219–26

Thames H D, Kuban D, Levy L B *et al* 2010 The role of overall treatment time in the outcome of radiotherapy of prostate cancer: an analysis of biochemical failure in 4839 men treated between 1987 and 1995 *Radiother. Oncol.* **96** 6–12

Tuleasca C, Paddick I, Hopewel J W *et al* 2019 Establishment of a therapeutic ratio for gamma knife radiosurgery of trigeminal neuralgia: the critical importance of biologically effective dose (BED) versus physical dose *World Neurosurg.* **134** e204–e213

Wenzl T and Wilkens J J 2011 Modelling of the oxygen enhancement ratio for ion beam radiation therapy *Phys. Med. Biol.* **56** 3251–68

Wigg D R 2008 *Applied Radiobiology* (Madison, WI: Medical Physics Publication Corporation)

Wyatt R M, Beddoe A H and Dale R G 2003 The effects of delays in radiotherapy treatment on tumour control *Phys. Med. Biol.* **48** 139–55

IOP Publishing

Quantitative Radiobiology for Proton Therapy

Bleddyn Jones

Chapter 3

Medical and surgical considerations that influence radiation tolerances, including interpretation of clinical trials

The clinical factors that contribute to radiotherapy outcomes are discussed. These include the effect of surgery and other medical conditions in increasing normal tissue toxicity, and which can be interpreted as a separate biological effective dose (BED). The degree of necessary dose and BED reduction is also considered.

Some of the pitfalls inherent in particle therapy clinical trials, their ethical aspects, patient follow-up deficiencies and clinical outcome data analysis are also discussed, since these are all relevant to particle therapy.

3.1 Introduction

The radiotherapy physics textbooks do not normally consider the practical influence of important medical factors in decision-making. A brief chapter is included here, which is designed to alert the non-medical reader (and medical readers embarking on their responsibilities) to some of the most important factors that could alert the clinician to change a treatment plan and influence the choice of the prescribed dose. Also, it is necessary to understand how radiation side-effect data are allocated, as well as how legal decisions as to whether radiation has caused tissue damage are taken. Medical physicists may be involved in correlating treatment plan dose distributions with patient outcomes, and academic physicists may be unaware of the practical difficulties inherent in such analysis as well as many of the terms in use.

3.2 Surgery

Radiotherapy is often preceded by surgery, which can vary in extent and in its effects on residual normal tissues. Cancers can be partially removed (sometimes referred to as partial excision) or 'debulked', but surgery is often radical in intent (a term which

doi:10.1088/978-0-7503-6209-2ch3

implies that total excision or removal is attempted with the aim of achieving cure). Where there is a risk of tumour regrowth due to residual cancer cells not removed by surgery, radiation can be given to reduce this risk, often with use of lower doses than would be given to an intact tumour. More uncommonly, surgery may follow the use of radiotherapy, for salvage of recurrent tumours or after tumours have been shown sufficient volume reduction to render them operable.

Surgery can be very prolonged, with retraction and stretching of normal tissues sufficient to causing local tissue hypoxia. Dissection planes are cauterised using diathermy to stop bleeding, so there is inevitable devascularisation of normal tissues. Healing occurs by the process of scar formation, which itself can strangulate (or obliterate) fine blood vessels and nerves. Consequently, and since radiation can cause late vascular damage, it is not surprising that the combination of surgery and radiation can lead to normal tissue injury of various kinds and to various degrees. Abdominal surgery, for example, can cause fibrotic adhesions to form, resulting in fixation rather than mobility of the small bowel. In this way, a fixed bowel loop can remain in the same daily position rather than move in and out of a radiation field if mobile, so that the bowel loop is exposed to a full rather than a partial dose.

In many body sites it is not advisable to give the full tissue tolerance dose of radiation after radical surgery, because of the enhanced risk of developing severe complications.

Operating in previously irradiated tissues is also more hazardous, since the tissues are thickened due to the presence of scar tissue, with fragile blood vessels that appear years after radiotherapy, resulting in prospects of delayed healing and wound breakdown accompanied by devitalisation of tissues and functional effects.

In principle, there is a dose-equivalent effect from surgery. For example, in Hodgkin's disease there appears to be a biological effective dose (BED) penalty of 17.7 $Gy_{[3]}$ in terms of abdominal radiation tolerance if the abdominal cavity has been explored (called a laparotomy procedure), so the BED needs to be lowered by this amount in order to achieve the same effect (Jones *et al* 2006).

In BED terms, the effect of surgery can be expressed as a combined BED, consisting of the sum of BEDs due to radiotherapy (RT) and surgery (SX) as

$$\mathrm{BED(RT)} + \mathrm{BED(SX)} = \mathrm{BED\ (COMBINED)}.$$

Radiation treatment planning should always consider the nature and location of previous surgery, by close inspection of the operative notes and, where possible, direct conversation between the radiation oncologist and the surgeon regarding the approach taken and the true extent of dissection, as well as the exact three-dimensional position of a tumour before its removal and what further tissue (such as a graft of fat or muscle) that may have been placed in or around that position.

It can be difficult to separate the true cause of complications when combined sequential treatments are given, but it is normal practice to classify a complication as being caused by radiation even if surgery has also been used, and even if that complication could occur in the absence of radiation. Because of this, radiation side effects can in some instances be exaggerated.

Unintended radiation overdosage can be life changing, causing severe disabilities, and in extreme cases can be lethal.

3.3 Cytotoxic chemotherapies

Similarly, chemotherapies of various kinds can be given before, during and after radiotherapy courses. Again, tissue radiation tolerance may be adversely affected and in principle a BED equivalent of chemotherapy can be estimated. For example, the use of a relatively mild combination of three drugs, called CMF (cyclophosphamide, methotrexate and 5-fluoro-uracil), is associated with a BED equivalent of 6.5 $Gy_{[3]}$ in terms of its contribution to chest wall fibrosis after radiotherapy for breast cancer. Similarly, the contributions are additive, so

$$\mathrm{BED(RT)} + \mathrm{BED(CHEMO)} = \mathrm{BED(COMBINED)}.$$

Other more complex formulations are available for chemotherapy radiosensitisation effects and the concomitant use of other treatments used for cytostatic effects, as in Jones & Dale (1999), Jones *et al* (2003), Plataniotis & Dale (2013) and Jones & Dale (2005).

3.4 Age and other medical conditions

It is increasingly recognised that late-developing vascular insufficiency causes many of the classical radiation side effects. Progressive obliteration of small vessels with changes in their morphology and function is characteristic, with subsequent deterioration of nutrition and oxygenation of tissues. The increasing prevalence of vascular disease with age, or the long-term effects of medical conditions that adversely influence tissue vasculature, such as hypertension, atherosclerosis, diabetes mellitus and other chronic inflammatory conditions, can also reduce radiation tolerance. Tissue damage, be it from direct radiation effects or indirect vascular effects resulting in chronic hypoxia, will cause scarring (or fibrosis). Medical conditions which predispose to scarring of tissues, such as rheumatoid arthritis and other autoimmune conditions, can also reduce tissue tolerance. Even older patients show a 3.6 $Gy_{[3]}$ change in tolerance for fibrotic effects after chest wall radiotherapy for breast cancer. The three examples of tolerance reduction, due to surgery, chemotherapy and age, can be found in Jones *et al* (2006).

The deposition of scar tissue is known as fibrosis: this can occur after surgery, radiation or other pathologies, and it is sometimes difficult to allocate the dominant cause when two or three of these factors coexist. Severe or repeated infection can also cause tissue damage sufficient to cause fibrosis and, again, if there has been previous radiation exposure, then tissue breakdown can occur. Because of chronic hypoxia in 'heavily' irradiated tissues, there is a predilection for infection by anaerobic organisms (those bacteria that thrive in low-oxygen-tension conditions).

The very young may also exhibit reduced tolerances, with marked growth disturbance following radiation therapy. They also may live longer and so develop more late effects of radiation including malignant induction.

3.5 Reductions in prescribed dose

A clinical decision to reduce the prescribed dose must be taken if there is an adverse medical history, including the extremes of age, extensive previous surgical procedure (s), chemotherapy and/or other molecular-based therapies. In some instances it may be decided that radiotherapy is contraindicated, but where it is decided to proceed the risk is often reduced, in standard forms of radiotherapy, by changing the dose, as shown in tables 3.1 and 3.2.

These dose reductions cover a range of up to and around a 20% reduction in BED; particle therapy dose reductions might be considered similarly, although in some instances the reduction in integral dose and the almost complete sparing of dose to some specific organs at risk (of special concern) may influence the decision further so that the full dose (or BED) will continue to be advised. This will depend on the actual clinical circumstances and the advice of an astute and competent physician.

Chapter 12 later includes re-treatments where the assessment of normal tissue tolerance varies with time following a first course of radiotherapy, and included a flexible BED of 0%–20% BED. The extent of BED reduction might be, say, 5% for age, 5%–10% for chemotherapy of various kinds and 10%–20% for surgery. These may be added to a limit of 20% in the graphical user system used, although further reductions can be done if thought to be clinically advisable.

Table 3.1. BED and EQD-2 values (rounded to the nearest 2 Gy) for brain and spinal cord tissues where $\alpha/\beta =$ 2 Gy.

	50 Gy in 25#	46 Gy in 23#	45 Gy in 25#	40 Gy in 20#
BED ($Gy_{[2]}$)	100	92	85.5	80
(% change)		(−8%)	(−14.5%)	(−20%)
EQD-2* (Gy)	50	46	42	40
(% change)		(−8%)	(−14.5%)	(−20%)

Table 3.2. BED and EQD-2 values (rounded to the nearest 2 Gy) for other normal tissues where $\alpha/\beta = 3$ Gy.

	60 Gy in 30#	56 Gy in 28#	50 Gy in 25#	50.4 Gy in 28#
BED ($Gy_{[3]}$)	100	93.33	83.33	80.64
(% change)		(−6.7%)	(−16.7%)	(−19.4%)
EQD-2* (Gy)	60	56	50	48
(% change)		(−6.7%)	(−16.7%)	(−19.4%)

3.6 Interpretation of the case histories and literature

On the whole, if a patient has had radiation exposure in the past to an anatomical region where there is now a significant medical problem, the cause is usually allocated as radiation induced in publications. However, in medico-legal work, the cause has to be proven 'on the balance of probabilities' (see Jones 2019) and in instances where the radiation dose is considered to be too low and another competing pathology capable of such tissue changes is present, then negligence cannot be admitted. The situation with particle therapy is more complex, since further questions would need to be asked: Could the assumed RBE or inaccurate Bragg peak dose placement considerations be causative? This would need to be balanced by considering whether the treatment indications, its delivery and overall conduct would have been supported by a responsible group of practitioners (this is known as the Bolam principle), although this can sometimes be overridden by new scientific evidence. The author is not aware of any such cases at the present time, but they could arise in the future. The use of BED and its linkage to risk may be important in the assessment of individual cases.

3.7 Clinical trials

These vary in intent from basic dose searching to identify efficacy and also side effects (or complications), when they are termed phase I and II. Phase III studies are normally randomised to compare a standard treatment with a new therapy and represent the highest level of evidence.

Prior evidence may be sufficient to suggest that only improvements can occur, in which case one-tailed probability levels can be used to test the null hypothesis, but normally two-tailed statistics should be used. In particle therapy, tumour control might be increased if the dose is escalated beyond that of the control, although in recent times the newer focussed forms of photon therapy are quite capable of delivering the same high dose. The really vexing question is concerned with the two main uncertainties in particle therapy, namely dose or Bragg peak positioning accuracy and reliability, and the appropriateness of the RBE value used. Dose positioning errors lead not only to dose changes but also LET and consequently RBE changes, and can be expected to reduce tumour control and potentially increase normal tissue complications. The RBE uncertainty can produce either reduced tumour control if the prescription RBE exceeds that of the tumour being treated (since the dose will be reduced), or enhanced tumour control if the prescription RBE is less than that of the tumour (as dose would be increased). Also, an incorrectly low allocation of RBE to a critical normal tissue could result in a higher risk of complications.

The terms local tumour control, disease-free interval, or even biochemical control (for instances where tumour mass can be monitored by assay of a blood-borne chemical signal such as prostate-specific antigen from prostate cancer) are sometimes used as end points, as well as patient survival, although the latter index can include local failure and salvage due to other treatments; time to first recurrence can sometimes be used to overcome the effect of later treatments. Actuarial statistics can be applied to all these measurements, where the index of survival is corrected for loss of patients due to death or lack of follow-up due to a variety of reasons. Differences in outcomes can be tested by simple *t*-tests at specified time points or over a cumulative period of time by the log-rank test, but there are other alternatives.

For side effects, there is less uniformity since there are a number of different categorical scoring systems for each region/organ of the body. Crude percentages of a specific complication grading are often presented, but more sophisticated actuarial time series are preferred. Changes in the incidence of rare side effects can be quickly tested by simple Poisson statistics. For example, from a sample of 100 patients, if the expected incidence is 1 but a study finds an incidence of 6 patients, the probability of this being due to chance is given by $\frac{1^6 . e^{-1}}{6!} = 0.00052$. This is low and unlikely to be due to chance. If, on closer inspection, it is found that three of these patients with complications had another significant predisposing cause (such as prolonged and difficult surgery with devascularisation), and one other had widespread vascular complications of diabetes, then only two clear-cut cases of toxicity due to radiation alone remain. The probability is then $\frac{1^2 . e^{-1}}{2!} = 0.184$, which fails to be significant at the $p = 0.05$ level. In contrast, a 1% finding when the expected incidence is 6% yields a lower p-value of 0.01487, which passes the 5% significance test.

In most instances non-parametric statistical tests are normally used for the various categorical results. There are several risk-related statistical end points in use, and in some instances quality of life may be fused with the survival end point (for example, the percentage survival at 5 years in the absence of any documented grade 3 or 4 toxicity). Simulations of such an approach may lead to statistically significant findings even if there are lower numbers of patients in a trial (Jones 2006). Textbooks of medical statistics should be consulted for further details.

3.8 Ethical issues

Much has been written about ethical considerations in particle therapy. There are enthusiasts who believe that treatment outcomes can only improve after particle therapy, but others insist that in many situations the randomised control study is essential to produce persuasive results that are independent of physician-related and other forms of bias (such as fitness to travel for therapy), which can influence outcomes. The guiding precept in such situations is that there should be true equipoise between the standard and test treatments. Outstandingly good results from non-randomised studies may sometimes be convincing, but with any new treatment that contains intrinsic uncertainties, which may increase or reduce effectiveness, the randomised study should always be preferred. Further details on the opposing opinions are given in Sheehan *et al* (2014) and Jones *et al* (2014).

Randomisation would be one way of potentially deciding how should RBE best be allocated. The present author has suggested randomly allocating certain classes of proton therapy patients to either the standard 1.1 RBE (for all tissues and doses) or alternatively to an RBE of 1 for radiosensitive tumours (as in children and lymphoma patients) with a higher RBE of 1.2 for any critical normal tissue. Such a trial would be important since at the present time it is difficult to separate if failure of tumour control and/or increased toxicity is due to dose placement or RBE allocation. Radiosensitive tumours form a very special case since their RBE are likely to be less than 1.1, so they may be underdosed by the standard approach.

3.9 Mixed end points

It has been suggested that since particle therapy is mainly concerned with reducing tissue side effects, combined local control and toxicity end points could be used, as suggested already above. Such an approach is only valid if the tumour control remains constant or improves while side effects are reduced. In principle, such an approach—using, for example, an end point such as the percentage of uncomplicated recurrence free patients, or say 'the % recurrence free with grade 1 toxicity', or even a disease-free survival corrected for adverse complications which reflects useful quality of life (these are referred to as quality adjusted)—can reach statistical significance for a smaller group of patients than would otherwise be the case in the example presented by Jones (2006).

3.10 The importance of follow-up

Cancer patients ideally require meticulous follow-up appointments to assess their progress, with a detailed interview to check on symptoms, general examination and special examination of the relevant anatomical region, although some health services appear not to be funding follow-up adequately. Various investigations including radiological techniques may be required. In general, the capture of relevant information is best when the patient attends the hospital where they were treated and also by a medical doctor who specialises in the area of the body which has been treated. Although effective questionnaires and regular communications with physicians and surgeons at remotely located hospitals can suffice, there can be under-reporting of the true incidence of side effects. It is often the case that when patients develop serious complications they seek help from other medical specialists, who do not necessarily inform the original treatment centre. Particle therapy has been especially prone to this, since over the past 30 years many patients in the pioneering centres were referred from long distances and often from different countries and continents. Modern IT communications can help in this respect, but there remain serious legal obstacles to the electronic transfer of medical data.

3.11 Publication bias

Under-reporting of medical research has been termed publication bias, and is now a well-recognised phenomenon. It remains to be determined as to why so many proton therapy centres have not published large and comprehensive reports of treatment effectiveness. This may be due to a number of reasons, such as lack of resources for analysis, disappointing results, difficulties in analysis of complex patients and where follow-up data may be incomplete. There may also be a tendency for journal editors and reviewers to reject what may be regarded as non-significant results or trials based on inadequate numbers. For example, the present author has advised acceptance of several submitted ion beam papers for publication only to find that they had been rejected by other reviewers, sometimes when the research was unique and provided some 'proof of principle', although based on relatively small numbers of patients. It is vital that the results of new technologies applied in medicine are published with care. Another potentially misleading form of publication is where acute (early) side effects are only considered. These may be lower for newer radiation techniques and for particle therapy, but this does not necessarily mean that the late tissue complications (which may accrue over 2–10 years or more) will also be reduced; indeed, some categories of late complications may increase with time. Non-medical readers have to understand that acute reactions are those which occur mainly in surface or lining tissues (skin, gut, etc.) where cell turnover times are rapid, whereas late reactions occur in more stable tissues due to the slow onset of late vascular damage. It is also pertinent to point out that late-reacting tissues probably have a higher RBE than the acute-reacting tissues, so some late-reacting tissues may be more at risk following particle therapies if the RBE allocation has been incorrect. At low clinical dose per fraction, the RBE is inversely related to tissue α/β ratios: these ratios differ considerably between acute (10–30 Gy) and late-reacting normal tissues (2–3 Gy).

In order to overcome some of the above difficulties, it is suggested that data analysis and trial organisation should be arranged on a national or international, or even global basis. This is because each individual centre may treat only 500–1000 patients per year, but with, say, 20–30 different types of tumour indications. This means that individual centres may not accumulate patients quickly enough to produce sufficiently larger numbers of patients in each tumour class for analysis. National databases would accumulate data faster, and for rare conditions international databases would be necessary. Countries with smaller populations could also contribute in this way. Furthermore, if national databases could identify individual cases with unexpected outcomes and then reconstruct the treatment plans using Monte Carlo–based simulations, for LET, inter-track distances and possible ranges of RBE, extremely useful information would be obtained for correlative purposes to identify which of the existing predictive models are the most suitable and in what clinical circumstances. In some respects, a single global centre could assist in checking such information from different national or international sources, using the latest Monte Carlo codes. In this respect, it may also be prudent to have quality assurance checks internationally or globally, as used to exist for fast neutron therapy trials. A single dedicated reference laboratory for particle therapy dosimetry would also be helpful, perhaps working in cooperation with existing international bodies like the International Atomic Energy Agency, the radiation division of the Bureau of Units and Measurements (Paris) and the particle physics simulation and IT expertise that exists in CERN (Geneva).

References

Jones B 2006 Implications of quality adjusted survival for clinical trials in radiation oncology *Br. J. Radiol.* **79** 353–5

Jones B 2019 Use of radiobiology in medical jurisprudence, with particular reference to delays in diagnosis and therapeutic onset *Br. J. Radiol.* **92** 20190672

Jones B, Cominos M and Dale R G 2003 Application of biological effective dose (BED) to estimate the duration of symptomatic relief and repopulation dose equivalent in palliative radiotherapy and chemotherapy *Int. J. Radiat. Oncol. Biol. Phys.* **55** 736–42

Jones B and Dale R G 1999 Inclusion of molecular biotherapies with radical radiotherapy: modeling of combined modality treatment schedules *Int. J. Radiat. Oncol. Biol. Phys.* **45** 1025–34

Jones B and Dale R G 2005 The potential for mathematical modelling in the assessment of the radiation dose equivalent of cytotoxic chemotherapy given concomitantly with radiotherapy *Br. J. Radiol.* **78** 939–44

Jones B, Dale R G and Gaya A 2006 Linear quadratic modelling of increased late normal tissue effects in special clinical situations *Int. J. Radiat. Oncol. Biol. Phys.* **64** 948–53

Jones B, Howick J, Hopewell J and Liew S M 2014 Response to 'Position statement on ethics, equipoise and research on charged particle therapy' *J. Med. Ethics.* **40** 576–7

Plataniotis G A and Dale R G 2013 Radio-chemotherapy for bladder cancer: contribution of chemotherapy on local control *World J. Radiol.* **5** 267–74

Sheehan M, Timlin C, Peach K *et al* 2014 Position statement on ethics, equipoise and research on charged particle radiation therapy *J. Med. Ethics* **40** 572–5

IOP Publishing

Quantitative Radiobiology for Proton Therapy

Bleddyn Jones

Chapter 4

Treatment planning and further medical perspectives

The essential aspects of the treatment-planning process are described along with the definitions of target volumes encompassing not only the tumour but the inevitable adjacent normal tissues in order to include microscopic tumour cell extension beyond the 'visible' tumour. The consequences of uncertainties in the relative biological effect (RBE) values used, and consequently of dose, in each of these separate volumes are considered. The trade-off or compromises involved in treatment-plan selection are described. Simple equations are given to match the constraint of a nearby critical normal tissue structure, including an allowance for RBE uncertainties in the normal tissue and tumour. Some authors advocate using the product of linear energy transfer (LET) and dose (rather than RBE itself). When this suggestion is tested against ion-beam cell surviving fraction data sets, it is found that the LET-dose product is not sufficiently robust for all possible situations. Surrogates of RBE should be used with great caution, although treatment-planning techniques that optimise the placement of the highest RBE values within the tumour target and the least in the critical normal tissues should be encouraged.

4.1 Introduction

It is essential to describe the treatment-planning process, while also including important medical and surgical factors which can influence the radiation tissue tolerances referred to in the previous chapter. The non-medical reader will then be aware of reasons why a clinician may change a treatment plan and the prescribed dose. Also, it is necessary to understand how radiation side-effect data are allocated. Physicists may be involved in correlating treatment-plan dose distributions with patient outcomes, and academic physicists may be unaware of the practical difficulties inherent in such analysis.

doi:10.1088/978-0-7503-6209-2ch4

The present author is aware that readers from different academic and vocational backgrounds require some basic explanations to help them better understand the context of some important practical dilemmas in radiation oncology.

4.1.1 Treatment-planning processes

Radiation treatment planning must be appreciated as being only a part of the overall management of cancer, which consists of epidemiology, screening, diagnosis, clinical assessment including physical examination, pathological confirmation, imaging studies and determination of tumour grade and stage and any other molecular-based information which may influence treatment. Then, the actual treatment may consist of surgery, radiotherapy, chemotherapy (cytotoxic, hormonal) and other approaches, either alone or in combinations determined by past experience and evidence. Especially important is the past medical history and age of the patient in the determination of an overall treatment strategy. These factors may also influence radiation tolerance, which is an assessment of how much radiation the tissue can tolerate, especially if other significant medical conditions coexist. There may even be past exposures to radiation to consider, as well as the often deleterious effects of surgery. Some of these points will be expanded upon in later sections.

After the decision has been taken to proceed with radiotherapy, the overall treatment plan is commissioned by experienced radiation oncologists, who are medically qualified but trained to assess, care for and supervise cancer patients requiring radiotherapy. Their role includes defining the radiation treatment volume (s), and allocating an appropriate total dose and its fractionation (number of separate treatments) over a designated period of time (the overall treatment time). They may alert the patient and treatment staff about possible contingencies; important dose constraints for important normal tissue doses are defined, often as dose limits with or without volume considerations (expressed as the % volume of a tissue that may receive a recommended dose limit, for example the V-20, the volume which receives a minimum dose of 20 Gy).

Needless to say, these normal tissue constraints frequently influence the tumour dose, which is often termed the prescribed dose, analogous to a medical prescription of a drug, which has to be under the control of a qualified practitioner.

The subtleties that follow are important. The target volume definitions recommended by the ICRU are essential to understand. According to Report 78 of the ICRU (2010), the visible tumour volume is called the gross tumour volume (GTV); the further volume, which includes a margin for microscopic tumour extension, is called the clinical target volume (CTV); and a further margin, which compensates for daily shifts in positioning of the patient relative to the beam, movements during treatment and penumbral beam effects, is called the planning target volume (PTV). In practice, the CTV is determined by clinical risk factors and can include a margin of 0.5–3 cm in some or all directions around the tumour, depending on its microscopic features (histological class, degree of differentiation and molecular markers). The CTV to PTV margin is often around a further 1 cm, but this can also vary with position in the body, the expectation of physiological movement, etc.

It is essential to know that the normal tissues situated around a cancer do frequently include infiltrating tumour cells which cannot be detected on imaging studies. From clinical and pathological experience, it is known that certain types of tumour have more invasive propensities than others. Tumours considered to be relatively or completely benign have low invasive or no invasive potential, respectively. The CTV may also extend to include lymph node groups situated several centimetres away from a primary cancer, which may also harbour metastatic (or escaped) cancer cells. Thus the radiation oncologist faces the same dilemma as a surgeon as to how much tissue should be removed in the case of surgery, or 'sterilised' of cancer cells with radiation, and what will be the effects on the patients if the normal tissue is rendered functionless. Surgeons are in a more fortunate position since they can use biopsies taken for immediate processing, which can advise them as to the effectiveness of their tissue dissections. No such aid is available for the oncologist, but surgical data backed by pathological evidence on the distance of spread is sometimes available, although often incomplete, along with data from recurrence patterns after previous radiotherapy. This critical problem is to some extent made less uncertain by better definitions of the tumour edge, its disturbance of local vascularity such as permeability and blood flow changes that may reflect infiltration, as well as tumour metabolic activity by image fusion of CT (photon-based), MRI (magnetic-resonance-based) and PET (positron-emission-based) scans, although the latter is prone to time-related fluctuations of perfusion of the delivered radioisotope, as can any perfusion-based study using contrast agents.

It is important to realise that the volume of normal tissue treated beyond a tumour can exceed that of the tumour itself. For instance, consider a spherical tumour 2 cm diameter with an additional 2 cm (linear) CTV 'margin' beyond it.

The volume of normal tissue is

$$\frac{4}{3}\pi 3^3 - \frac{4}{3}\pi\,.1^3 = \frac{4}{3}\pi\ 8 = 33.51\ \text{cm}^3,$$

whereas the tumour volume (the second term in the above equation) provides a volume of 4.19 cm^3.

As may be expected, this discrepancy increases further with tumour volume and the marginal distance used.

For a 4 cm diameter tumour where for this particular situation only a 1 cm margin is required, then the volume of normal tissue included is

$$\frac{4}{3}\pi 3^3 - \frac{4}{3}\pi\,.2^3 = \frac{4}{3}\pi\ 19 = 78.59\ \text{cm}^3.$$

This exceeds the tumour volume (again, the second term of the last equation), which is only 33.51 cm^3.

It is very often the case that for even small margins of 1 cm, the volume of normal tissues treated to the full dose will exceed that of the tumour itself, as shown in figure 4.1.

One can now appreciate that the normal tissue volume included in the full-dose region can be substantial, as may be the case if a critical organ at risk (OAR) is

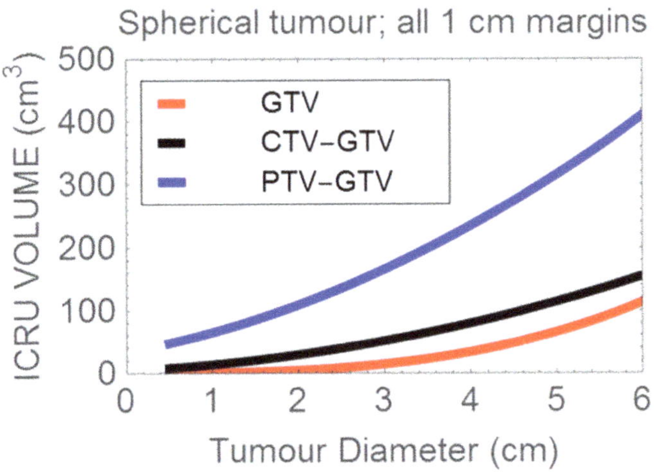

Figure 4.1. Plot of the three ICRU tumour volumes, with 1 cm margins between the GTV and CTV and between the CTV and PTV. Beyond the GTV, each volume is obtained by subtracting the neighbouring smaller volume, to show how much normal tissue is included between each volume.

situated close to, but outside, or partially inside the PTV margin. This may be especially relevant in particle therapy where a prevalent relative biological effect (RBE) disadvantage due to raised linear energy transfer (LET) could in some instances be sufficient to overcome the degree of dose sparing of the OAR.

This clinical relevance of the normal tissues within the PTV and those close to it will depend on the functional importance of the tissue, its ability to regenerate or not. The brain tissue is so often critical, but even there some areas are relatively 'silent' in that they may involve areas that perceive sensory perception of limited importance, compared with precious areas that govern speech (the prefrontal cortex) or total vision (such as the optic chiasm). Other examples include the white-matter tracts which carry the neurological impulses that transmit motor signals, or in the reverse direction, direct sensory input to the central and processing brain. The criticality of the spinal cord, or optic chiasm, is a good example where severe radiation injury results in paralysis of movement of the limbs, and other diverse functions such as sensory loss, bladder and bowel incontinence, with impotence in males. In contrast, one can accept functional loss or depletion of some tissues such as skin (which if treated to a critical depth and volume can effectively regenerate, and if sometimes severely damaged can be replaced by plastic surgery 'skin grafting' techniques); the liver—if healthy—is a tissue that can regenerate in three-dimensional space and so the margin becomes less relevant; if the tumour arises in muscle, then the surrounding tissue will be muscle, which is radioresistant compared to many other tissues. The primary tumours that arise in muscle and other connective tissues of the body are called sarcomas: depending on their location, most soft-tissue sarcomas arising in muscle will not usually confer much motor deficit due to radiation beyond that already achieved by prior surgery. In this limited discussion it must be pointed out here that the sensitivity to an increment in LET with particle therapy may be greater in late-reacting tissue, with slower cellular turnover kinetics, than in more acute-reacting tissue, which exhibit short cellular turnover times.

A further issue that can surprise some academic physicists is that—not infrequently—the primary target volume has no tumour on imaging, since it has been removed (or excised) surgically. There may be, at best, some imaging features of a tumour cavity and the operative path taken by the surgeon in some instances. The surgical 'tumour bed' and surrounding tissues may be harbouring residual tumour cells and require radiotherapy, usually to a lower dose than that required for an intact tumour, in order to reduce the chance of recurrence. In such cases the entire treatment volume is composed of normal tissues.

From the above considerations it can be appreciated that the zonal definition of risk should be dependent on the tumour type and not the technique used to treat it. So often in radiotherapy, a new technique—perhaps with greater accuracy of photon delivery, for example—is accompanied by the temptation to use a reduced tumour margin. Disrespect by the physician for the true CTV may frequently lead to tumour-edge recurrences (i.e. tumours regrowing within their margin distance).

Physicists may like to think of the tumour infiltration as being similar to electron probability clouds around the atomic nucleus.

Now that the CTV has been more fully considered, there is a further volume to be added: the PTV. This is necessary to account for daily setup errors and movements of tissues during treatment such as due to breathing in the case of thoracic and upper abdominal organs, where shifts of 1–3 cm are commonly encountered. This extra margin is not tumour dependent like the CTV, but is amenable to careful reductions by use of more meticulous and reproducible immobilisation techniques. Breath-holding can be used, with physiotherapy training, but the more sophisticated technique of respiratory gating can be used, or the breathing tracked continuously with on-line feedback to change beam collimation or positioning. Particle therapy is not so forgiving as x-ray-based treatments as far as PTV dose compliance is concerned, because of the sharp dose falloff associated with Bragg peaks; although these may be similar for some highly focussed x-ray techniques, there is always an exit dose with most rotational techniques. The highest risk of PTV non-compliance is with particle therapy pencil beams, where there is always the possibility of the Bragg peak region being misplaced, when the tumour and adjacent tissue is moving. Many research groups have addressed this problem and it was first tackled—using protons—by Japanese clinicians and scientists in the context of treating hepatomas in the liver around 25 years ago. Modern linear accelerators for x-ray treatments have cone-beam CT scan facilities which can assess the treatment accuracy on a daily or less frequent basis. Ultrasound techniques can also be used to check field limits and depths to a certain extent, together with the best possible radiographer skills. For conventional radiotherapy, the linear accelerator (LINAC) x-ray beam position quality assurance includes use of a portal imaging facility, where the transmitted x-ray is captured beyond the patient and checked for accuracy against what was intended relative to the local bone anatomy. This is not possible during particle therapy because the energy deposition ends with the proton Bragg peak in most cases, or with the relatively small fragmentation tail of ions heavier than helium. Test doses of protons or ions at a much higher energy than required for the treatment could be used for this purpose (proton radiography) but the accelerator must then have higher-energy delivery capabilities. Protons can be used in this way in areas of the body with shorter tissue thickness such as the head and neck region, but not in the chest or pelvis without higher-energy availability. However, the receptive detector technology is not yet commercially available. The considerable advantages of proton radiography include the fact that the absorbed dose throughout the thickness of the body is far less than that deposited by an x-ray beam, and also the proton scatter by tissue is less than that from even megavoltage x-rays, so the tissue resolution is better.

4.1.2 The important interaction of RBE issues with the marginal target volumes

There is a real concern in charged-particle therapy (CPT) that the RBE is high in normal tissues as far as their late effects, mediated by vascular damage, is concerned, and especially so at low doses per fraction. This has the implication that if the RBE used in the tumour prescription is applied to all other tissues, and is lower than the RBE in the normal tissue of concern, then overdosage could occur in the normal tissues included in the CTV and PTV. This may not be problematic in some clinical situations, such as the liver where the surrounding tissue regenerates, or in examples such as connective tissue muscle or fat. The impact of a higher than anticipated RBE in a more precious tissue may be very important, however, as would be the case for anatomical locations such as critical areas of the brain, spinal cord, bowel, heart, etc. This situation can be expressed as an inequality for general simplification purposes, where

If RBE [NT, Late] > RBE [Prescription], then the bioeffects may be greater.

This situation can be opposed by dose reduction, but this may carry the risk of underdosage of infiltrating tumour cells. Another potential approach would be to increase the dose per fraction in order to reduce the late-effect RBE—as well as its variation with the α/β ratio (discussed in chapter 2)—although again care would be required to ensure an adequate tumour cell eradication dose.

It is instructive to study the ICRU volumes given in table 4.1 and also in Jones (2015), and to consider the implications of dose allocations to each volume with respect to later outcomes (tumour control and normal tissue complications). A significant change in the RBE may override initial expectations. Readers may wish to construct their own table in particular treatment situations and vary the RBE assumption in each category.

4.1.3 Comparative planning studies

Comparative planning studies compare CPT with x-ray techniques—and, perhaps in the future, several different ion beams as well—in order to assess the dose distributions and choose the best overall treatment plan. CPT patient selection will undoubtedly be based on such an approach, especially if coupled with comparative predictions of tumour cure probability (TCP) and normal tissue complication probability (NTCP). The Netherlands has an agreed system for doing

Table 4.1. Dose status for each ICRU volume and likely clinical outcome changes produced by CPT compared with megavoltage photon radiotherapy

Dose status	Tumour control in GTV and {CTV+PTV}	{CTV+PTV} side effects	OTV side effects
GTV↑, {CTV+PTV}↑, OTV↓	Much better[c]	Worse[a]	Better
GTV↑, {CTV+PTV}=, OTV↓	Better[c]	Equal[b]	Better
GTV=, {CTV+PTV} =, OTV↓	Equal[b]	Equal[b]	Better
GTV=, {CTV+PTV}↓, OTV↓	Worse[d]	Better	Better or worse

[a] In some cases, reduced doses outside {CTV+PTV} may allow better radiotolerance due to less late vascular insufficiency in the OTV. Also, this row condition may be acceptable in a non-essential tumour-bearing tissue, or for a small volume of essential tissue with little risk of subsequent functional change.
[b] An equal outcome exists only if RBE is correct.
[c] In some instances (the radiosensitive tumour classes), tumour control will be very high with x-rays and there will be no gain in tumour control from dose escalation using any form of radiotherapy. These tumours may also have a lower RBE than 1.1, in which case the tumour control probability will be reduced if an RBE of 1.1 is used.
[d] Reductions in dose to CTV and PTV can occur due to range uncertainties and tissue movement, sometimes exacerbated by the use of scanned beams. The clinician may decide to extend the PTV and/or increase the local dose, depending on the tissue contained in the PTV and as a trade-off for gains in the OTV.
Where ↑ is an increased dose, = is the 'equivalent' dose and ↓ is a reduced dose for the CPT. OTV is the volume of the body outside the PTV.

this for proton therapy patient selection and its funding. Such an approach was considered to be an advance over the standard evidence-based medicine criteria, which demanded high-level evidence from actual treatments, preferably in the context of randomised control trials. This type of exercise could produce erroneous predictions if the RBE assumptions are incorrect. Furthermore, NTCP models are notoriously unreliable and based on very simple physical representations of complex normal tissues so that volume-related changes can be misleading. However, with reasonably correct allocations of RBE, in principle it should be possible to predict photon equivalent doses and volumes and relate these to existing photon data relating dose volume and risk. There is a real need to develop better systems in this respect, where well-verified LET-RBE models can be linked to dose per fraction effects and applied with existing low-LET radiobiological parameters such as the α/β ratio.

The RBE issues in comparative planning studies can also apply to the tumour RBE. If, for example, the actual tumour RBE is less than the prescription RBE, then tumour underdose could occur, with possible reduced tumour control depending on the extent of underdosage. In proton therapy, RBE values lower than 1.1 are predicted in tumours known to be very radiosensitive to conventional (low-LET) radiotherapy. These include the lymphomas and many childhood tumour types. Although their RBEs may be in the 1.03–1.05 range, there would be a potential significant reduction in dose, which could exceed the ICRU recommendation of a 5% lower dose limit within the PTV. This may seem to be a trivial change, but it should be remembered that a 5% reduction of dose may prove to be significant if added to the already existing 5% guideline. This could also be compounded by small errors in dose delivery, Bragg peak positioning, etc., resulting in a recurrent tumour. In such circumstances it may be best not to use a conventional RBE for the tumour prescription, as long as the various normal tissue tolerances are respected. These tolerance doses are usually lower than the tumour prescribed dose for such radiosensitive tumours, so there is a reasonable scope for such a policy in the treatment of these tumours where cure rates are high and quality of life is at a premium.

4.1.4 Trade-off situations in comparative treatment planning

Some good examples would be in the treatment of lung cancer or with oesophageal cancer, where an additional safety margin could be applied around a tumour to at least ensure 100% dose (rather than 95%) to cover the CTV and PTV. This would only be reasonable if there is an acceptable increase in the V-20 index (this refers to the volume of lung that receives over 20 Gy, the dose limit beyond which lung function can be impaired due to reduced gas exchange). The V-20 would need to remain less than what would be achieved with x-ray/photon techniques. The gas exchange loss following the alternative of surgical lobectomy or pneumonectomy should always be kept in mind, although in many examples of more unusual lung cancers the option of surgery has been rejected not only because of tumour stage (or size) but also because of the histological class. Similar arguments can be made for margins around primary liver cancers (hepatomoas), pancreatic cancers, renal cancers (hypernephromas) or any situation where a small amount of additional parenchymal tissue may be sacrificed without major loss of function.

Another option in this type of situation is to express the V-20 or any other such index which might determine overall normal tissue tolerance, in terms of another RBE-adjusted dose. It is important to ascertain if the treatment-planning system (TPS) is producing a 20 Gy physical dose volume statistic or an RBE-weighted one. If the latter is assumed and, for example, if the late-effect RBE of lung tissue in the mid spread-out Bragg peak was considered to be 1.3 rather than the 1.1 used in the TPS, then one could consider the V-20 to be actually a V-23.64 (where 23.64 is $20 \times 1.3/1.1$).

4.1.4.1 Changes in the treatment plan

During radiotherapy the treatment plan and dose prescription is occasionally modified, and for good reasons. These include the following:

1. Severe acute reactions causing medical complications and other causes of treatment interruption such as accelerator breakdowns, inter-current illness, failure to attend due to inclement weather or other causes.
2. Errors in treatment delivery (sometimes manifesting as severe acute reactions if overdosage occurs and a lack of acute reaction at an appropriate time with under-osage). These may occur due to dose-calculation errors, or be due to

changes in body anatomy such as weight loss or weight gain, which can result in under- or overdosage and which may require correction. Rarely, the treatment field position is incorrect and so a compensatory plan is necessary. The remaining treatment may require a recalculation of the dose per fraction using biological effective dose (BED) equations.

3. Further information such as examination of the patient or new imaging studies reveal tumour spread or its expansion from whatever cause (e.g. cystic degeneration or bleeding, with fluid accumulation within the tumour).
4. Adaptive therapy defines a more flexible approach for modifying treatment plans on a deliberate basis according to information gained by serial imaging such as tumour shrinkage rates, shifts of normal tissue, etc.

More detailed examples of the above are given in the chapters already referred to, with some worked examples that illustrate the additional pitfalls which exist with charged hadrons in BED equations. It should also be noted that particle beams are more sensitive to changes in body anatomy, due to misplacement of Bragg peaks, which may change the LET and RBE, as well as dose. X-ray/photon-based treatment is much more forgiving not only in physical dose placement but also in radiobiological terms, as will be shown later.

4.1.5 How to accommodate assumed errors in RBE

Later in this book, in chapters 8 and 9, the relationships between LET and RBE will be discussed, but in the present context it is assumed that there is a lack of information, or a range estimate, as to what the most appropriate RBE might be. If models that link LET and RBE are not used, but if changes of RBE are to be respected in critical tissues such as the central nervous system, the following approach might be used.

Essentially, the easiest way of taking variations in proton RBE into account will be to assume worst-case scenarios in the critical normal tissue of interest, and to use a larger RBE than that used in the planning process, where at the present time all RBEs are 1.1. If the normal tissue tolerance constraint is, say, a dose of 54 Gy, and the plan provides 51.5 Gy-RBE, then if the RBE could be as high as 1.2, then the adjusted dose will be $1.2/1.1 \times 51.5 = 56.2$ Gy-RBE, which exceeds tolerance; if the RBE was even higher at, say, 1.25 or 1.3, then the respective Gy-RBE values would be 58.52 and 60.87, which significantly exceed the constraint and carry an enhanced risk of toxicity.

Such an approach may be all that is necessary, but it does not include the tumour RBE. A more sophisticated approach might be to use both tumour and normal tissue RBEs, as in the approach taken by Jones *et al* (2011). As throughout this book, subscripts of L and H are used for low- and high- LET radiations, respectively. If the tumour dose per fraction at the prescription point is z_H for high-LET and z_L for low-LET radiations, then since RBE is the ratio of the low- to high-LET single doses (or dose per fraction) necessary for a given biological isoeffect, then the required value of z_H in the high-LET case may be found from the RBE specific to the tumour volume ($\mathrm{RBE_{tum}}$) by

$$z_H = \frac{z_H}{\mathrm{RBE_{tum}}}. \tag{4.1}$$

Equation (4.1) represents the isoeffective dose conversion required when the fraction number is the same for both the high- and low-LET cases. In most forms of radiotherapy, but especially in CPT, a degree of physical normal tissue sparing is expected for normal tissues outside the PTV, such that the physical dose (d_H) to a critical region of normal tissue (e.g. the maximum or modal dose given to a clinically relevant normal tissue point or volume according to local anatomical constraints) is given by

$$d_H = z_H \times P_H, \tag{4.2}$$

where P_H is the physical sparing factor of the high-LET radiation, that is the fraction of the tumour dose (z_H) delivered to the normal tissue. Ideally, P_H should be as low as possible. For low-LET the associated sparing will likely be less, i.e. the physical sparing factor (P_L) will be greater than P_H. For example, if a vertebral tumour is given a dose z_L by low LET or z_H by high LET, the dose at the surface of the spinal cord a few millimetres away might be $P_H \times z_H = d_H$ in the high-LET case and $P_L \times z_L = d_L$ in the low-LET case.

Using equations (4.1) and (4.2), the normal tissue high-LET dose per fraction, d_H, can be converted back to an equivalent low-LET dose per fraction, d_{Leq}, by use of the normal tissue RBE ($\mathrm{RBE_{norm}}$), to give

$$d_{\mathrm{Leq}} = z_H \times P_H \times \mathrm{RBE_{norm}}. \tag{4.3}$$

Then, by substituting z_H from equation (4.1):

$$d_{\mathrm{Leq}} = z_H \times P_H \times \frac{\mathrm{RBE_{norm}}}{\mathrm{RBE_{tum}}}. \tag{4.4}$$

For the low-LET radiation the normal tissue dose is

$$d_{\mathrm{L}} = z_L \times P_L, \tag{4.5}$$

where P_L is the physical sparing factor for the low-LET radiation and $P_H < P_L$ in most circumstances. Combining equations (4.4) and (4.5) and rearranging the terms leads to

$$\frac{d_{\mathrm{Leq}}}{d_L} = \frac{P_H}{P_L} \times \frac{\mathrm{RBE_{norm}}}{\mathrm{RBE_{tum}}}, \tag{4.6}$$

which can be rewritten as

$$S_0 = \frac{P_H}{P_L} \times \frac{\mathrm{RBE_{norm}}}{\mathrm{RBE_{tum}}}, \tag{4.7}$$

where $S_0 = d_{\mathrm{Leq}}/d_L$ represents the combined physical and radiobiological sparing. S_0, which could also be called the biological sparing advantage factor, needs to be as small as possible for particle therapy to have an advantage over conventional x-ray therapy. It is clear that the precise value of S_0 will not only depend on the physical dose sparing ratio, but will also be highly sensitive to errors made in estimating RBE for both tumours and normal tissue, especially as the RBEs are themselves dependent on fraction size, intrinsic low-LET radiosensitivites and tissue cell kinetics. To give an S factor 'inclusive of error terms' (S_I), the errors in RBE values may be incorporated as multiplicative terms on the normal tissue and tumour RBEs values (defined as Error_d and Error_Z, respectively), resulting in

$$S_I = \frac{P_H}{P_L} \times \frac{\mathrm{RBE}_{\mathrm{norm}}}{\mathrm{RBE}_{\mathrm{tum}}} \times \frac{(1 \pm \mathrm{Error}_d)}{(1 \pm \mathrm{Error}_z)}. \tag{4.8}$$

The error term can simply be treated as a factor from 0 to 1 or as a percentage change. For example, if the recommended RBE weighting factor is 3, while actually it is 1.5 in a particular tissue of interest, this represents a 50% error, whereas if the actual RBE is 6, there is a 100% error. In equation (4.8), such an error of 50% would be included as a factor 0.5, an error of 30% as 0.3, etc.

In this way, it can be seen that the errors in RBE if in the wrong 'direction' can impose a higher demand on treatment planning. For example, applying 20% errors to equation (4.8):

$$S_{w,20\%} = \frac{P_H}{P_L} \times \left(\frac{\mathrm{RBE}_{\mathrm{norm}}}{\mathrm{RBE}_{\mathrm{tum}}} \times \frac{(1+0.2)}{(1-0.2)}\right), \tag{4.9}$$

or

$$S_{w,20\%} = \frac{P_H}{P_L} \times \left(\frac{\mathrm{RBE}_{\mathrm{norm}}}{\mathrm{RBE}_{\mathrm{tum}}} \times \frac{3}{2}\right). \tag{4.10}$$

By substituting S_0, the S value assumed prior to the consideration of RBE errors (equation (4.7)), then:

$$S_{w,20\%} = S_0 \times \frac{3}{2} \tag{4.11}$$

Thus for S_0 to be maintained in the case of $S_{w,20\%}$, the high-LET physical dose sparing factor, P_H, would have to be reduced by one-third:

$$S_{w,20\%} = \left(P_H \times \frac{2}{3}\right)\frac{1}{P_L} \times \left(\frac{RBE_{norm}}{RBE_{tum}} \times \frac{3}{2}\right) \Rightarrow S_{w,20\%} = S_0. \tag{4.12}$$

Further discussions and examples are given in Jones *et al* (2011).

4.1.6 The product of LET and dose

It has recently been suggested in international meetings that the product of LET and dose can be used to replace RBE. This product cannot fully represent the likelihood

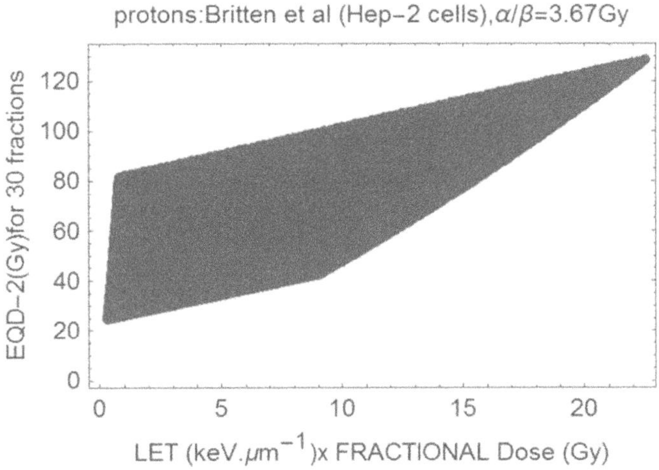

Figure 4.2. EQD-2 and variable LET-fractional dose product phase space for the Hep-2 cellular data of Britten *et al* (2013).

of biological effects, especially since RBE varies inversely with dose itself. The product's physical units are not meaningful (energy released/distance × energy absorbed/mass) and is seen to be insufficiently discriminating in figure 4.2, where the product is plotted against the equivalent dose in 2 Gy fractions for an isoeffect based on the BED concept applied to the proton cell survival data of Britten *et al* (2013), using the proton LET model described in chapters 8 and 9. The large phase space occupied shows that the use of the product may produce erroneous predictions, despite the overall trend showing a positive correlation. Further details are given in Jones (2017a).

The same can be deduced from the plots of the same product against surviving fraction for ion beams in figures 4.3(a)–(c), where the overlap is often significant even in the case of substantial changes in the surviving fractions.

4.1.7 Some final caveats and suggestions

Many studies and some national programmes for proton therapy selection have been based on treatment planning with estimation of TCP and NTCP, with use of an RBE value of 1.1 in all tumours and tissues. Although this may appear to be very scientific, many inherent errors may result in an incorrect decision, especially when full prescribed doses are to be given to brain tissues on the margin of a tumour. Not only are volume-related normal tissue models susceptible to error, but TCP and NTCP models require assumptions on clonogen numbers, and also the use of a constant RBE will result in dose discrepancies. The simplest and best method may be to use BED only with or without or EQD-2 assessments together with a flexible RBE parameter (Jones 2017b), and to link this to risk-based models (Jones 2022), as discussed further in chapters 8, 9 and 10.

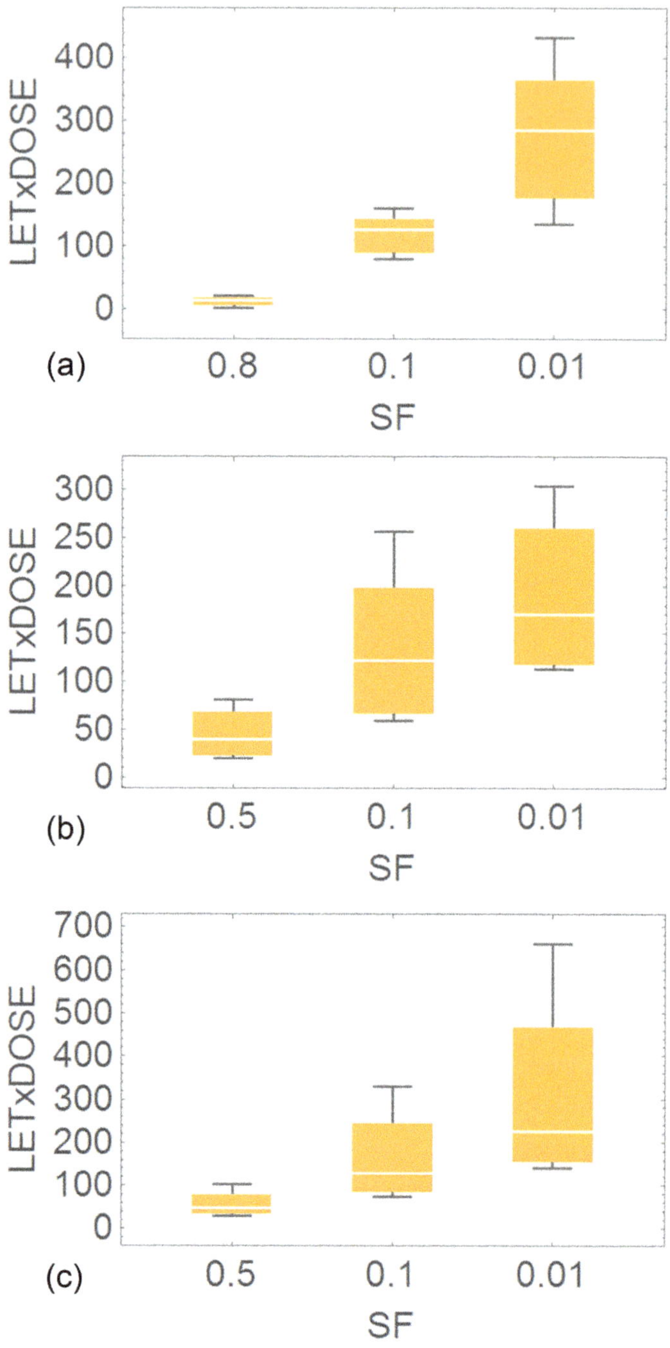

Figure 4.3. (a) Data of Barendsen human T cells exposed to deuterons and helium ions. (b) Weyrather *et al* data for carbon ions using CHO cells. (c) Weyrather *et al* (1999) data using V-79 cells.

References

Barendsen G W 1968 Responses of cultured cells, tumours and normal tissues to radiations of different linear energy transfer *Curr. Topics Radiat. Res. Q.* **4** 293–356

Britten R A, Nazaryan V, Davis L K *et al* 2013 Variations in the RBE for cell killing along the depth-dose profile of a modulated proton therapy beam *Radiat. Res.* **179** 21–8

ICRU 2010 *Prescribing, Recording, and Reporting Proton-Beam Therapy (Report 78)* (Bethesda, MD: International Commission on Radiation Units & Measurements)

Jones B, Underwood T C and Dale R G 2011 The potential impact of RBE uncertainty on charged particle treatment prescriptions *Br. J. Radiol.* **84** S61–9

Jones B 2015 Towards achieving the full clinical potential of proton therapy by inclusion of LET and RBE models *Cancers (Basel)* **7** 460–80

Jones B 2017a Clinical radiobiology of proton therapy: modeling of RBE *Acta. Oncol.* **56** 1374–8

Jones B 2017b Proton radiobiology and its clinical implications *Ecancermedicalscience* **11** 777

Jones B 2022 Risk assessment for proton therapy in the central nervous system by assuming small increments in RBE *Radiat. Phys. Chem.* **200** 110213

Weyrather W K, Ritter S, Scholz M and Kraft G 1999 RBE for carbon track-segment irradiation in cell lines of differing repair capacity *Int. J. Radiat. Biol.* **75** 1357–64

IOP Publishing

Quantitative Radiobiology for Proton Therapy

Bleddyn Jones

Chapter 5

Historical development of radiotherapy: what was learned from fast neutrons including their linkage with proton relative biological effect

The empirical advances in radiotherapy are summarised since they are relevant to particle therapy. The reasons for the development of neutron therapy, and why this treatment did not produce the expected gains in tumour control relative to normal tissue toxicity, are discussed. Neutrons did not have 'tissue-sparing' Bragg peaks, and the constant neutron relative biological effect (RBE) tumour prescription values did not adequately respect the probable higher RBE values in late-reacting tissues with low α/β values. The increase in RBE as dose falls along a beam would also contribute to greater toxicity than in a similar megavoltage photon beam.

A better understanding of fast neutron experiments and therapy, due to better methods of analysis, offers important insights into the problems that can occur in proton therapy, especially since neutron ionisation effects in living tissues are mainly caused by recoil protons. For this reason, neutron studies can represent the worst-case scenario in proton beams and reflect the RBE values in the proton Bragg peak region. Neutron RBEs can be estimated from the energy profiles of their recoil protons, and further considerations regarding the range of recoil protons can give insights into the conditions which determine the peak RBE values near LET_U, including a better understanding of the effective LET_U value around 30.5 keV μm^{-1}, where the RBE decreases with further increases in linear energy transfer (LET). Recoil proton energies within a neutron beam can be used to estimate neutron RBE and provide substantially higher LET_U values for protons, although particle ranges relative to cellular dimensions will influence the lower proton-beam LET_U found in proton beams, but not in neutron beams where release of protons occurs stochastically along the neutron tracks, which include all intracellular locations. In a proton beam, energy inefficiency starts where the proton ranges become less than 1 cell diameter (when the LET is around 30.5 keV μm^{-1}); energy inefficiency within a

doi:10.1088/978-0-7503-6209-2ch5

neutron beam starts when the intracellular range is much shorter (at a recoil proton LET of around 62.5 keV μm^{-1} produced by neutrons with energies near 2 MeV).

It is also possible to deduce the effective single neutron energy for RBE effects within a neutron beam with a specific maximum energy.

5.1 Introduction

The following brief description of the historical development of radiotherapy is necessary in order for readers from some backgrounds to understand the present dilemmas facing decision makers. It explains some of the problems associated with technical development (most of which have been beneficial), but the example of fast neutrons contains important lessons in radiotherapeutics, and which are relevant to particle therapy today.

5.2 A brief synopsis

The discovery of x-rays and natural radioactivity were soon followed by their application in medicine. Diagnostic imaging became widespread within a few decades; radiotherapy of cancer, as an alternative to surgery, became increasingly important and remains so. Technical developments were mainly based on the achievement of higher photon energies, which increased the range or tissue depth while also, for megavoltage photons, reducing the skin, or entry dose, before attaining full secondary electronic equilibrium. Improvements in dosimetry and computational interactions yielded further advances in medical diagnosis, including nuclear medicine (radioisotope emissions), computerised tomography (CT scans), positron emission applications, as well as imaging advances from other branches of physics (magnetic resonance imaging and ultrasound). All these imaging techniques have been used to further improve radiotherapy targeting and have made it possible to superimpose radiation depth dose curves in three dimensions on a relevant scan or even a combination of fused scan images.

During World War II an important advance was made by Frank Ellis, who realised during an air raid that the local beam intensity could be varied[1]: this was achieved by introducing a wedge-shaped medium (initially wood and later metal) to attenuate the beam along its axis in order to produce more homogenous doses around a target when multiple beams were used and where the anatomical shape of the body would distort the regular profile of the beam. These became known as wedge filters, and compensators were a further extension wherein small areas of the beam were made to pass through tailor-made thicknesses of metal, which were based on the thickness of tissue to be traversed.

[1] Ellis was asked by his physicist to go to the deeper end of the air-raid shelter, which was better protected since there were a greater number of sandbags above that section than over the entrance region: it was explained that the roof was effectively wedge-shaped, the thin end being over the entrance. Ellis remarked that they should use similar principles in radiotherapy to overcome the problem of curved anatomical surfaces, and they started drawing diagrams of what was necessary. So, in some respects, Goering's Luftwaffe bears some responsibility for this important development. Ellis told this to the present author at a special dinner given by the British Institute of Radiology to commemorate his 100th birthday.

Naturally occurring radioisotopes were used in an increasingly controlled manner with excellent results if the radioactivity could be concentrated within a cancer; the use of rare and manufactured isotopes and various methods of enhancing their localisation continue to be developed. The best example is thyroid cancer, which, although rare, has distinct subtypes each with different propensities to trap iodine. Cure rates are very high for the avid iodine-trapping cancers, even when these have spread to distant parts of the body. Sealed radioisotope sources also became important for applications where the sources could be placed within or close to many forms of primary cancers, and remain is use.

During the 1950s and 1960s external radiation beams progressed to the mega-voltage energy range by use of cobalt-60 (^{60}Co) units and later increasing use of linear accelerators (LINACS), after the potential of the cavity magnetron had been fully realised for radar applications, to an extent that the already existing cyclotron accelerators were only rarely used, for proton acceleration onto beryllium targets to produce fast neutrons for clinical studies.

Along with the computing advances mentioned above, during the 1990s it became possible to shape each individual beam in order to match the clinically defined target by introducing variable strips of metal in the accelerator collimation system. This became known as conformal radiotherapy. A UK randomised clinical trial showed that normal tissue side effects were reduced due to the large reduction in normal tissue volume irradiated to a high dose, but without a reduction in prostate cancer tumour control with long-term analysis (Dearnaley *et al* 2014). The beam-control possibilities were improved further by using a multi-leaf collimator to vary the beam intensity along its profile: this became known as intensity-modulated radiotherapy, which further improved the degree of conformity to the defined target volume[2]. Although the UK was slow to adopt this technique, randomised studies were also performed to confirm the improved normal tissue sparing of defined organs, such as the parotid gland while treating head and neck cancer (Nutting *et al* 2011). In order to achieve the best available conformity index around the immediate vicinity of the target volume, it was necessary to use more individual beams, and with the differential attenuation used the net effect was to increase the amount of tissue exposed to medium or lower doses, with some potential for causing more subtle later effects such as cancer induction or late vascular effects over time periods of 5–30 years. More recently, developments include robotically controlled small LINACs, offering rapid changes in the beam direction and intensity modulation of small beamlets, which can further improve the conformity index and be used with more precise body immobilisation techniques and state-of-the-art image-guidance

[2] Conformity index (CI) refers to a single-figure assessment of the merit of a planned dose distribution compared to an ideal situation where the radiation dose is completely uniform (or where the target volume dose is totally achieved), with or without a desired reduction of dose to further volumes of normal tissue. There are many variants of CI in use for this purpose, some of which may be misleading in some situations, since they tend to be defined with certain techniques in mind. The reader should consult widely before selecting any particular one system. For particle therapy the situation is more complex due to LET and dose inhomogeneity, and the main advantage is a dose reduction or no direct dose in some tissues, reflected more by the integral dose in the region outside the target volume limits.

techniques. These treatments, depending on the dose distributions achieved, can be given in fewer treatments (hypofractionation) or even in a single session (often referred to as radiosurgery).

More recently, there has been an expansion in cyclotron or synchrotron acceleration to deliver protons and light ions for cancer therapy. These positively charged particles have Bragg peaks whose tissue depths are energy dependent. Appropriate energy selection can be tailored to detailed tumour imaging so that energy deposition can occur in the selected cancer volume and its immediate surroundings.

In comparison with the best available photon beams, charged particles offer reduced entrance doses and no direct dose beyond the target. However, when more than one beam is used and with pencil (or raster) intensity-modulated beams, good to excellent tumour conformity can be achieved. Yet, the degrees of freedom of angular selection are considerably reduced, and even if expensive gantries are available the degree of conformity in the immediate tumour region may not be as good as with some photon techniques, though the integral dose (that is, the dose over the entire part of the body being irradiated) can be substantially reduced. Thus the medium to low dose volume is reduced and more tissue tends to receive no direct radiation than would be the case with all modern photon techniques. One drawback is that skin sparing can be sub-optimal compared to LINACs or electrons when protons are used for volumes near to the skin surface.

Both radioisotopes and charged-particle beams rely on preferential radiation dose distribution, respectively, due to sharp inverse square dose falloff with distance and the Bragg peak effect.

Research studies showed that the biological effects of radiation varied not only with dose but with dose rate, the degree in which the dose can be split in time (fractionation), the chemical environment of the cells (some chemicals protecting and others sensitising radiation by influencing the yield of free radicals) and also the 'quality' of the radiation. The latter refers to the LET characteristics of a radiation, which depends not only on the nature of the radiation (e.g. photon or hadron), its energy (lower energies confer higher LET) and nuclear charge.

A major question that remains to be completely settled is whether the increase in LET may be disadvantageous to some normal tissues situated very close to the tumour, depending on the anatomical region being treated and the decisive relative biological effect (RBE) allocation. This is taken further in chapters 7–11.

5.3 Neutron therapy

Many current authorities tend to be dismissive of the history of fast neutron therapy, because of its disappointing clinical outcomes, often interpreted as being 'bad press' for radiotherapy in general and especially for any form of particle therapy emerging from a cyclotron. This is unfair for several reasons, as shown in the outline provided below, with special reference to their physical properties (uncharged and similar in some respects to photons) but with high-LET features.

Fast neutrons cause most of their ionisation by forming recoil protons as well as some nuclear fragments, so their radiobiological features, including their RBE

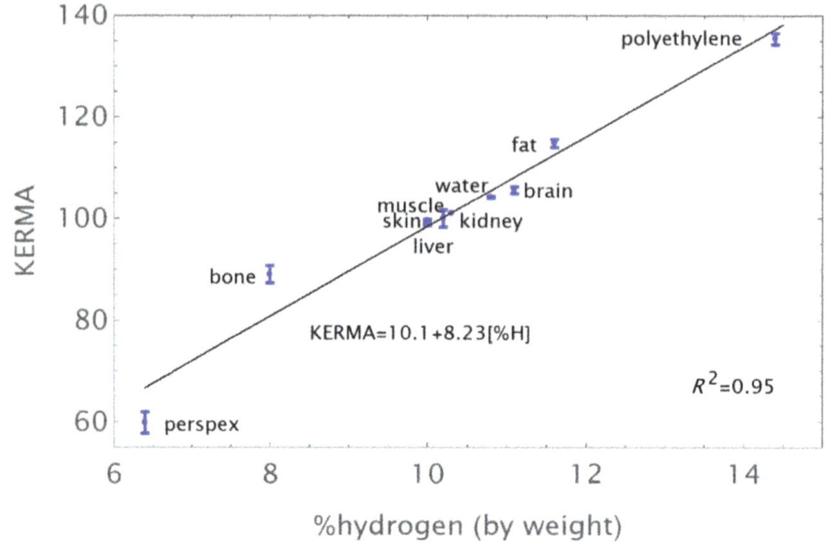

Figure 5.1. Plot of the relationship between the percentage of hydrogen (by weight) and relative values of KERMA for various materials and tissues exposed to five different fast neutron beams. The skin and liver have almost identical KERMA, and is shown as a square. Modified from Jones, with inclusion of standard error bars and with least-squares fitted equation. Tissues with a high fat content, such as the white matter of the nervous system, will consequently receive a higher dose than other soft tissues with a lower fat content. Adapted from Jones (2020). CC BY 4.0.

values, will be similar to those of a proton beam in the Bragg peak region where the LET and dose increase substantially. Another important feature is that the kinetic energy released per unit mass (quantified as KERMA) is proportional to the hydrogen content of the substance or tissue being irradiated. This can be seen in figure 5.1.

This fact has not been sufficiently appreciated within the proton therapy community until recently, although it was predicted as explained in the previous edition of this book (see references in chapters 7–9). Indeed, RBE values in the fast neutron range have been found at the end of spread-out Bragg proton peaks (SOBPs) in the human lung, and there is concern about nervous tissues (references are provided in chapter 1).

Fast neutron therapy of cancer started optimistically on the basis of limited *in vitro* experimental evidence of more efficient cell killing per unit dose, but unfortunately the clinical results were disappointing. The history of neutron therapy illustrates the frustrations encountered when partial scientific knowledge is used in an attempt to improve the treatment of a complex biological condition such as cancer: the sterilisation of cancer cells in a laboratory experiment is considerably easier than the elimination of a malignant tumour situated close to essential organs/ tissues of the body. In the context of future radiotherapy developments, particularly the use of proton- and ion-beam therapy, this history is highly relevant.

Scientists such as Gray *et al* (1940) had shown that it was possible to achieve the same level of biological effect with a lower dose of neutrons than with gamma or x-rays. Such a difference is quantified by the RBE, the ratio of the doses of the two forms of radiation required to produce the same biological effect. Fast neutron RBE values of 1.5–5 were found in a variety of biological systems (e.g. bacteria, plants and transplanted animal cancers). The immediate inference was that neutrons would be ideal for cancer therapy; yet the first human experimental treatment in the USA showed marked toxicity, because the relationship between the exposure dose and RBE had not yet been identified. Gray remained sceptical, and realised that in the three spatial dimensions encountered within the human body, neutrons could cause more problems because of the RBE: he knew that RBE varied inversely with dose, so that dose falloff with distance along a neutron beam would inevitably be accompanied by higher RBE values in normal tissues beyond any cancer target. His opinion had devastating personal and other organisational consequences for radiobiology and radiotherapy, especially in the UK[3]. Gray believed that neutrons were an important tool for research, for the investigation of high-LET effects, but not necessarily in treatment. He was eventually proved correct, and the wealth of fast neutron experimental data (much of it performed in the UK) probably provides the best insights into high-LET phenomena, especially the inverse dose per fraction effect on RBE, especially marked in late-reacting tissues as compared to acute tissue effects.

Further interest arose because of the discovery that high-LET radiations, e.g. fast neutrons, with increased clustering of ionisation events along micrometre distances of their tracks are less dependent than x-rays on the presence of oxygen to produce cell death (oxygen essentially amplifies low-LET ionisations by increasing the yield of reactive free radicals in solution). The previous work of Gray and others had shown that many cancers contained zones of very low oxygen tension, which were considered an important cause of radioresistance. To overcome this problem, high-pressure oxygen (HPO) was used in experimental radiotherapy, with impressive results. In the UK, it was developed in Hammersmith, and the initial results in animal experimental systems were impressive (Gray *et al* 1953). In clinical practice HPO had many disadvantages, since patients had to be placed within HPO tanks or chambers, and there was no overall improvement in patient survival, although some tumour types were better controlled (Henk *et al* 1977). An attractive alternative to

[3] Dr Constance Wood, Medical Director of Radiotherapy, dismissed Gray from his post as Director of Radiotherapy Physics at the Hammersmith Hospital, where important groundbreaking work had been done on describing the cell cycle and other biomedical advances. Wood had a distinguished clinical background and had used some of her personal inheritance to jointly fund the development of the first LINAC in Europe, in partnership with Metropolitan Vickers, who manufactured radar and other defence-related equipment. She later regretted her decision, based on her own conviction that neutrons were the way forward for radiotherapy. In order to salvage Gray's career, a new laboratory was created for him on the Mount Vernon Hospital site in Northwood, London, and it even bore his name. The rest is history since the Gray laboratory, funded by some UK cancer charities, the MRC and with impressive contributions by The Scott of Yews Trust, became the world-leading laboratory for radiobiology research (Jones & Hendry 2017). It is interesting to note that of the long list of distinguished scientists who had been Fellows of Trinity College Cambridge, only Newton and Gray have SI units named after them.

HPO was the use cyclotrons to accelerate protons—to around 20 MeV or higher—colliding with beryllium targets to produce fast neutrons with high-LET properties and so a reduced cell-killing oxygen dependency within cancers. It was argued by the neutron enthusiasts that the HPO chambers would no longer be necessary.

The UK Medical Research Council (MRC) funded three important sequential projects to investigate fast neutron therapy:

1. At Hammersmith, clinical studies were conducted with initial promise using a geometrically limited fixed horizontal beam. But, despite clear evidence that the neutron RBE was inversely related to dose per fraction in a wide variety of animal tissues, the clinical dose prescriptions used a fixed RBE. So, the dose plan took no account of the increase in RBE in normal tissues beyond the tumour, which received lower doses than those prescribed to the tumour. Initial attempts at randomised trials involved control patients treated with x-rays or cobalt beams at other hospitals without defined protocols so that a wide range of doses, including some that were unsuitable, were used. Suffice it to say that much was learned on how to conduct cancer trials properly.
2. Secondly, at Edinburgh, stricter 'in-house' randomised trials were carried out comparing megavoltage x-rays (with superior tissue penetration) and relatively poorly penetrating fast neutrons, but for both radiation classes the beams could be rotated on a gantry. However, the tumour control rates were disappointing and were accompanied by enhanced normal tissue toxicity.
3. Thirdly, at Clatterbridge (Liverpool), an extended fast neutron energy (obtained using 64 MeV protons) produced depth doses equivalent to 5 MeV x-rays in randomised trials, some of which were jointly undertaken with research in Seattle (USA).

Taken together, these trials showed that neutrons conferred no clinical advantage, as summarised by Duncan (1994). In other countries, relatively low-energy neutrons had been tried without recourse to formal trials and with little convincing success, although one small randomised trial, reported by Laramore *et al* (1993), showed benefits for neutrons in the control of unresectable cancers of the parotid gland; but it is possible that a higher dose of x-rays or electrons in the control arm might have produced the same result, by matching the actual tumour RBE, which was probably higher than that used in the prescription since most parotid tumours are slow growing. Relatively superficial cancers of the nasal cavities and nearby sinuses were also thought to be better controlled, although there was always concern that neutrons were particularly damaging to the tissues of the underlying brain, where it had been identified that the RBE was around 5 rather than 3.

In retrospect, neutron therapy failed to match its original promise for the following physical and radiobiological reasons:

- Routine absorbed dose computations did not include the highly efficient neutron capture by hydrogen, resulting in higher energy release in hydrogen-rich tissues such as brain white matter and fat, which surrounds most important organs and is closely associated with their blood supply.

- Dismissal of the well-established finding of RBE variations in different tissues and its important increase with a falling dose, which mitigates the effect of a reduction in physical dose beyond a cancer.
- The appreciation that RBE also varies with cell proliferation rate, so that slow-growing cells have higher values. It is the slow-growing cells that make up the majority of normal tissues and contribute to the severe tissue damage at extended time periods after irradiation.

The considerable literature on neutron radiobiology was summarised by Bewley (1989) and remains relevant to proton therapy. More recent mathematical modelling, which included RBE within biological effective dose (BED) equations, showed that neutrons would only have improved therapeutic results in the case of very superficial cancers with little normal tissue coverage (Dale & Jones 1998). Further information is available in a more recent publication (Jones 2021).

5.4 More recent developments based on neutron studies

Fast neutron radiobiology studies had already shown high RBE values which varied inversely with dose, reductions in oxygen enhancement ratio (OER) and cell cycle phase dependency, with greater fraction insensitivity. Extended analysis of the fast neutron experiments at Hammersmith and Clatterbridge continued in more recent times, providing many informative reports as in Carabe-Fernandez *et al* (2007, 2010), Jones (2010) and Jones *et al* (2011), which model the well-recognised inverse dose per fraction and RBE effects, using the RBE_{max} and RBE_{min} concepts, as defined in chapter 2, in different tissue classes represented by their characteristic α/β ratios. For example, early-reacting tissues such as the acute oesophageal mucosal reaction show almost no change in RBE with dose per fraction, whereas later reactions in various tissues such as skin, lung and kidney show greater changes in RBE with dose per fraction. In accord with linear-quadratic model theory (see Appendix A at end of this chapter), RBE_{max} is inversely related to the α/β ratio (see figure 5.2(a)) while RBE_{min} is directly proportional to the square root of α/β (see figure 5.2(b)). By using these relationships, for the most criticial low α/β (late-reacting) tissues their RBE at low dose is highest, but these have the lowest RBE at high dose when compared with more rapid proliferating biosystems with high α/β ratios, which have a 'flatter' response, as shown in figure 5.3(a).

By rescaling figure 5.3(a) to match a 1.1 proton RBE, for $\alpha/\beta = 10$ Gy (the value of the predominant jejunal crypt *in vivo* assay used to achieve this RBE in mid-SOBPs), it is possible to predict as a first approximation what the RBE values would be at other doses and for different tissue types, as shown in figure 5.3(b). Again, there is a crossover effect where for large dose per fraction, the RBE values are lowest in the tissues with low α/β values, the reverse of that found at low dose per fraction. At 2 Gy per fraction, the α/β of 2 Gy characteristic of central nervous tissue is around 1.2. It is noted here that such a crossover effect is reliant on using the RBE_{max} and RBE_{min} limits; other radiobiological models of proton- and ion-beam therapy which do not use these limits will not predict such effects, especially at high dose.

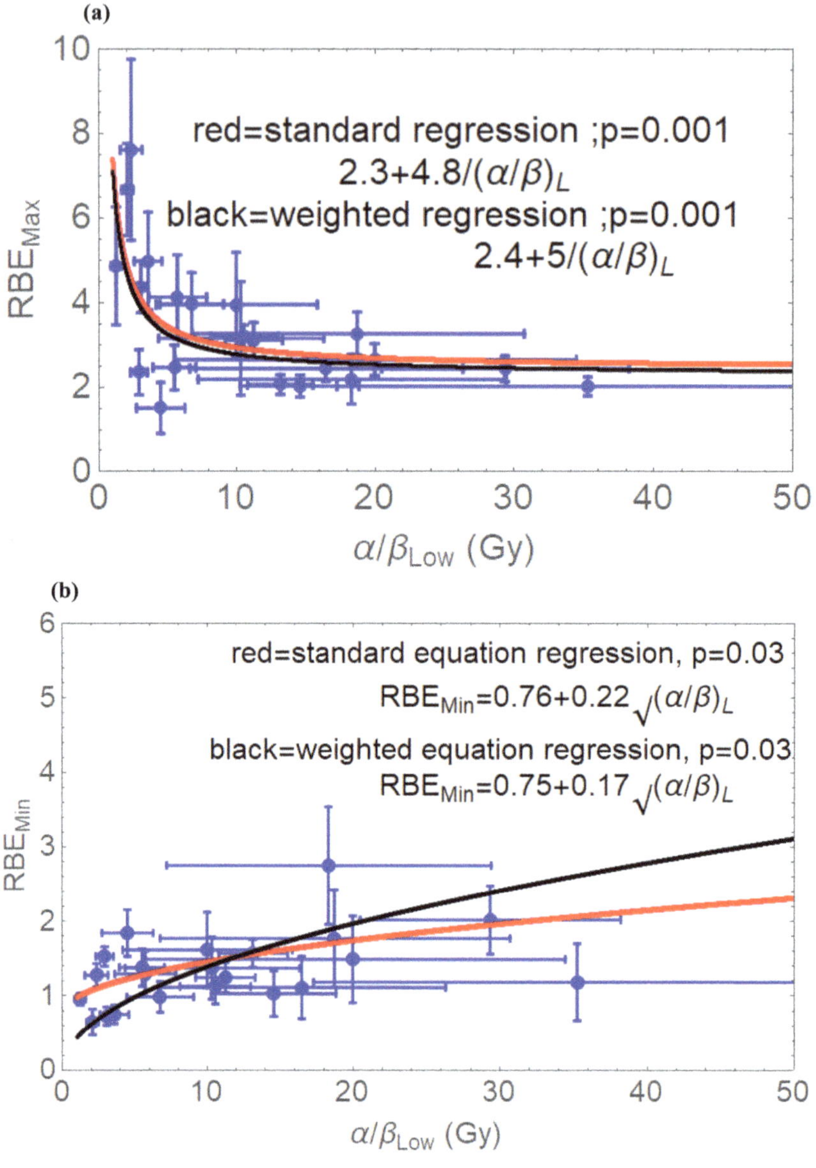

Figure 5.2. (a) and (b): Plots of (a) RBE_{max} and (b) RBE_{min} against the reference low-LET α/β ratio. Adapted from Jones *et al.* (2011). Copyright (2014) The British Institute of Radiology. Published by Oxford University Press.

Another consequence of the fact that the overall RBE is controlled by RBE_{max} and RBE_{min}, and that these parameters are, respectively, inversely and directly related to the reference radiation α/β ratio or its square root (see Appendix A of this chapter), then a practical RBE for a clinically used dose cannot be assumed to be only related to RBE_{max}. Mathematical models that predict RBE from the inverse or reciprocal value of α/β must be incomplete. A better approach, shown in chapters 8

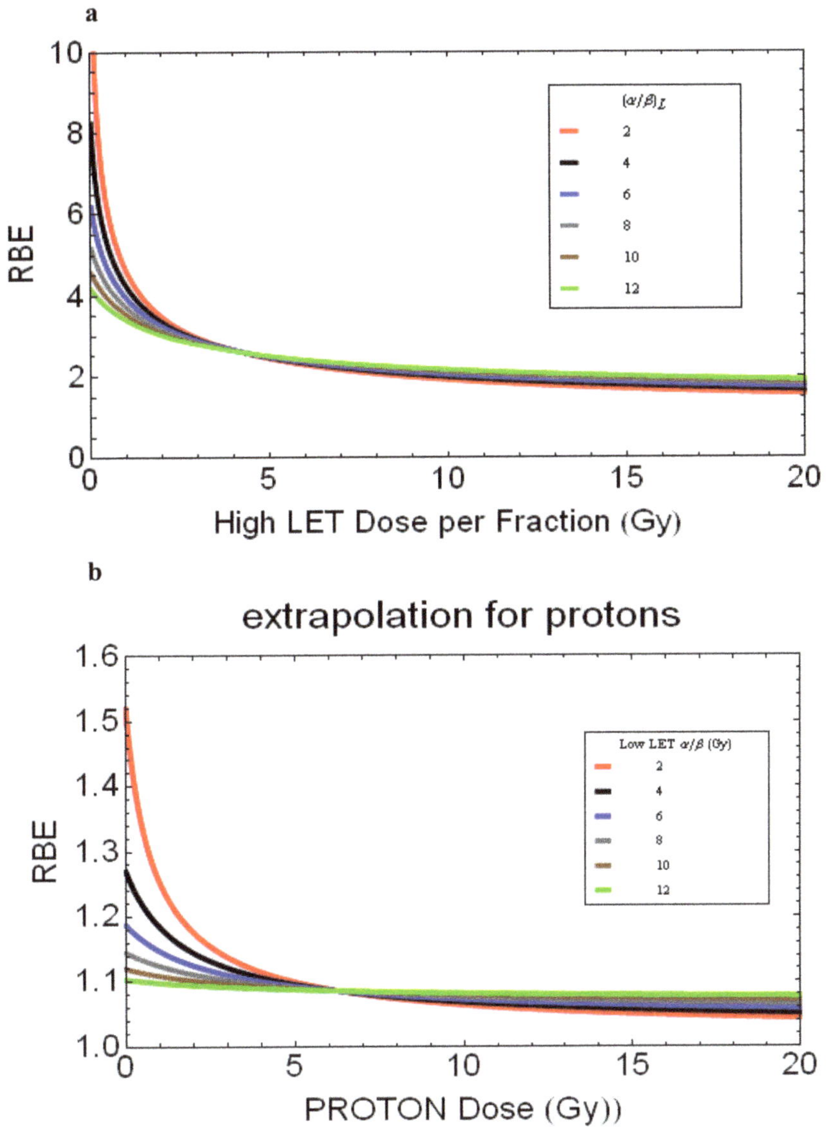

Figure 5.3. (a) and (b): Relationship between (a) fast neutron dose per fraction and RBE for different α/β ratios, and (b) the transformation of the above to provide a near-flat response for α/β of 10 Gy to simulate proton data, as discussed in chapters 7 and 9. The red curves suggest how brain and spinal cord tissues may behave ($\alpha/\beta = 2$ Gy), followed by a gradual change in α/β to faster-growing systems such as many rapidly growing tumour types and acute-reacting normal tissues ($\alpha/\beta = 10$ Gy).

and 9, enable separate modification of α and β with increasing LET, and consequently allow the RBE to be related to the reciprocal of α/β at low dose, but to be dependent on $\sqrt{(\alpha/\beta)}$ at high dose, with a gradual transition between these two limits with change of dose.

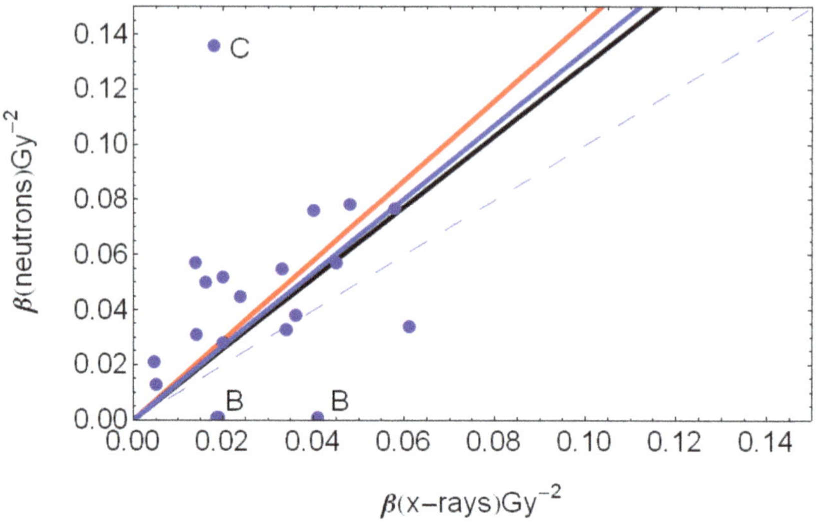

Figure 5.4. Plotted data of the β-parameter for x-rays and neutrons. Cell lines labelled C and B were excluded due to known radiation repair deficiencies and extreme values, β being difficult to measure when α is high. Reproduced from Jones (2010). Copyright (2014) The British Institute of Radiology. Published by Oxford University Press.

Warenius and colleagues (Warenius & Britten 1994, Warenius *et al* 1994) identified that the respective rank order of radiosensitivities for photons and neutrons were not the same. This is a consequence of the above transition between RBE_{max} and RBE_{min} and other effects such as the saturation or reduction of RBE increments with increasing intrinsic (photon) radiosensitivity. This is discussed further in chapter 9 with estimations of what might be expected for protons.

It has also been shown that the LET values produced by fast neutrons increases the α radiosensitivity parameter by a factor of 3.17, but the β parameter increases as $1.59\sqrt{\beta}$ on average. Previously, it was thought that β did not increase with LET (as evidenced in meticulous experiments involving only one cell line, the V-79 cell line by Chapman 2003); but the Clatterbridge *in vitro* neutron data set contained over 20 cell lines, and the increase in β can be seen in figure 5.4 (Jones 2010).

There now remain very few advocates for neutron therapy in the world. In fact, the only promising development for neutrons is arguably boron neutron capture therapy—a complex binary therapy that involves a low-dose exposure to thermal or epithermal neutrons which are selectively captured by boron-labelled molecules taken up by rapidly growing tumour cells. The reaction creates more intense localised ionisation by generating an alpha particle and a lithium ion, with tissue ranges of only around 10 μm (around one cell diameter). Some pilot studies have shown promise in highly malignant brain tumours or for recurrent tumours, although in uncontrolled, highly selected patients (Kageji *et al* 2014, Lim *et al* 2015). Further discussion is beyond the scope of this book.

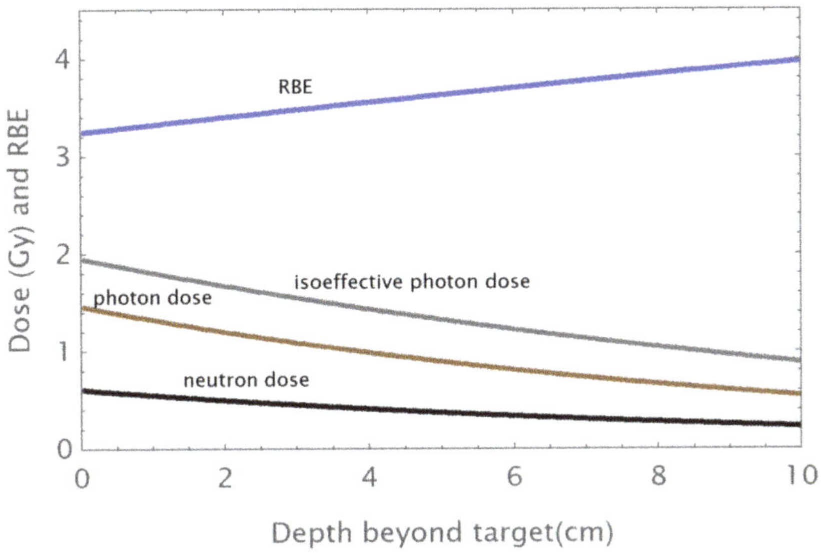

Figure 5.5. Plot of tissue depth distance beyond a target volume and neutron dose, with estimated photon equivalent dose and RBE. The assumptions made were an exponential attenuation coefficient of 0.1 cm^{-1}, $RBE_{max} = 5$, $RBE_{min} = 1.3$, intrinsic photon $\alpha/\beta = 3$ Gy, in a multiple field arrangement where only a single exit dose is considered.

Following the clinical fast neutron trials, the UK funding authorities decided not to invest in further ambitious radiation projects, and as a result a general decline in radiotherapy research followed, although the Clatterbridge cyclotron was successfully adapted for proton therapy in the eye. There emerged a clinical scepticism regarding the use of cyclotrons in radiotherapy and high-LET radiations in general. In other countries, more progress was achieved using charged-particle therapy (protons or light ions) produced from cyclotrons or the larger synchrotrons. Some of these countries had no prior experience of high-LET radiations in the form of neutrons.

The extensive late tissue side effect of fibrosis (scarring) was prominent around neutron-treated volumes. Although the falloff of dose was broadly the same in the Clatterbridge trials, the reduction in neutron dose beyond a target volume will result in an increased RBE because of the inverse relationship between RBE and dose per fraction. Figure 5.5, which follows the dose falloff with distance beyond a target volume, uses the RBE BED isoeffect equations to estimate the equivalent photon dose and also provides the operative RBE value. It can be seen that the RBE becomes progressively larger with increasing depth due to the lower dose per fraction, which drives the equivalent photon dose to be higher than the actual photon dose. The latter is higher than the neutron dose by a value determined by the single (or constant) RBE used in the prescription process, in this case an RBE of 2.43. Thus the tissue effect will be the same as if the higher dose of photons had been used.

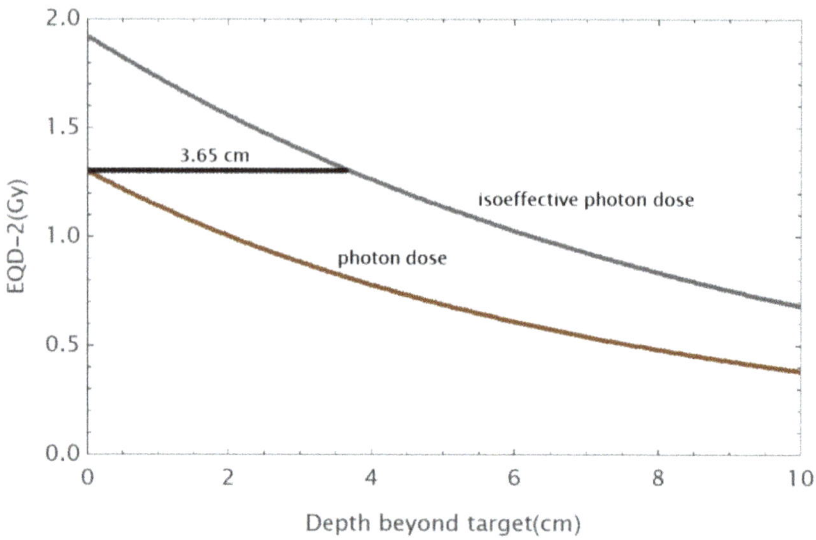

Figure 5.6. Plots of equivalent dose in 2 Gy fractions for a fractional exposure, based on figure 5.5. The brown curve is the simulated photon exit dose from a single beam and the grey curve the isoeffective photon dose provided by the fast neutron beam.

These results can be converted into BED estimates and then to EQD-2 (the equivalent dose in 2 Gy fractions) for each fraction, as displayed in figure 5.6, where it can be seen more clearly than in figure 5.5 that there is a 'triangle' of unintended excess dose over the first 3.65 cm beyond the target which is caused by the neutron RBE. This excess dose might contribute to fibrosis development since there will be a greater volume of tissue exposed to a higher than intended dose. The dose-volume effect on normal tissue tolerances is substantial, as discussed in chapters 3 and 4. Over this initial distance of 3.65 cm from the target volume, the mean EQD-2 for the photon beam is 1.03 Gy per fraction, but the equivalent mean EQD-2 of the neutron beam is estimated to be 1.59 Gy per fraction. This excess dose will probably make a significant contribution to fibrosis development since there will be a greater volume of tissue exposed to a higher than intended dose. The dose-volume effect on normal tissue tolerances is substantial, as discussed in chapters 3 and 4, although there is no adequate predictive model, which is probably a consequence of the local vascularity pattern having different spatial distributions according to the precise anatomical location.

A major radiotherapy research question over the next few decades will be whether carbon ions are superior to protons in specific cancers, because of better beam ballistics and dose localisation and/or the apparent greater reduction in the oxygen effect. Suit *et al* (2010) have pointed out that since even the neutron studies did not show a convincing overall local tumour control improvement, it should not be expected that carbon ions will provide improved efficacy since the oxygen effect dependency is greater for spread-out carbon-ion peaks than for fast neutrons (OER ratios of around 1.8–2 compared with 1.6–1.8, respectively).

The process of reoxygenation in tumours during radiotherapy, lasting a week or more, may be the reason why hypoxic radioresistance is not especially important; dose escalation for hypofractionation may also overcome initial hypoxia. But it is intriguing that identification of tumours with slow reoxygenation kinetics may yet be important since high-LET therapy and dose escalation may be important. Again, the reality of treating tumours *in situ* appears more difficult than the *in vitro* treatment of cells, for many reasons.

5.5 Estimation of neutron RBE from neutron energy

Further analysis of the important Clatterbridge neutron-photon data sets and other detailed RBE studies by Hall *et al* (1975) was written during the COVID-19 pandemic by the present author (see Jones 2021), where many further references can be found. To predict the neutron RBE, it was assumed that recoil proton energies of around 50% of the neutron energy would be mainly responsible for RBE effects, and on this basis a predictive model was constructed, which is described below.

It is known that roughly half the dose due to megavoltage neutrons is due to recoil (elastically scattered) protons, mainly from hydrogen atoms in the biological systems or in water. The remaining half consists of 10%–35% from nuclear recoils (elastic neutron scattering) and 35%–40% from neutron-generated light ions (including protons, deuterons, tritons, ^{3}He and alpha particles). Each of these ionic species will have their own LET–RBE relationship. Furthermore, the neutron energies in most beams form part of a spectrum, and consequently the neutron products will also have their related energy distributions.

The present report describes a tentative and approximate method for estimating fast neutron RBE values by considering elastically scattered recoil proton energies and their LET values and assumes a proportional averaged higher LET contribution from all other ionic products including non-elastic (nuclear) scattering.

A diagram of the nuclear events which lead to the radiobiological change in the α parameter is shown in figure 5.7.

The link between neutron energy, proton recoil energy and LET is obtained by listing outputs of LET for proton kinetic energies (assumed to be half those of the relevant neutrons) in liquid water by using the SRIM software package (see Jones 2021). The outputs form a non-linear relationship, the obtained function F[Pr]LET, to express proton recoil LET with changes in neutron kinetic energy (NKE) by the sum of three-exponential functions as

$$\mathrm{F[Pr]LET} = 73.55\mathrm{e}^{-1.64\,\mathrm{NKE}} + 21.05\mathrm{e}^{-1.65\,\mathrm{NKE}} + 5.04\mathrm{e}^{-0.016\,\mathrm{NKE}}. \tag{5.1}$$

This function was fitted to SRIM-estimated proton energies, as shown in figure 5.8.

Hall *et al* (1975) showed that for quasi-monoenergetic neutrons, the maximum neutron RBE was around 0.4 MeV. A neutron kinetic energy of 0.4 MeV, when inserted in equation (5.1), provides a recoil proton LET_U value of 62.88 keV $\mu\mathrm{m}^{-1}$.

It was then shown that only the ratio of the proton recoil LET values at any energy divided by the proton recoil energies at LET_U is necessary in order to map

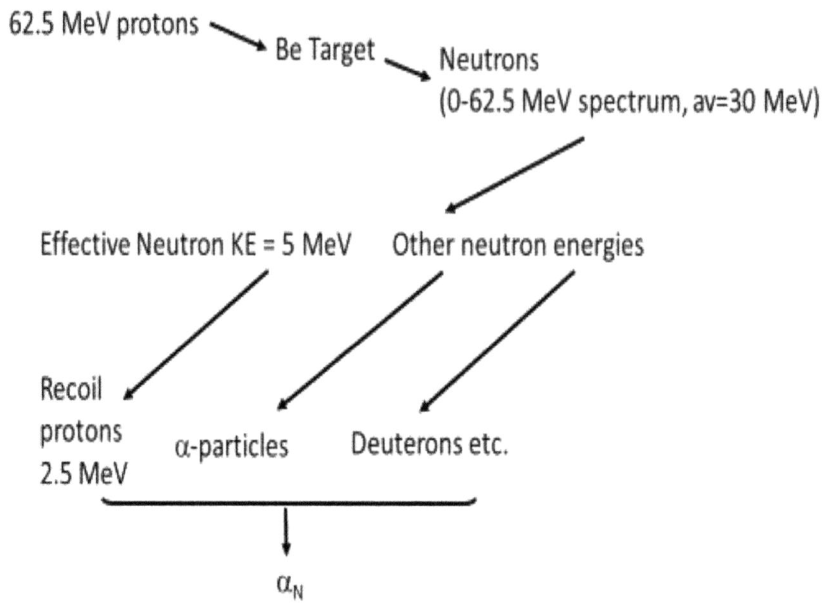

Figure 5.7. A summary of the typical energy relationships that contribute to the biological effectiveness via the α radiosensitivity parameter. Reproduced from Jones (2021). © The Author(s). Published by IOP Publishing Ltd. CC BY 4.0.

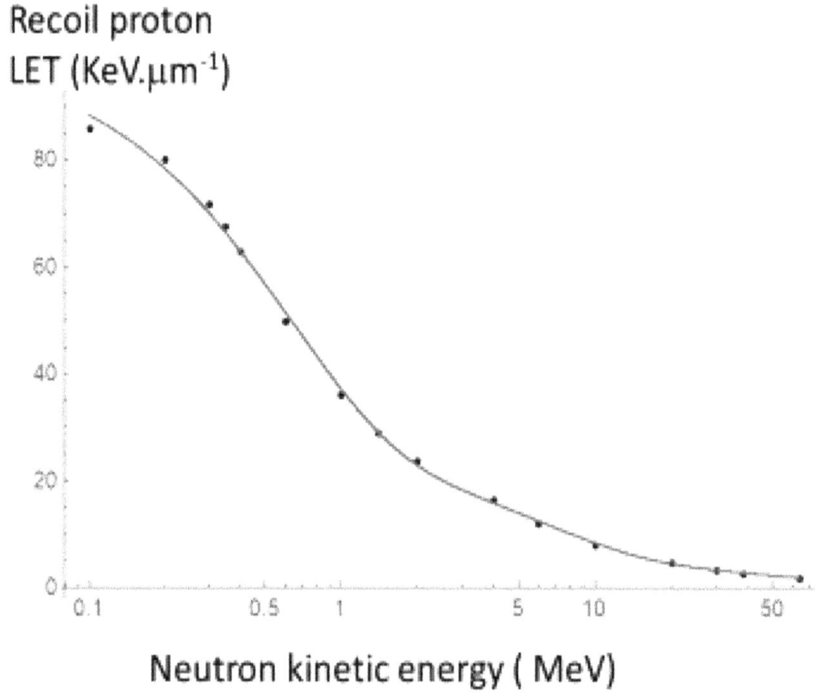

Figure 5.8. The curve given by equation (5.1), which expresses recoil proton LET as a function of neutron kinetic energy, is plotted with data points obtained using the SRIM software for protons in water. Reproduced from Jones (2021). © The Author(s). Published by IOP Publishing Ltd. CC BY 4.0.

any neutron energy onto the proton LET curve shown in figure 5.1. The relative proportion of proton recoils to the LET of the other ions generated is not necessary for these scaling procedures.

Thus the fractional LET will be

$$\text{Fractional LET} = \frac{\text{F[Pr]LET}}{\text{LET}_U[\text{Pr}]}, \tag{5.2}$$

where LET_U will be the specific value for protons, estimated above to be around 62.88 keV μm^{-1}.

This fractional LET method has been used in previous publications for proton- and ion-beam modelling (see chapters 8 and 9), which assumes that the increment of radiosensitivity with LET is linear. Also, the same method can be used for neutron α and β parameters, as in the following.

The α term at any neutron energy (α_N) becomes

$$\alpha_N = \frac{\text{F[Pr] LET}}{\text{LET}_U[\text{Pr}]}\alpha_U - \alpha_C, \tag{5.3}$$

where α_C is the reference radiation α value.

The same form of equation can be used for β, with similar symbolism, namely

$$\beta_N = \frac{\text{F[Pr] LET}}{\text{LET}_U[\text{Pr}]}\beta_U - \beta_C. \tag{5.4}$$

The model described above can be applied easily in a short basic programme (see Appendix B) and was then applied to simulate the Hall RBE data sets for monoenergetic neutrons, as shown in figures 5.9(a)–(d).

The relationship between the maximum neutron energy NE_{max} (within an energy spectrum) and the effective neutron energy (NE_{eff}) which determines the RBE can be fitted by a linear function ($R^2 = 0.97$; $p < 0.01$) as

$$NE_{\text{eff}} = 0.087NE_{\text{max}}. \tag{5.5}$$

The data and fitted line are shown in figure 5.10, which shows one anomalous point where there is insufficient data about the actual beam energy spectrum.

The resulting relationship between RBE and NE_{eff} is shown in figure 5.11.

The present study suggests that the LET_U value of protons is around 62–63 keV μm^{-1}, which is considerably larger than the value of 30.4 keV μm^{-1} derived from the data of Belli *et al* (2000), and upon which some proton models are based, as discussed in chapter 9. Various authors have suggested higher values around 60–80 keV μm^{-1} or higher, as reviewed by Friedrich *et al* (2013) and also found in the later discussion in Jones & Hill (2020), but many experimental groups included an increasing proportion of deuterons in order to maintain particle range; deuterons probably have a higher LET_U value. The Belli *et al* (2000) data set contained protons only, and it is possible that their range was limited in comparison with the average cellular thicknesses of 6–7 μm found using confocal microscopy, whereas when the experiments took place a thickness of 4 μm was measured using older optical

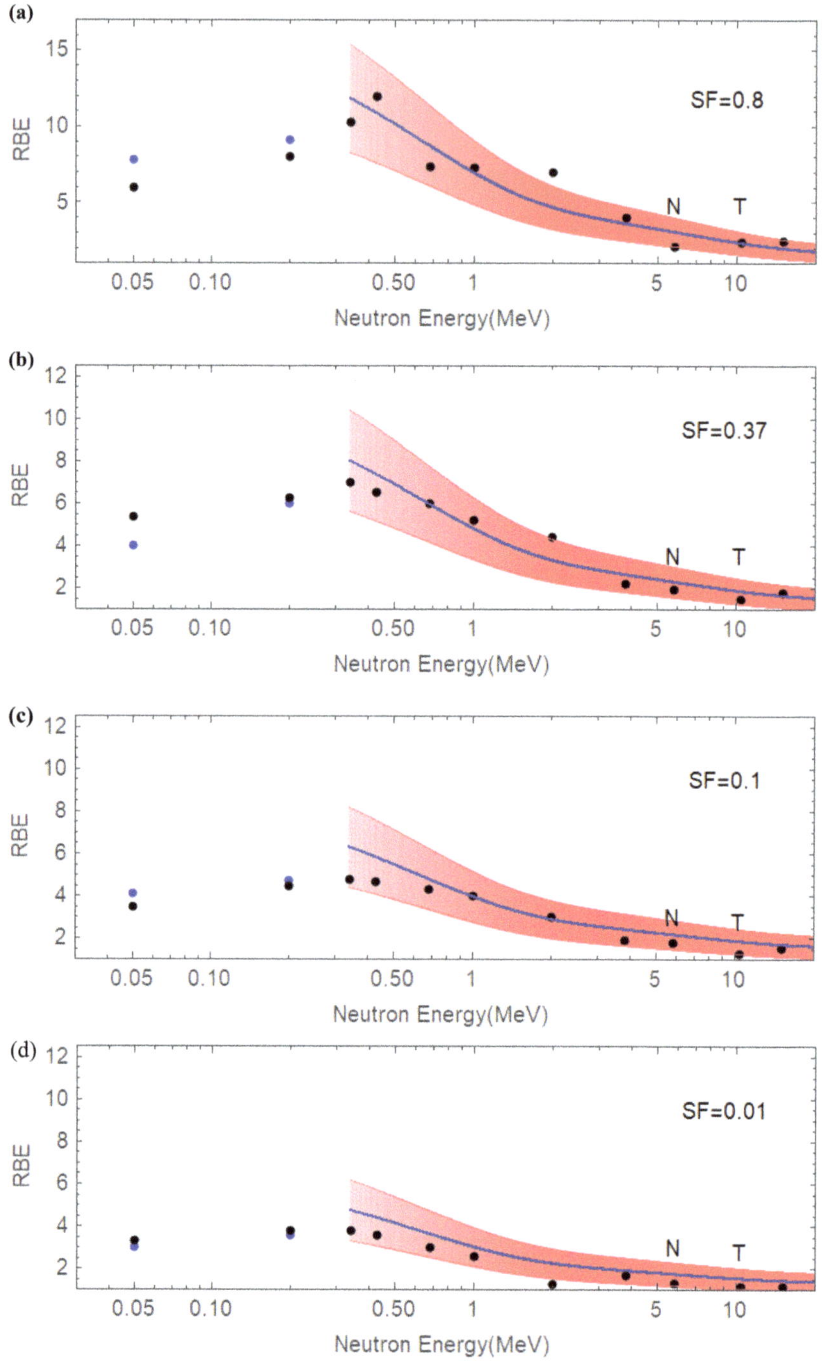

Figure 5.9. (a)–(d): The Hall data set RBE values at cell survival fractions of 0.8, 0.37, 0.1 and 0.01 are shown as black dots, the plotted modelled providing the blue curve and dots (with 95% confidence limits given by the shaded area surrounding the curve). Reproduced from Jones (2021).

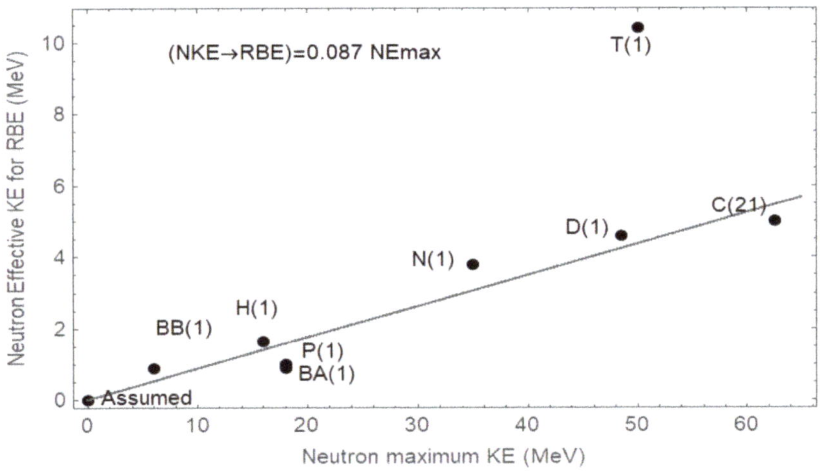

Figure 5.10. The relationship between neutron maximum kinetic energy in a beam and the effective neutron energy for bioeffectiveness. The individual beam codes are for the following cyclotrons: T = TAMVEC, C = Clatterbridge], D = Detroit, N = NRL (Washington), H = Hammersmith, followed by the fission sources at P = Petten, B(A) = Brookhaven (full spectrum), and B(B) = Brookhaven (using a late converter assumed to have max energy of 6 MeV). An assumed (0, 0) coordinate point was also used to obtain the slope. For further details see Jones (2021).

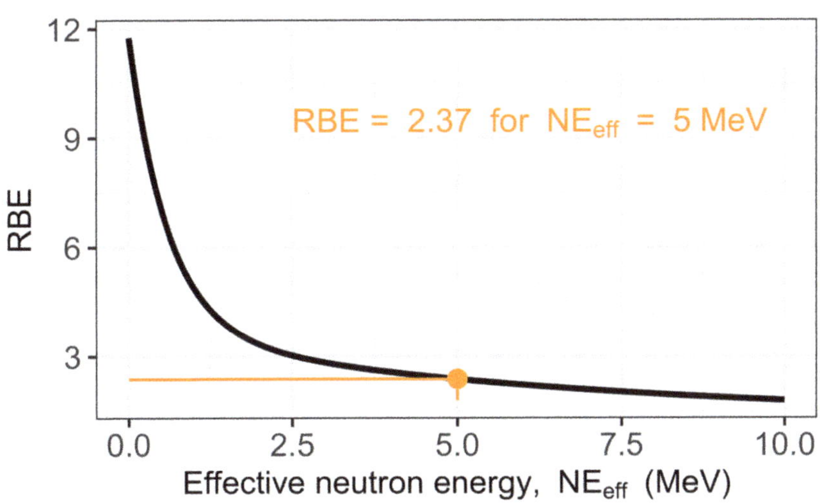

Figure 5.11. Plot of RBE as a function of effective neutron energy for different radiosensitivity ratios (α/β) and reference photon dose, d_{low}. Note that a reference low LET $\beta = 0.03$ Gy^{-2} is used for the reference radiation. The access link for changing the other input parameters is https://josh-will-moore.shinyapps.io/InteractivePlots_Jones_IOP/. Credit: Joshua Moore.

methods (Dr P O'Neill, personal communication). Thus if proton energies increase beyond 30.4 keV μm^{-1} they may fail to reach cellular nuclei, so the RBE is likely to reduce with further increases in LET. This may now explain the Belli *et al* (2000) results where a linear increase is not maintained beyond 30.4 keV μm^{-1}. In contrast, fast neutrons can release recoil protons at any distance, so there would be no physical consequences to the limited tissue range, since the recoil could be released very close to or within a cell. This also implies that proton experiments will always have this limitation, so that a direct demonstration of the true LET–RBE turnover point may not be possible, but only inferred indirectly by using recoil protons. However, for clinical RBE estimations the data of Belli *et al* (2000) should still be used as it reflects the reality of a proton beam.

What are the implications for proton therapy? Will predictions of RBE need to be lowered? This may not be necessary, since in the course of the present study it was found necessary to assume a much higher value of α_U than in previous studies, which results in the predicted proton RBE values being similar. For example, a 30.4 keV μm^{-1} LET_U value with LET values of 1, 2, 3, 5 and 10 keV μm^{-1}, respectively, gives estimated RBE values of 1.08, 1.18, 1.27, 1.44 and 1.82, whereas a 62.88 keV μm^{-1} LET_U value, with a larger α_U value by a factor of 1.7, gives estimated RBE values of 1.07, 1.15, 1.23, 1.38 and 1.7. These estimates are based on the conditions where a high RBE can be expected using 1.8 Gy per fraction of protons and reference radiation radiosensitivities given by $\alpha = 0.06$ Gy^{-1} with $\alpha/\beta = 2$ Gy as used elsewhere, as in chapter 9. Although these are reasonably similar results, this higher value of LET_U may not be appropriate for a proton beam, since protons with energies corresponding to a LET of around 60–70 keV μm^{-1} cannot reliably penetrate most V-79 mammalian cells, but neutrons of 0.4 MeV will do so, releasing their recoil proton within a cell. Thus the 30.4 keV μm^{-1} proton LET_U, found by experiment, should continue to be the value used for a proton beam; with this value it is not necessary to apply the 1.7 times correction to α_U, since there will inevitably be a mix of energies, for reasons mentioned above, which will modify pristine Bragg peaks to become spread-out peaks with lower averaged LET values.

More complex Monte Carlo simulations of proton RBEs are available in some institutions, as described in Jones (2021). Considerable theoretical Monte Carlo simulation work would be required to implement these seemingly useful neutron RBE values into present proton- and ion-beam treatment-planning systems, taking into account all the necessary physical interactions, to provide LET and dose maps, although a more simple formulation as described above may be sufficient to give useful working information. Further experimental studies are also indicated since some of the available data sets considered above contain a limited number of cell lines and neutron energies and the non-linear effects found by McNally *et al* (1984) for neutron and photon mixtures may apply. Studies that use multiple cell lines with a wide range of monoenergetic fast neutrons obtained are indicated to confirm possible higher RBEs predicted to occur at energies beyond the range of monoenergetic (0.2–15 MeV) and effective energies obtained from beams (with maximum energies as high as 62.5 MeV), which are considered in the present work. It would be ideal to perform experiments where neutrons and proton/ion beams can be delivered simultaneously to the same cells. Perhaps some physics institute with sufficient beams in close proximity and the available beam time might allow such work to be done.

Although fast neutron radiotherapy use has declined because of inadequate evidence of therapeutic benefit (Jones 2020), neutron production in proton and other ion beams are potentially important (whether produced from interactions with collimators, filters, etc., or arising within the patient due to interactions mainly with water). The use of raster scanned pencil beams has reduced the former effect but cannot eliminate the latter.

Neutron exposures are of greater concern not only in the nuclear industry for workers' radioprotection purposes, but also in high-altitude and transpolar air travel, as well as outer-space travel exposures of cosmic rays with secondary neutron production.

5.6 Some important conclusions

- There can be no complacency about x-ray radiotherapy, as some patients continue to develop severe, chronic and debilitating side effects, so that prescribed doses are often limited by clinical decisions taken regarding the probability of such complications in each individual.
- It is important that the same mistakes made with neutrons are not repeated with charged particles.
- Radiobiological testing should be sufficiently comprehensive, including many cell lines of various radiobiological characteristics, and not just a few or one.
- In retrospect, better radiobiological modelling would have alerted clinicians of at least some of the adverse features.
- All new forms of radiotherapy need to be tested in high-quality centres, using the best input from physics, biology and medicine.
- The experimental fast neutron database remains important and has implications for proton therapy because neutrons mainly ionise by forming recoil protons.
- More work is required to produce realistic LET and RBE contributions from secondary neutron formation in proton beams.
- Useful neutron RBE estimates can be obtained rapidly by consideration of the recoil proton energy and dividing this by the LET_U value.
- It is suggested that a proton LET_U value of 30.5 keV μm^{-1} should continue to be applied for clinical proton beams, but 62.5 keV μm^{-1} for neutron beams.
- The effective neutron energy which determines the RBE is around 0.085 of its maximum energy.

Appendix A

RBE_{max} and RBE_{min} act as multipliers of the low-LET α and β parameters. By considering low and high dose limits, these parameters have the following identities (the subscripts L and H refer to low- and high-LET radiations, respectively):

$$RBE_{max} = \frac{\alpha_H}{\alpha_L}, \tag{A.1}$$

so that

$$\alpha_L = \frac{\alpha_H}{R_{max}} \tag{A.2}$$

and

$$RBE_{min}{}^2 = \frac{\beta_H}{\beta_L}, \tag{A.3}$$

so that

$$\beta_L = \frac{\beta_H}{RBE_{min}{}^2}. \tag{A.4}$$

Equation (5.2) is divided by equation (5.4), then

$$\frac{\alpha_L}{\beta_L} = \frac{\alpha_H}{\beta_H}.\frac{RBE_{min}{}^2}{RBE_{max}}. \tag{A.5}$$

Rearrangements of this last equation allow RBE_{max} and RBE_{min} to be expressed as

$$RBE_{max} = \frac{\alpha_H}{\beta_H}.\frac{RBE_{min}{}^2}{\left(\frac{\alpha_L}{\beta_L}\right)} = \frac{Q}{\left(\frac{\alpha_L}{\beta_L}\right)} \tag{A.6}$$

and

$$RBE_{min} = .\sqrt{\frac{\alpha_L}{\beta_L}.\frac{RBE_{max}}{\frac{\alpha_H}{\beta_H}}} = S\sqrt{\frac{\alpha_L}{\beta_L}}, \tag{A.7}$$

where

$$Q = \frac{\alpha_H}{\beta_H} \cdot RBE_{min}{}^2 \tag{A.8}$$

and

$$S = .\sqrt{.\frac{RBE_{max}}{\frac{\alpha_H}{\beta_H}}}. \tag{A.9}$$

Appendix B

Here is provided brief Mathematica code for estimation of RBE for monoenergetic neutrons (between 0.4 MeV to a limit of around 20 MeV) when the reference low-LET dose is known.

(Where 'letc' is reference LET, 'nke' is the neutron kinetic energy, 'au' and 'bu' are α_U and β_U, 'prlet' is proton recoil LET; 'letu' is LET_U, 'dc' is the reference radiation dose and 'dn' the neutron dose; and 'an' and 'bn' are α_N and β_N.)

```
letc=1;ac=0.106; bc=0.0236;
au=1.7 10.57/3.92 (1−Exp[−3.92 alow]);
bu=0.05 (1−Exp[−50 blow]);
prlet=73.55 Exp[−1.64 nke]+21.05 Exp[−0.165 nke]+ 5.04 Exp[−0.016 nke]
letu=157;dlow=insert dose of reference radiation;
an=ac+(prlet-letref)/(letu-letref)(au-ac);
bn=bc+(prlet-letref)/(letu-letref)(bu-bc);
dn=1/(2 bn) (−an+√(an²+4ac.bn.dc+4 bn bc dc²)
rbe=0.2+dc/dn
```

If the neutron dose is known, then one can use equation (A.9) to obtain the isoeffective reference radiation dose at the penultimate step.

References

Bewley D K 1989 *The Physics and Radiobiology of Fast Neutron Beams* (Bristol: Institute of Physics Publishing)

Belli M, Bettega D, Calzolari P *et al* 2000 Inactivation of human normal and tumour cells irradiated with low energy protons *Int. J. Radiat. Biol.* **76** 831–9

Carabe-Fernandez A, Dale R G and Jones B 2007 The incorporation of the concept of minimum RBE (RBE_{min}) into the linear-quadratic model and the potential for improved radiobiological analysis of high-LET treatments *Int. J. Radiat. Biol.* **83** 27–39

Carabe-Fernandez A, Dale R G, Hopewell J W, Jones B and Paganetti H 2010 Fractionation effects in particle radiotherapy: implications for hypo-fractionation regimes *Phys. Med. Biol.* **55** 5685–700

Chapman J D 2003 Single-hit mechanism of tumour cell killing by radiation *Int. J. Radiat. Biol.* **79** 71–8

Dale R G and Jones B 1998 The assessment of RBE effects using the concept of biologically effective dose *Int. J. Radiat. Oncol. Biol. Phys.* **43** 639–45

Dearnaley D P, Jovic G, Syndikus I *et al* 2014 Escalated-dose versus control-dose conformal radiotherapy for prostate cancer: long-term results from the MRC RT01 randomised controlled trial *Lancet Oncol.* **15** 464–73

Duncan W 1994 An evaluation of the results of neutron therapy trials *Acta Oncol.* **33** 299–306

Friedrich T, Scholz U, Elsässer T, Durante M and Scholz M 2013 Systematic analysis of RBE and related quantities using a database of cell survival experiments with ion beam irradiation *J. Radiat. Res.* **54** 494–514

Gray L H, Mottram J C and Read J 1940 Some experiments upon the biological effects of fast neutrons *Br. J. Radiol.* **13** 371–88

Gray L H, Conger A D, Ebert M, Hornsey S and Scott O C A 1953 The concentration of oxygen dissolved in tissues at the time of irradiation as a factor in radiotherapy *Br. J. Radiol.* **26** 638–48

Hall E J, Novak J K, Kellerer A M *et al* 1975 RBE as a function of neutron energy: I. Experimental observations *Radiat. Res.* **64** 245–55

Henk J M, Kunkler P B and Smith C W 1977 Radiotherapy and hyperbaric oxygen in head and neck cancer. Final report of first controlled clinical trial *Lancet* **2** 101–3

Jones B 2010 The apparent increase in the β-parameter of the linear quadratic model with increased linear energy transfer during particle irradiation *Br. J. Radiol.* **83** 433–6

Jones B, Underwood T C, Carabe-Fernandez A and Dale R G 2011 Further analysis of fast neutron relative biological effects and implications for charged particle therapy *Br. J. Radiol.* **84** S11–8

Jones B and Hendry J 2017 Professor Jack Fowler and Sir Oliver *Scott Br. J. Radiol.* **90** 20160904

Jones B 2020 Clinical radiobiology of fast neutron therapy: what was learnt? *Front. Oncol.* **10** 1537

Jones B 2021 Fast neutron energy based modelling of biological effectiveness with implications for proton and ion beams *Phys. Med. Biol.* **66** 045028

Jones B and Hill M A 2020 The physical separation between the LET associated with the ultimate relative biological effect (RBE) and the maximum LET in a proton or ion beam *Biomed. Phys. Eng. Exp.* **6** 055001

Kageji T, Nagahiro S, Mizobuchi Y *et al* 2014 Boron neutron capture therapy (BNCT) for newly-diagnosed glioblastoma: comparison of clinical results obtained with BNCT and conventional treatment *J. Med. Invest* **61** 254–63

Laramore G E, Krall J M, Griffin T W *et al* 1993 Neutron versus photon irradiation for unresectable salivary gland tumors: final report of an RTOG-MRC randomized clinical trial *Int. J. Radiat. Oncol. Biol. Phys.* **27** 235–40

Lim D, Quah D S, Leech M and Marignol L 2015 Clinical potential of boron neutron capture therapy for locally recurrent inoperable previously irradiated head and neck cancer *Appl. Radiat. Isot.* **106** 237–41

McNally N J, de Ronde J and Hinchliffe M 1984 The effect of sequential irradiation with x-rays and fast neutrons on the survival of V79 Chinese Hamster cells *Int. J. Radiat. Biol. Relat. Stud. Phys. Chem. Med.* **45** 301–10

Nutting C M, Morden J P, Harrington K J *et al* 2011 Parotid-sparing intensity modulated versus conventional radiotherapy in head and neck cancer (PARSPORT): a phase 3 multicentre randomised controlled trial *Lancet Oncol.* **12** 127–36

Suit H, Delaney T, Goldberg S *et al* 2010 Proton vs carbon ion beams in the definitive radiation treatment of cancer patients *Radiother. Oncol.* **95** 3–22

Warenius H M, Britten R A, Browning P G, Morton I E and Peacock J H 1994 Identification of human *in vitro* cell lines with greater intrinsic cellular radiosensitivity to 62.5 MeV (p–>Be+) neutrons than 4 MeV photons *Int. J. Radiat. Oncol. Biol. Phys.;* **28** 913–20

Warenius H M and Britten R A 1994 *In vitro* studies of intrinsic cellular radiosensitivity following 4 MeV photons or 62.5 MeV (p–>Be+) neutrons. Potential implications for high LET therapy *Acta. Oncol.* **33** 241–9

Chapter 6

Fractionation modelling

Dose fractionation can be used to modify radiation effects, mainly due to changes in cellular repair, repopulation and reoxygenation, and the modifications differ markedly between normal acute and late-reacting tissues, as well as between different classes of tumours.

The principles of how to model fractionation effects in radiotherapy are discussed. This is extended to high-linear-energy-transfer (LET) radiations, with worked examples of isoeffective fractionation calculations (using biological effective dose, BED, formulations with inclusion of relative biological effect, RBE, parameters) between low- and high-LET treatments, or between two different fractionated schedules of high-LET radiation. Since RBE will vary with dose per fraction, it is essential to include a variable RBE within the necessary equations.

Also, the benefits or detriments of different fractionation regimes can be compared by use of the BED concept. Differential calculus can be applied to higher-LET radiations than conventional photons in order to obtain maximal tumour cell kill while maintaining the same constraint in terms of normal tissue BED.

6.1 Introduction and background radiobiology

The term 'fractionation' refers to the splitting of a dose into separate treatment 'fractions', or treatment sessions. This is an important part of the treatment prescription. The splitting process carries further consequential implications on the overall treatment time, depending on the inter-fraction time interval used. Fractionation is important because it can be used to either improve clinical outcomes, or alternatively to achieve closely similar outcomes at reduced financial cost. For example, a greater degree of fractionation of the same total dose reduces most late normal tissue side effects, whereas the same biological end point can be achieved by two very different fractionation schedules provided total dose is changed to accommodate the degree of fractionation used. Time is a further

doi:10.1088/978-0-7503-6209-2ch6

parameter within the radiotherapy prescription, since the overall treatment duration is related to the number of fractions multiplied by the average inter-fraction interval. Increasing the time normally reduces acute normal tissue reactions, but the use of too closely spaced fractions can enhance all normal tissue effects. Fractionation is often referred to as 'time-dose-fractionation'.

There is a large literature on fractionation of conventional x-ray (photon)-based therapy, which varies from relatively simple qualitative considerations to more complex mathematics. The process of fractionation includes key variables, which are in most situations under medical control: the dose per treatment (d), the number of treatments (n), the total dose D ($or\ n \cdot d$) and the overall treatment time (t). In general, when n is increased, d decreases (to an extent that D almost always increases) in order to preserve the same bioeffect. This occurs due to sub-lethal radiation damage repair between fractions: the greater the fractionation, the greater the opportunity for repair between fractions. It follows that cells which have defects in damage recognition or repair pathways, as found in mutated tumour cells, will be more radiosensitive and less fraction sensitive. Prolongation of t may also require increases in d or n, or both, in order to preserve a biological isoeffect such as to match tumour cell repopulation with time in the case of tumours that contain rapidly dividing cells, or normal epithelial tissues that contain rapidly growing cell populations. The relative magnitude of these changes vary in different normal tissues and tumours, depending on their biological properties:

- Slow proliferation states, associated with a high repair capacity, have a high fractionation sensitivity; that is, a large change in effect follows a small change in d. These conditions are characterised by a low α/β ratio. Examples will include late-reacting normal tissues and slowly proliferating tumours.
- Fast proliferation states, associated with a lower repair capacity, have a lower fractionation sensitivity; that is, a much smaller change in effect follows a small change in d. These conditions are characterised by a high α/β ratio and are typically found in acute-reacting tissues and rapidly proliferating tumours.

Although there have been many attempts to characterise fractionation 'rules' in terms of equations, the most successful and widely used model is that of the linear quadratic (LQ) model of radiation effect, which contains α and β radiosensitivity parameters, and for fractionation studies the α/β ratio is important since it is essentially inversely related to fractionation sensitivity, although the terms are sometimes used synonymously.

The term hypofractionation may require clarification: this essentially refers to a shift in fractionation to larger doses per fraction than 2 Gy by using fewer numbers of fractions. The converse is hyperfractionation, where doses below 2 Gy are used. These terms can be confusing to some readers. Accelerated fractionation refers to dose schedules which deliver greater than 2 Gy (of conventional radiotherapy photons or x-rays) per day, independently of the number of fractions per day or week.

6.2 A brief history of fractionation

6.2.1 Radiobiology

Fowler (1984) summarised the extensive work on fractionation experiments and their analysis, emphasising the dominance of the dose per fraction effects on total dose requirements when compared with overall time for experimental acute skin reactions: as dose per fraction reduces, a greater number of fractions is required which allows sufficient time for greater amounts of repair between these fractions; time-related effects are related to cellular repopulation, which is a slower process. Fowler also applied LQ theory, originally an empirical description in the 1940s of the yield of lethal chromosomal events with dose per cell by Douglas Lea (1962), to the study of isoeffective doses (Douglas & Fowler 1976) using an algebraic reconfiguration of the LQ model in the form of a fractionation effect (FE) plot.

The linear quadratic effect, E (or yield of lethal chromosomal aberrations in terms of Lea's findings), is expressed in fractionated form as

$$E = n(\alpha d + \beta d^2). \tag{6.1}$$

It follows, if $D = nd$, that

$$\frac{1}{D} = \frac{\alpha}{E} + \frac{\beta}{E}.\ d. \tag{6.2}$$

This transformation to linearity allowed Douglas & Fowler (1976) to study isoeffective doses in their FE plots of $1/D$ against d. By taking the ratio of the intercept to the slope, they showed that α/β ratios differed for acute and late effects. They also, importantly, showed that α/β values were far higher for fast neutron fractionation experiments, including in pig skin, which closely resembles human skin in radiation tolerance. This finding correlated with the fact that increased fractionation does not require as great a change in total dose as in the case of x-rays (photons) to preserve an isoeffect.

The time effect, measured as the additional radiation dose required to maintain the same degree of skin reaction, progressively increased after a finite time delay: this was due to repopulation of skin commencing only after radiation damage expression, which leads to the concept of accelerated repopulation in early-reacting tissues (Denekamp 1973). It is therefore inappropriate to use a power-law model for such an effect since the change in isoeffective dose with time requires a variable slope, even on a logarithmic plot. For tumour control, Fowler *et al* (1974) found an optimum overall time in an experimental tumour while maintaining a normal tissue (skin) isoeffect. This achievement was attributed to effective tumour reoxygenation at the optimum overall time since equally high tumour control was found at much shorter overall times either by the addition of metronidazole (as a hypoxic cell sensitiser) or by using fast neutrons (due to their reduced dependency on oxygen for cell killing, often referred to as a reduced oxygen enhancement ratio, or OER). At longer overall times than the optimum time tumour control was progressively reduced, probably due to tumour cell repopulation.

During the 1980s further progress included the detailed analysis of Withers, that acute-reacting tissues (by then characterised by high α/β values) required little change in total dose with increasing fractionation, whereas late-reacting tissues (with low α/β ratios) required more substantial changes in total dose: the form of the relationship, with an asymptotic limit at very small values of d (and large n) was compatible with LQ theory (Withers 1985). Towards the end of the decade several advances were made, including the following:

1. Inclusion of a repopulation factor alongside the LQ surviving fraction equation (by Dale 1989 and Fowler 1989), which allowed different fractionation schedules to be compared. Fowler could then argue that clinical outcomes with quite different fractionation schedules could be broadly equivalent.
2. Evolution of the LQ model to the biological effective dose (BED) concept, following the original idea of Barendsen and subsequent important adaptations by Dale and Fowler. This allowed calculation of isoeffective (or equieffective) treatment schedules, ranking of different fractionation schedules, addition of multiple phases of treatment by different radiation modalities or different fractionation patterns, different dose rates (Jones *et al* 2001, Fowler 2010) and eventually the inclusion of relative biological effect (RBE) limits, as originally described by Bewley, in BED equations for high-linear-energy-transfer (LET) radiations (Jones *et al* 2006, Carabe-Fernandez *et al* 2007), and which allow a variable or flexible RBE to change with dose per fraction, as will be shown later.

6.2.2 A synopsis of clinical fractionation

Accounts of the history of fractionation are available in Thames & Hendry (1987), with a good description of the failure of power-law fractionation models in the clinic.

Progress in clinical fractionation was made by careful empirical practice and observation. Following the lead of Regaud in France, who used very-low-dose-rate radium applications, Coutard noted that protraction and hyperfractionation of teletherapy to high total doses produced a substantial reduction in both acute and late effects of therapy while maintaining the desired tumour effect.

The advent of megavoltage radiotherapy, with improved depth dosage, led to further and more formal studies, such as the studies at the Hammersmith Hospital. There, patients were treated in trials which varied the total doses, but the overall time remained constant since the number of fractions was fixed at 20. The results effectively confirmed that small increments in dose per fraction and total dose caused both enhanced toxicity and tumour control. A general trend emerged: cancer centres in the north of England, Scotland and Canada favoured daily hypofractionated radiotherapy at 2.5–3.3 Gy per fraction in 15–20 fractions over 3–4 weeks, while those in the south of England favoured the French/American approach of conventional daily doses of 1.8–2 Gy given in 30–35 fractions (five fractions per week) over 6–7 weeks.

Almost alone, St Thomas' Hospital in London used six and 12 fraction radical treatments based on fractionation schedules previously used in hyperbaric oxygen (or HBO) trials. The present author started his radiotherapy experience there. Although the department received considerable criticism for this policy, especially from the USA and the radiobiology community, clinical results were impressive in some body sites. For example, prostate cancer treatments were given to a dose of 30–36 Gy in six fractions over around 16–18 d (Collins *et al* 1991), and it is now, some 50 years later, that the recent PACE-B trial preliminary results have shown that a five-fraction schedule using the stereotactic body radiation therapy (or SBRT) technique to a dose of 36.25 Gy is very effective (Tree *et al* 2022), and further press releases suggest that the preliminary results are maintained at 5 years. The key to the St Thomas' Hospital results was that small rectangular field sizes were used after tumour debulking by trans-urethral resection, and the dose prescribed, which varied inversely with field size, was the maximum dose in the midplane of the treatment volume, accepting the fact that the tumour would receive lower doses elsewhere.

The concept of hyperfractionation combined with acceleration emerged in the early 1980s and followed advances in the understanding of the radiobiology of cell killing, repair processes and repopulation effects.

Because of persistent economic constraints in the provision of radiotherapy facilities, there remains considerable interest in the use of relatively hypofractionated radiotherapy, especially for delivery of sub-radical doses in an adjuvant setting, such as pre-operative rectal cancer or after wide excision of a primary breast cancer. The UK START breast cancer trial was designed to test daily 2 Gy fractions against larger fraction sizes over the same overall treatment time, and showed broadly similar effects (Haviland *et al* 2013).

The importance of fractionation in radiotherapy cannot be doubted, because of its clinical impact. Increasing the number of fractions n, along with a reduction in d, inevitably increases t if, say, only a maximum of five fractions a week are to be given: this will allow acute-reacting normal tissues (such as epithelial surfaces, skin, oesophagus, intestine) to tolerate radiation treatment better, since the increase in elapsed time will allow more cellular repopulation to occur. Exactly the same will occur with particle therapy, so that for large treatment volumes containing epithelial surfaces that can repopulate within a month, longer treatment courses tend to be given in order to spare acute effects. The opposite, overintensification of dose in time, can cause very severe acute effects that can lead to so-called 'consequential' late effects in tissues, as well as being very unpleasant to the cancer patient.

The situation with late tissue effects is different. In their case, increasing fraction size will have a more deleterious effect for x-rays (photons) than for positively charged particles (PCPs): the former will require a larger reduction in total dose to maintain an isoeffect, whereas the latter will not require as great a change in total dose and so can be given in fewer fractions.

Late effects and very-slow-growing tumours generally require no time-correction factor, unless treatment is very protracted or if multiple fractions per day (MFD) are used. For MFD, incomplete repair (IR) equations are required, especially for three fractions or more per day. IR is likely to be reduced for high-LET radiations compared with low-LET radiations, since IR is included within the LQ model by linkage to the β parameter and not the α parameter, which increases to a greater extent than β with LET, as explained previously. Another issue with IR is fraction duration, t_f: difficult to deliver techniques allow short but significant interruptions of treatment (due to gantry rotation, reimaging, etc.). This also applies to some modern photon techniques such as Gamma Knife and linear accelerator treatments such as Cyber Knife. This is because there are principally two repair half-times: the best estimates remain those in the rat spinal cord, namely the first component is fast (half-time = 0.19 hr) and the second slower (half-time = 2.16 hr) with close to 50% of damage associated with either form of repair (Pop *et al* 2000). It has been shown that many treatments with prolonged t_f values can result in a significant reduction in BED per fraction (Hopewell *et al* 2012). It can be argued that all fractional durations longer than 30 min should be recorded for later analysis. Ion-beam treatments such as the large 40–44 Gy-eq single fractions given for early-stage lung cancer in older Japanese patients can in some instances take over 2 hr to deliver (Karube *et al* 2016). The intervals of time within a fraction that allow repair to continue between 'pulses' of treatment will affect low-LET therapy to a greater extent than high LET. Also, tumours and tissues with a high α/β are less sensitive to dose rate and IR effects than their low-α/β counterparts where extension of t_f produces a greater reduction in BED. More detailed work is required on this topic in the context of hadrontherapy, using the prospective data recorded in ion-beam centres to be eventually correlated with clinical outcomes.

It must always be remembered that a small increment in dose per fraction beyond that prescribed and if deposited in normal tissue can lead to enhanced tissue damage due to the non-linear effects associated with the LQ model. This has been termed 'double trouble', at 2 Gy per fraction, and this effect is enhanced when dose per fraction increases further beyond 2 Gy in hypofractionated radiotherapy, when it is called 'treble (or triple) trouble' (Jones *et al* 2000, 2001). It follows that increasing hypofractionation (larger doses per fraction) must be given with caution with respect to dose homogeneity, and individual calculations should be done since RBE effects will also complicate this effect, as shown later in this chapter.

Much could be written here on the economic advantages of hypofractionation: fewer treatments of larger doses per fraction allows greater throughput of patients per year, reduced individual patient costs and inconvenience, with greater utility within society, bearing in mind strong competition for finite healthcare resources. Such potential advantages can only be pursued if outcomes, in terms of tumours controlled and cured along with satisfactory quality of life statistics, either match expectations or can be proven to be superior to other more expensive approaches. The use of adjuvant therapies, either conventional or experimental, must also be considered with fractionation trials, since they may overcome certain disadvantages (e.g. cetuximab on tumour repopulation for longer schedules, new anti-metabolites which reduce oxygen consumption and permit rapid tumour reoxygenation prior to short schedules).

Also, it remains to be shown if protons can be delivered in hypofractionated form as safely as can be achieved with carbon ions. It is perhaps paradoxical that the majority of patients treated with protons had eye melanomas, treated in four large fractions to 52–54 Gy doses, using 'small fields'. The large and protective volume effect will tend to favour larger fractions for small target volumes as long as non-essential tissues are included in the tumour–normal tissue margin. Our inadequate, though improving, knowledge of the mathematical relationship between normal tissue volume and radiotolerance may yet provide safer guidelines in the future.

Since most randomised fractionation trials have shown only marginal differences, it is likely that higher gains will only be achieved by treatment individualisation, or at least treatment determination according to an analytical formula based on predictive assays and other information. Random-sampling simulations of virtual trials, using radiobiological modelling where treatment is allocated according to radiobiological characteristics such as radiosensitivity and repopulation, produce considerably greater gains in tumour control probabilities while respecting normal tissue tolerance (Jones & Dale 2000); this represents personalisation of treatment, and the scope for this approach is perhaps even greater in the case of particle therapy.

6.3 Modelling of fractionation

6.3.1 LQ modelling of fractionation in high-LET radiations with inclusion of RBE

In comparison with conventional x-ray-based fractionation experience, detailed fractionation experiments using high-LET radiation have only a 50 year history. They show reduced dependency on FEs compared with low-LET radiations:

$$\mathrm{RBE} = \frac{d_L}{d_H}, \tag{6.3}$$

where the subscripts L and H refer to low and high LET, respectively.

Now, when the fractionation schedule changes, the numerator d_L changes with fractionation to a greater extent than d_H. The low-LET numerator dose changes because of repair occurring between fractions, but the denominator (d_H) is less susceptible to changes in fractionation. This is because high-LET radiations form more clustered, locally complex damage within DNA, which is more difficult or impossible to repair. As such, there is lesser repair between fractions in the case of high-LET radiations compared with low-LET radiations. This must also be understood in terms of the single fraction experiment, where there is no opportunity for repair between fractions. With increasing LET, the increases in the α radiosensitivity parameter exceed those of the β parameter: this means that the ratio of α_H/α_L should always exceed β_H/β_L. Now, since α_H/α_L is $\mathrm{RBE_{max}}$ (the RBE at near-zero dose where β-related cell kill is negligible) and $\sqrt{(\beta_H/\beta_L)}$ is $\mathrm{RBE_{min}}$ (the RBE at high dose where β-related cell kill predominates). It follows that a reduction in dose per fraction will increase the RBE towards the $\mathrm{RBE_{max}}$ limit; conversely, as dose increases the RBE will approach the lower $\mathrm{RBE_{min}}$ value. It can also be appreciated that the yield of complex lethal chromosomal aberrations per unit dose increases with LET, so the same biological end points can be achieved with lower doses, where the α-related cell-killing mechanism predominates, rather than the β-related mechanism. This again means that radiations that have high LET and RBEs will be associated with reduced fractionation sensitivity, since it is the β-related damage that is susceptible to sub-lethal damage repair.

This original description of RBE was convenient to radiobiologists, since RBE could be measured from the defining ratio given in equation (2.4); but this led to an oversimplified view of RBE, indeed of almost trivial complexity. In fact, RBE is a highly complex parameter, depending on multiple variables including particle mass, energy, charge, target volume (and its depth), dose, beam contamination (e.g. with neutrons, gamma rays, etc.) and the radiobiological characteristics of the tissue/tumour being targeted (repair capacity, proliferative status—linked to the low-LET α/β).

For simplification and to obtain greater clarity in understanding the radiobiological principles, the text below contains RBE parameters without reference to specific LET values. Some of the methods for estimating RBE_{max} and RBE_{min} from LET are given separately in chapters 8 and 9, and can be used to provide these RBE parameters for individual calculations.

6.3.2 BED equations

The BED equations that include RBE have already been given in chapter 2. They will now be used to illustrate FEs.

The BED equation can be modified for hadrontherapy (Jones *et al* 2006, Carabe-Fernandez *et al* 2007) as

$$\mathrm{BED} = D_H\left(\mathrm{RBE}_{\max} + \frac{\mathrm{RBE}_{\min}^2\, d_H}{\alpha/\beta}\right). \tag{6.4}$$

The basic BED principle can also be extended to provide EQD-2 equations, which express the dose required for a defined biological or clinical end point when the dose is given in 2 Gy fractions: EQD_2 is simply the BED divided by $(1 + 2/(\alpha/\beta))$.

The function of the α/β ratio is to act as a coefficient which controls the fractionation sensitivity. When the fraction size is changed, the resulting total dose needs to be modified in order to provide a constant BED (and the same bioeffect). It is important to understand that different tissues and tumours can possess quite different α/β ratios, so that they respond differently to different changes in dose fractionation (for further details, see chapter 2).

When the two limits of RBE are used, the α/β ratio must be the same as that for the low-LET (x-ray) case, and this parameter will now be less important in influencing the BED when d_H is changed, compared to the standard low-LET equation, especially when RBE_{max} is large. The percentage BED increment with dose per fraction is consequently larger for low-LET treatments compared to higher-LET treatments.

This equation when used to equate with a low-LET schedule allows the RBE at any intermediate dose to vary between the RBE_{max} and RBE_{min} values used.

6.3.3 Converting a specific low-LET BED fractionation to that for high LET, when the low-LET α/β ratio is known, but with no change in overall treatment time

It is then possible to pursue isoeffect calculations using the equality low-LET BED = high-LET BED:

$$D_L\left(1+\frac{d_L}{\left(\frac{\alpha}{\beta}\right)_L}\right)=D_H\left(\mathrm{RBE}_{\max}+\frac{\mathrm{RBE}_{\min}{}^2\,d_H}{\left(\frac{\alpha}{\beta}\right)_L}\right). \tag{6.5}$$

The major advantage here is that the α/β ratio used throughout this equality is that of the low-LET α/β, which is well established for some tissue types, e.g. brain and spinal cord, although it is necessary to know the likely values of RBE_{max} and RBE_{min}. In important clinical scenarios these RBE parameters should be sufficiently large to produce conservative values of dose per fraction for the protection of normal tissues with low α/β values, yet sufficiently low in the case of fast-growing tumours with large α/β ratios.

6.3.3.1 Worked example

It is decided to design a clinical trial which provides the same BED for late brain effects as 60 Gy in 30 fractions of megavoltage x-rays, using either 10 or 15 fractions of carbon ions, which are assumed to have RBE_{max} values of 6 and RBE_{min} of 1.25. Find, also, the dose required if given in 2, 3 or 4 Gy fractions. The brain α/β is 2 Gy. Compare the results with an assumption that dose is modified by constant RBE factors of (a) 3 and (b) 4, regardless of the magnitude of dose. (Caveat: The parameters and numbers used here are chosen for the convenience of those using pocket calculators.)

The BED for x-rays is

$60(1 + 2/2) = 120\ \mathrm{Gy}_{[2]}$.

And this BED must now equate with the high-LET BED such that

$120 = nd_H(\mathrm{RBE}_{max} + \mathrm{RBE}_{min}{}^2 d_H/k)$, where k is from now on the low-LET α/β ratio.

So, for $n = 10$, $d_H = 1.65$ Gy and $n = 15$, $d_H = 1.16$ Gy.

If doses (d_H) of 2, 3 or 4 Gy fractions are to be given, the solution of the above equation provides $n = 7.9$, 4.79 and 3.29. These are not close to integer values. Rounding off to the nearest fraction would be inappropriate, resulting in under- or overdosage. Consequently, it is best to use the former approach, which calculates the dose per fraction.

Now, if the ‘overall RBE’ is a constant at all doses, it has a purely dose-modifying function, so that each d term in the BED equation is multiplied by RBE. Then we must solve for d_H in

$120 = nd_H\,(\mathrm{RBE} + \mathrm{RBE}^2 d_H/\mathrm{k})$, (or $120 = nd_H\,\mathrm{RBE}(1 + \mathrm{RBE}d_H/\mathrm{k})$).

So that for RBE = 3, $n = 10$, $d_H = 1.33$ Gy and $n = 15$, $d_H = 1.04$ Gy.

And for RBE = 4, $n = 10$, $d_H = 1.00$ Gy and $n = 15$, $d_H = 0.78$ Gy.

These results show the critical dependency of the RBE model (fixed versus flexible) for the assumptions used.

6.3.4 Overall fractionation differences between low- and high-LET radiations

The solution of the isoeffect equations given above (equation 3.6 is solved for d_L and the result divided by d_H to provide the RBE at any value of d_H) can be used to show how low-LET (figure 6.1) and high-LET (figure 6.2) fractionation influences the total dose required to maintain a tissue isoeffect. The change in total dose with number of fractions (and consequently dose per fraction) is much greater for the low-LET megavoltage x-rays. The dependency on tissue α/β can also be seen, with a pronounced flattening of the relationship after a few fractions only for the high-LET radiation: the change over the first few fractions indicates the shift from reliance on RBE_{min} for the first few fractions to a greater dependency on RBE_{max} after that. There appears to be little change in total dose after the 4–6 fraction schedules, with only marginal changes after 10–20 fractions. These modelled examples are typical of the pioneering fast neutron experiments. Similar proton-beam isoeffects are given in chapter 9.

In PCP therapy, it is important to remember that these considerations apply to the high-LET part of the beam; FEs corresponding more closely to the low LET will be found where there are only entry beams that are distant from the Bragg peak regions. Thus if, say, the skin and rib dose (mainly low LET) determine tolerance for a lung cancer treatment, as is the case in Japan, then fractionation will continue to have an important function. The incidence of rib fractures with large single doses remains of concern, and this would probably fall with modest further fractionation since the ribs are not in the very-high-LET region. Three-dimensional LET, dose and BED plans will ideally be required. LET-based treatment plans have already been generated, although in the head region (figure 6.3).

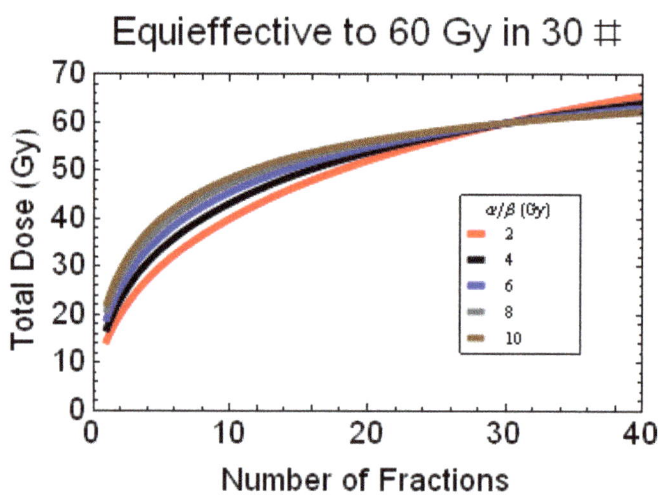

Figure 6.1. Total dose and number of fractions (of different fraction sizes) for megavoltage x-rays.

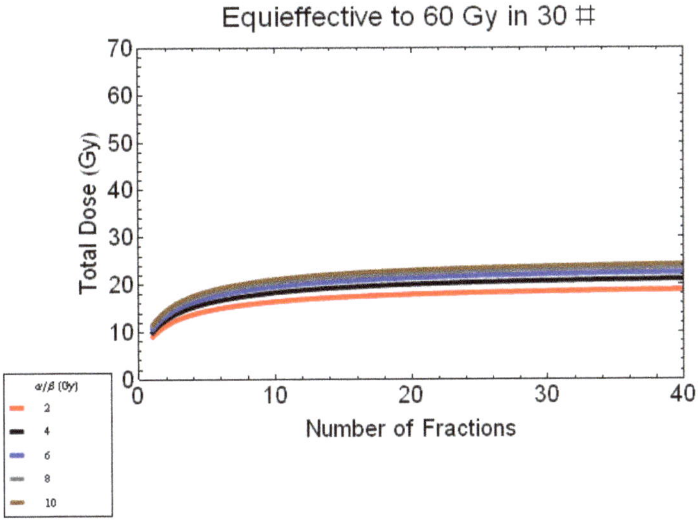

Figure 6.2. Total dose and number of fractions (of different fraction sizes) for carbon ions or fast neutrons assuming $RBE_{max} = 6$ and $RBE_{min} = 1.25$.

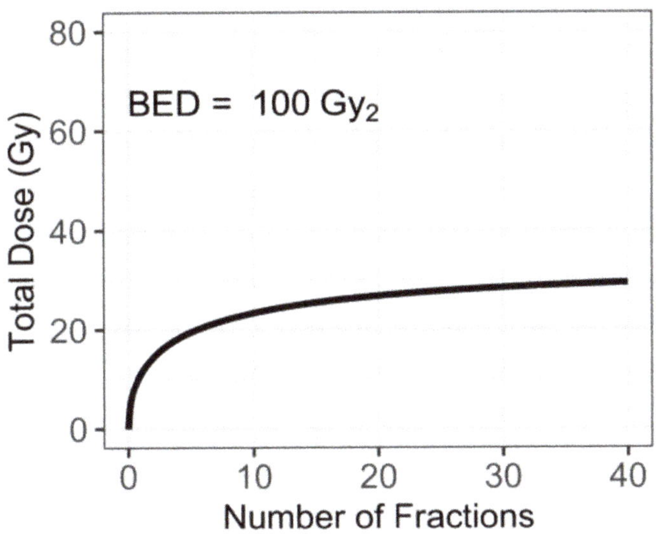

Figure 6.3. Interactive plot of total dose, (D), for a given number of fractions, (N), with variation of α/β and RBE parameters available on link https://josh-will-moore.shinyapps.io/InteractivePlots_Jones_IOP/: eee figure 9.4 for guidance on selecting maximum and minimum RBE values for different LET conditions.

6.3.5 Boost doses

In radiotherapy it is often the case that treatment is given in phases, typically beginning with wider field arrangements, often to cover regional lymphatic tissues, but ending with a boost dose to a smaller volume (the tumour itself with appropriate infiltrative margins); with x-ray-based intensity-modulated radiation therapy (IMRT) the boost can be given simultaneously with the wider field. Sometimes different radiation modalities are used for each phase: for example the larger initial treatment could be given by megavoltage IMRT, followed by the final phase using either brachytherapy, electrons, or proton/ion beams.

6.3.5.1 Worked example

A dose of 45 Gy in 25 fractions delivered by IMRT is followed by a carbon-ion boost, with the aim of giving a total tumour dose equivalent to 70 Gy in 35 fractions of megavoltage x-rays, but preserving a normal tissue isoeffect, equivalent to 40 Gy in 20 fractions. Find the dose per fraction required for a three-, four- or five-fraction boost for the same tumour control, but also give the normal tissue BED values for each case. The likely tumour α/β is 4 Gy with $RBE_{max} = 4$ and $RBE_{min} = 1.4$; the critical late normal tissue has a α/β of 3 Gy and $RBE_{max} = 4.7$ and $RBE_{min} = 1.3$, and the most relevant normal tissue volume receives a modal 72% of the IMRT dose and only 42% of the ion-beam dose.

The intended total tumour BED is $70\ (1 + 2/4) = 105\ Gy_{[4]}$.

The IMRT will provide a tumour BED of $45\ (1 + 1.8/4) = 65.25\ Gy_{[4]}$.

The deficit tumour BED to be provided is $105 - 65.25 = 39.75\ Gy_{[4]}$.

The allowed total normal tissue BED will be $40\ (1+2/3) = 66.67\ Gy_{[3]}$.

The IMRT will provide a normal tissue BED of $0.72\,45\ (1 + 0.72\,1.8/3) = 46.40\ Gy_{[3]}$.

For tumour boost dose per fraction find d_H for $n = 3$, 4 and 5 in:

$39.75 = nd_H\ (RBE_{max} + RBE_{min}{}^2 d_H/4)$.

For $n = 3$, then $d_H = 2.53$ Gy; for $n = 4$, then $d_H = 2.00$ Gy and if $n = 5$, then $d_H = 1.65$ Gy.

The normal tissue BEDs will be, for each dose per fraction:

$0.72 \times 45\ (1 + 0.72\,1.8/3) + 3 \times 2.53 \times 0.42(4.7 + 1.3^2 \times 2.53 \times 0.42/3) = 62.87\ Gy_{[3]}$.

$0.72 \times 45\ (1 + 0.72\,1.8/3) + 4 \times 2.00 \times 0.42\ (4.7 + 1.3^2 \times 2.00 \times 0.42/3) = 63.34\ Gy_{[3]}$.

$0.72 \times 45\ (1 + 0.72\,1.8/3) + 5 \times 1.65 \times 0.42\ (4.7 + 1.3^2 \times 1.65 \times 0.42/3) = 63.74\ Gy_{[3]}$.

All of these BED values are below the allowed 66.67 $Gy_{[3]}$, but it is instructive to note that the lowest normal tissue BED is found for the least number of fractions (and the highest dose per fraction), because of the effective fall of RBE with hypofractionation in this case when using the extreme limits of the RBE as parameters.

In other clinical situations, if normal tissue tolerance is exceeded, a BED calculation cannot provide the desired result for both the normal tissue and tumour, because their BEDs are separately governed by different α/β and RBE parameters. A compromise in dose selection is necessary and this will require detailed clinical discussion, perhaps accepting increased risks of either recurrence or toxicity, or even a modest amount of each. Typical examples were given in the previous report on unintended treatment interruptions.

6.3.6 Converting a specific low-LET BED fractionation to that for high LET, when the low-LET α/β ratio is known, but with a change in overall treatment time

The equations have been used previously to estimate compensatory doses for unintended treatment interruptions:

$$\text{BED} = D_L\left(1 + \frac{d_L}{\left(\frac{\alpha}{\beta}\right)_L}\right) - KT_L = D_H\left(\text{RBE}_{\max} + \frac{\text{RBE}_{\min}{}^2\, d_H}{\left(\frac{\alpha}{\beta}\right)_L}\right) - KT_H,$$

and where K is the low-LET BED dose equivalent of repopulation per day, K being defined as

$$K = \frac{0.693}{\alpha_{L.}\omega},$$

where ω is the operative cellular doubling time. K values are known for some tumour types and are sometimes used along with a lag (or delay) time until the onset of accelerated repopulation. In such cases (usually assumed for squamous cell and transitional cell cancers) the T values are reduced by the delay time T_K, which is usually assumed to be 21–28 d. It is advantageous that the low-LET K values can be used in this form, even within the high-LET side of the equation, but provided the RBE factors are included within the BED portion of the equation.

6.3.7 Alternative approach for isoeffect calculations in the case of two high-LET schedules

For two identical high-LET treatments, fractionation isoeffects can be calculated using BED equations that contain high-LET α/β ratios.

Thus for two isoeffective schedules of high LET, we have for N_1 fractions and N_2 fractions of dose d_1 and d_2:

$$N_{1H}(\alpha_H d_{1H} + \beta H d_1^2{}_H) = N_{2H}(\alpha_H d_{2H} + \beta_H d_2^2{}_H). \tag{6.6}$$

It is then permissible to divide throughout by α_H (and not α_L, as was previously the case) and obtain

$$D_{1H}\left(1 + \frac{d_{1H}}{\left(\frac{\alpha}{\beta}\right)_H}\right) = D_{2H}\left(1 + \frac{d_{2H}}{\left(\frac{\alpha}{\beta}\right)_H}\right). \tag{6.7}$$

In this case, the two RBE parameters $\text{RBE}_{\max}$ and $\text{RBE}_{\min}$ are no longer necessary. It would also be possible to use the single R_C conversion factor:

$$\text{where } R_C = \text{RBE}_{\max}/\text{RBE}_{\min}{}^2, \tag{6.8}$$

$$\text{This is because} \left(\frac{\left(\frac{\alpha}{\beta}\right)_H}{\left(\frac{\alpha}{\beta}\right)_L} \right) = \left(\frac{\left(\frac{\alpha_H}{\alpha_L}\right)}{\left(\frac{\beta_H}{\beta_L}\right)} \right) = \frac{\mathrm{RBE}_{\max}}{\mathrm{RBE}_{\min}{}^2}. \tag{6.9}$$

In the situation of comparing two identical high-LET radiations, so that equation (6.15) would become

$$D_{1H}\left(1 + \frac{d_{1H}}{R_C\left(\frac{\alpha}{\beta}\right)_L}\right) = D_{2H}\left(1 + \frac{d_{2H}}{R_C\left(\frac{\alpha}{\beta}\right)_L}\right), \tag{6.10}$$

which could also be used in this form along with the time factor corrections, as given below.

For unintended treatment interruptions, the most appropriate time and repopulation correction factors can be added for the case of tumour isoeffects. This is not necessary for late-reacting tissues. The equations are then

$$D_{1H}\left(1 + \frac{d_{1H}}{\left(\frac{\alpha}{\beta}\right)_H}\right) - K_H.\ t_{1H} = D_{2H}\left(1 + \frac{d_{2H}}{\left(\frac{\alpha}{\beta}\right)_H}\right) - K_H.\ t_{2H}, \tag{6.11}$$

where t_1 and t_2 are the respective overall treatment times for schedule 1 and 2, and K_H is defined as

$$K_H = \frac{0.693}{\alpha_{H.}\omega}. \tag{6.12}$$

Compared with the K values for low LET (K_L), there is little knowledge of K_H values in the literature. K_H can, however, be found from K_L by dividing by $\mathrm{RBE}_{\max}$ (which is α_H/α_L), that is

$$K_H = \frac{K_L}{\mathrm{RBE}_{\max}}. \tag{6.13}$$

A note of caution must be given about using RBEs based on total fractionated dose, since this approach can lead to confusion and potential errors. It is best to use RBE on a dose per fraction basis, which is consistent with cell survival curve theory and the original definition of RBE. It is recommended that individual dose per fraction RBEs be calculated and then total dose calculated. Where fraction numbers differ between low- and high-LET schedules this is especially important.

For example, let us suppose that a 10 Gy carbon-ion physical dose in five fractions produces the same late effect as a 50 Gy in 25 fractions photon dose—what is the RBE?

By taking each of the total doses, the RBE is $50/10 = 5$; and taking the delivered doses per fraction, the RBE is 2/2, which is absurd. However, by using the following procedure—based on corrected dose per fraction—a different answer is obtained.

The RBE denominator will be the high-LET dose per fraction, which is 2 Gy. The photon dose per fraction, if given in five fractions (rather than 25), which would match the same effect as 50 Gy in 25 fractions of photons, assuming a late effect $\alpha/\beta = 3$ Gy, and would be given by d in the following BED isoeffective doses:

BED (five fractions, unknown d) = BED (25 fractions, $d = 2$)

$5\,d(1 + \frac{d}{3}) = 50(1 + \frac{2}{3})$

$d = 5.73$ Gy, which is then used as the numerator of the RBE.

The RBE is then 5.73/2 = 2.87.

In situations where under- or overdose has occurred or in calculation of x-ray equivalent schedules the most reasonable estimates of the parameters should be used; clinicians may prefer to use the safest choices, such as a high RBE_{max} in tissues which are highly fraction sensitive for x-rays, such as the central nervous system (CNS). The general advice for such calculations in the case of x-rays has been published elsewhere (e.g. Joiner 2004, Jones & Dale 2008), but the additional effect of RBE must be included if there is any attempt to use (low-LET) x-ray tissue tolerances or x-ray tumour control data. The alternative approach is to use only high-LET α/β ratios within BED equations where the tolerance and tumour control BED values for the high-LET radiation are known.

6.3.8 Differences in exposure times

Significant reductions in BED estimations can occur if the treatment, by whatever technique, takes longer to deliver due to ongoing DNA repair. For example, this might be because of gantry rotations in proton therapy causing a longer total fraction time in comparison with a very rapidly delivered photon-based treatment. The beam downtime should always be taken into account, since repair is operative from the beginning of the exposure until the end of all exposures that contribute to a treatment fraction. Equations for such fractional protraction have been presented in chapter 2. In summary, if T is specified here as being the sum of n sub-fractional exposures each given in an averaged time t_f, with $(n - 1)$ intervals of averaged time g when no radiation is delivered, then $T = n.t_f + (n - 1)g$.

If biphasic repair is modelled with inclusion of the two necessary RBE parameters then the BED can be approximated as

$$\mathrm{BED} = x.\,D\left(\mathrm{RBE}_{max} + \frac{D}{k}.\,f\mu_1 T\mathrm{RBE}_{min}^2\right) + 1 - x.\left(\mathrm{RBE}_{max} + \frac{D}{k}.\,f\mu_2 T\mathrm{RBE}_{min}^2\right).$$

The repair functions are given in chapter 2 in connection with the dose-rate effect and T is then expressed as in the preceding equation above, which allows incorporation of parameters n, t_f and g.

It is essential to realise that an isoeffective proton- or ion-beam schedule can only be arrived at iteratively because of the complexity of the $f(\mu T)$ expressions and the variables which contribute to T.

6.3.8.1 Worked example

Find a proton dose per fraction which is isoeffective to a dose of 6 Gy using megavoltage photons given in a total fraction time of 8 min for a treatment close to the CNS, but with good sparing. Consider only the maximum possible dose that the CNS could receive (assumed to be the full prescription dose here, which will exceed standard tolerance).

The assumed proton parameters are $RBE_{max} = 1.4$ and $RBE_{min} = 1.04$, using only two fields with gantry rotation and setup intervals of 7 min for the second field, and a dose rate of 3 Gy min^{-1}. The following equations may be used when the field setup intervals within a fraction (with beam downtime) are relatively short.

First, assess the photon treatment BED.

The standard BED (uncorrected for treatment delivery time) is

$6\ 1 + \frac{6}{2} = 24Gy_{[2]}$,

But when corrected for an 8 min delivery time with biphasic CNS repair (the repair parameters are given in chapter 2) and simplified here, and where T is the total treatment time of the fraction:

$$x.\, 6\left(1 + \frac{6}{2}.\, f\, \mu T_1\right) + 1 - x.\, 6\left(1 + \frac{6}{2}.\, f\, \mu T_2\right) = 22.6Gy_{[2]},$$

The iterations for the proton treatments are based on a variable dose (d) in

$$x.\, d\left(RBE_{max} + \frac{RBE_{min}^2\ d}{2}.\, f\, \mu T_1\right) + (1 - x).\, d\left(RBE_{max} + RBE_{min}^2 \frac{d}{2}.\, f\, \mu T_2\right),$$

which provides BED values as follows:

$d = 5$ Gy, BED $= 20.5$ $Gy_{[2]}$; $d = 5.3$ Gy, BED $= 22.6$ $Gy_{[2]}$; $d = 5.5$ Gy, BED $= 24.0$ $Gy_{[2]}$, from which a dose of 5.3 Gy appears to be isoeffective.

What would the results have been if no time corrections were used?

The isoeffective dose would then be given by solving the equation

$$d\left(RBE_{max} + \frac{RBE_{min}^2\ d}{2}\right) = 24,$$

which provides $d = 5.5$ Gy.

The difference obtained is small at 0.2 Gy within one fraction, but could be larger according to special circumstances, e.g. longer proton treatments.

If given for a seven-fraction treatment course, the total BED estimates would be $24 \times 7 = 168$ $Gy_{[2]}$, if uncorrected, and $22.6 \times 7 = 158.2$ $Gy_{[2]}$ with a time correction.

If the CNS receives a maximum of 85% of the prescribed dose, then the photon single fraction dose yields a BED of 17.12 $Gy_{[2]}$ with a time correction, which gives a total BED of 102.7 Gy for the complete treatment.

6.3.9 RBE and dose per fraction: clinical implications

Early RBE experiments, especially studies using fast neutrons, with RBE values similar to carbon-ion therapy, showed that RBE reduced with increasing dose per fraction, leading to potential clinical dangers for small fractions, or higher than expected bioeffects despite high-LET dose falloff in normal tissues. Falloff of megavoltage x-ray dose causes a reduction in tissue dose per fraction; but falloff of high-LET dose beyond a target volume may be, at least partially, compensated for by a higher RBE.

It is instructive to study figure 6.3, which shows the relationship between dose per fraction of neutrons and RBE for tissues with different α/β ratios: the overall change in RBE with dose per fraction is much less for biosystems with a high α/β than for those with a low α/β.

This was compiled using parameters derived from a variety of fast neutron experiments *in vivo* and on human cancer cells *in vitro* (Jones *et al* 2011), already shown in chapter 5. Due to RBE_{max} being inversely related to the low-LET α/β, and RBE_{min} being linearly related to the square root of α/β, there is a crossing over of the RBE values such that biosystems with a low α/β have the highest RBEs at low doses but the lowest RBE at high doses. If a cell or tissue system does not have a clearly identified α/β ratio then the choice of dose per fraction around the crossover part of the curves would minimise RBE uncertainty.

There are important implications for clinical fractionation here, although these predictions must be better validated by further experimental studies. It is interesting to note that lowering the dose per fraction probably caused more toxicity in late-reacting tissues in UK neutron trials. Also, there are suggestions from the Japanese ion-beam centres that late side effects may be less prevalent with hypofractionated schedules. Such claims must, however, be subjected to prospective studies, since at present the hypofractionated regimens have the shortest follow-up times and so may show bias. However, these findings are compatible with a hypothesis that the rank order of RBE values can be reversed according to the dose level, as in figure 6.3. In the case of the brain, with the lowest α/β of 2 Gy, this may be important, since the therapeutic ratio might be improved by hypofractionation as long as the brain RBE at large doses would be sufficiently lower than the tumour RBE. This may already explain some excellent outcomes at Heidelberg and GSI for skull-base tumours compared with low dose per fraction protons in USA, although the shorter treatment time (<20 d) may also be operative in at least some tumours which may contain more rapidly growing clonogenic cells, as may be found after repeated surgery and long intervals of time between the original diagnosis and definitive therapy. In contrast, the Swiss Paul Scherrer Institute has used protons with low dose per fraction, but in their case their development of beam-scanning techniques permitted a more conformal physical dose distribution. All these results should eventually be subjected to rigorous comparative analysis using the BED with flexible RBE concept.

Major decisions are required in some European centres before carbon-ion dose per fraction is changed from a relatively fixed dose equivalent of around 3 Gy of photons to higher or lower doses.

The use of hypofractionation is increasing, with newer photon treatments based on robotic guided linear accelerator techniques (e.g. stereotactic ablative radiotherapy and others) or multiple cobalt sources (as in radiosurgery). The possibility that normal tissue late toxicities could be reduced by using hypofractionated PCP therapy compared to these other photon-based techniques would be a reasonable starting point for clinical trials at some future time, but they would need to be guided by better and more specific data on RBE, leading to improved BED estimates in order to have reasonably isoeffective comparisons. However, the conformity index of gantry-mounted fixed fields using particle therapy may not be as good as that achieved with photon-based techniques using a much more flexible geometrical delivery system, although the integral dose should be substantially lowered with particle-based therapy.

Present proton therapy practice requires some discussion here: the persistent use of a fixed proton RBE of 1.1, based on *in vivo* and *in vitro* experiments using rapid assays (Paganetti *et al* 2002, 2003), with a tendency to high α/β values, has a high chance of underestimating RBE values in late-reacting tissues and in slowly growing tumours, as well as overestimating the RBE in some very rapidly dividing systems such as cancers of childhood; the latter could lead to underdosage in long fractionated schedules (Jones *et al* 2012).

Examples of isoeffective dose plots for protons are provided in chapter 9.

6.3.10 Effects of regions of higher and lower dose per fraction relative to the prescribed dose for different fractionation patterns

The medical prescription refers to a volume of interest, normally the planning target volume (PTV), where the prescribed dose often refers (e.g. in photon therapy) to the dose at the field intersection or other representative point such that the PTV is allowed to have a variation of dose by as much as −5% to +7%. Normally these percentages (expressed as 95%–107% of the prescribed dose) do not deviate by these amounts, but with large field sizes and with difficult individual treatment geometry these figures are approached and rarely exceeded.

Homogenisation of dose has become increasingly possible due to intensity modulation in photon therapy and with similar approaches in PCP therapy due to beam-scanning and beam-weighting approaches. A deviation in dose will produce a changed biological effect, such that the surviving fraction will be multiplied each fraction; in the case of BED, which is derived as a logarithm, it allows the BEDs to be added for each fraction. For larger doses per fraction the biological deviation will be more significant, although fewer fractions are then given; for smaller doses per fraction the biological deviation will be smaller but will occur over a larger number of fractions.

Essentially, if x represents the change in dose, then the low- and high-LET BED will be, respectively,

$$\mathrm{BED} = xD_L\left(1 + \frac{xd_L}{\left(\frac{\alpha}{\beta}\right)_L}\right), \tag{6.14}$$

$$\mathrm{BED} = xD_H\left(\mathrm{RBE}_{\max} + \frac{\mathrm{RBE}_{\min}{}^2\, xd_H}{\left(\frac{\alpha}{\beta}\right)_L}\right), \tag{6.15}$$

where, for example, $x = 0.96$ for 96% of the prescribed dose (of 100%), and 1.05 for 105% of the prescribed dose, etc.

It is instructive to compare BED values for various values of x in low- and high-LET radiations, for two tumours or tissues with $\alpha/\beta = 4$ Gy and $\alpha/\beta = 8$ Gy, as shown in figures 6.4(a) and (b). A non-linear effect is apparent, probably caused by the complexity of PCP radiobiology, where the RBE is inversely related to dose, with RBE 'crossing-over' effects.

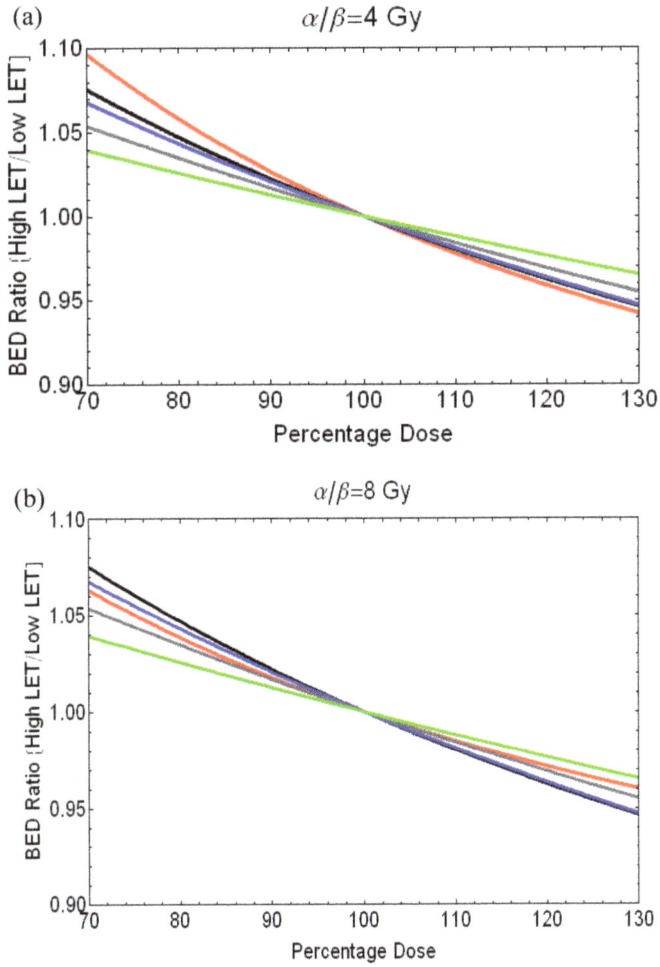

Figure 6.4. (a) and (b): Ratios of high-LET BED to low-LET BED are plotted against percentage dose deviation (the factor x expressed as a percentage), for a prescribed dose of 100%, and for different fraction numbers that provide isoeffective tumour control at the prescribed dose level for each fractionation schedule. The colour codes are red = 1, black = 4, blue = 10, grey = 20 and green = 37. The assumed RBE limits were $RBE_{max} = 3$; $RBE_{min} = 1.6$; and a low-LET α/β ratio of 4 Gy (a) and 8 Gy (b) as shown appropriate for conditions in the end of a spread-out Bragg peak for protons in the context of (a) a slow-growing tumour such as an adenocarcinoma and (b) a more rapidly growing human squamous cell cancer.

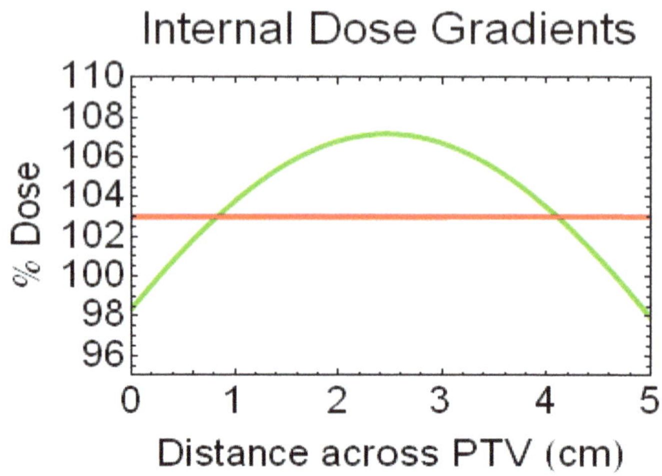

Figure 6.5. Percentage dose across a planning target volume (PTV) of width 5 cm for protons (red) and x-rays (green). This refers to a hypothetical treatment where there is non-uniformity of dose in the x-ray case and excellent uniformity of dose for the proton beam, although non-uniformity of LET may influence the proton effectiveness, as given by the ratios presented in figure 6.4.

These high-LET dose changes tend to oppose underdose (since the BED ratios exceed unity at doses below the prescribed dose) and also protect against overdose (where the ratios are lower than unity), although only partial protection is given.

So, high LET can be considered to be more 'forgiving' in these respects. However, when figures 6.6(a) and (b) are looked at closely, it can be seen that the α/β values change the order of these BED ratio plots for different fraction numbers, indicating the need for individual calculations of the BEDs in all cases.

It is important to note that the dose gradient across the tumour target volume may be different between an x-ray (photon) plan and a PCP plan, where greater uniformity can be achieved, although this is based on assumptions linking LET and RBE, as in the work of Kanai *et al* (1997) in Japan where, from the example of a single field, the distal dose is down-weighted because of the increased LET due to a greater number of Bragg peaks whereas the proximal part of the target contains more plateau dose regions with lower LET. Ideally, comparison of an averaged BED across the target volume should be used to compare high- and low-LET target volumes. Failure to do so may allow an advantage for either modality. For example, schematic proton (red line) and x-ray (green curve) dose distributions across a target volume are shown in figure 6.5. There is a dilemma as to what proton dose should be given to provide the same tumour control: should the proton dose be matched to the calculated average x-ray dose across the volume (as attempted here), rather than be close to the minimum or maximum x-ray dose? Techniques such as the uniform equivalent dose of Niemierko (1997) may be of use in this dilemma.

6.3.11 Taking RBE uncertainty into account in fractionation

A suitable method, using the index S_I, has been given in chapter 4. A further example is given here.

By applying 25% errors to the equation (4.8) in chapter 4, then

$$S_I = \frac{P_H}{P_L}\left(\frac{\text{RBE}_{\text{norm}}}{\text{RBE}_{\text{tum}}} \cdot \frac{1+0.25}{1-0.25}\right) = \frac{P_H}{P_L}\left(\frac{\text{RBE}_{\text{norm}}}{\text{RBE}_{\text{tum}}} \times 1.67\right). \tag{6.16}$$

Accordingly, it is necessary to improve P_H (the physical sparing ratio of the high-LET radiation) by 1/1.67 = 0.6 approximately, in order to maintain the same value of S_I, which would be a further challenge to the treatment planning physicist.

The situation is more difficult than the above for important normal tissues (or organ at risk, OAR) that extend into the PTV (in this case, $P_H = P_L$). For example, consider the optic chiasm (which carries visual information between eyes and brain), within the PTV of an adjacent tumour of the skull base, pituitary or supra-sellar region. The dose received by the OAR is then assumed to be the same as the tumour in the case of low-LET radiation; but if the OAR has a higher RBE than the tumour, then the OAR will be susceptible to radiation injury, depending on its tolerance level. The only way of reversing this adverse RBE condition would be to lower the BED by changing dose fractionation. In conventional low-LET x-ray (photon) radiotherapy, standard practice is to use a large number of fractions (often 30 or more). However, hyperfractionation of a high-LET treatment will lead to high RBEs; the alternative course of action would be to consider the opposite, hypofractionation, since the high-LET RBE is then lowered.

However, if the dose can be more selectively deposited in the necessary target volumes without clinically significant alteration in surrounding tissue function, then optimisation systems show that a higher dose per fraction can be of benefit, is economically more desirable and is easier for the patient.

Worked example of fractionation effects for critical normal tissue included in PTV.

A normal tissue such as the optic chiasm with $\alpha/\beta = 2$ Gy falls within the PTV of a slow-growing tumour with $\alpha/\beta = 4$ Gy. Assume tumour RBE limits of 4 and 1.4, respectively, with normal tissue RBE limits of 6 and 1.25. Ideally, the tumour should receive a dose equivalent to 72 Gy in 36 fractions of megavoltage x-rays and the tolerance of the chiasm is 50 Gy in 25 fractions with $\alpha/\beta = 2$ Gy.

Tolerance BED = 50(1 + 2/2) = 100 $\text{Gy}_{[2]}$.

Intended tumour BED = 72(1 + 2/4) = 108 $\text{Gy}_{[4]}$.

The estimated doses per fraction to preserve a tumour isoeffect equivalent to 72 Gy in 36 fractions for 5, 15, 25 and 35 fractions are 3.71, 1.52, 0.97 and 0.71 Gy. These schedules provide an OAR BED of 165.20, 163.60, 163.08 and 162.82 $\text{Gy}_{[2]}$, respectively.

It can be seen that the schedules with fewer fractions (and larger fraction sizes) produce the largest BED values in this case, so that the effect of a fall in RBE with dose per fraction does not 'rescue' the problem. Also, all BED values exceed tolerance. Also, if a lower dose then has to be given (at least to a part of the tumour adjacent to the OAR), it is necessary to check tumour BED values.

Then, for one, two, three, four, five and six fractions (considering the case of extreme hypofractionation) we have to maintain an isoeffect for the normal tissue tolerance level, d_H, doses of 8.11, 5.03, 3.74, 3.00, 2.51 and 2.17 Gy, respectively. These schedules give tumour BED values of 64.64, 65.10. 65.37, 65.56, 65.69 and 65.80 $Gy_{[4]}$, respectively. These are considerably less than the intended value of 102 $Gy_{[4]}$. It can be seen that, in this example, increasing the number of fractions improves the tumour BED. This is because the tumour α/β is larger than the OAR α/β.

If it is decided to undertreat part of the tumour PTV but accept a higher dose to the chiasm equivalent to 56 Gy in 28 fractions, then we obtain in 5, 10, 15, 20, 25, 30 and 35 fractions, tumour control BEDs respectively of 73.50, 73.92, 74.12, 74.23, 74.30, 74.36 and 74.40 $Gy_{[4]}$. Again, it can be seen that increasing fractionation is slightly better for tumour control, but it is interesting to note that the equivalent dose for conventional x-ray tumour control to 74 $Gy_{[4]}$ is 49.33 Gy in 2 Gy fractions.

Alternatively, if the number of fractions is further increased to 40, and we accept a reduced tumour BED of, say, 85 $Gy_{[4]}$, this can be achieved by a dose per fraction of 0.5 Gy, but this gives 127.8 $Gy_{[2]}$ as a late-effect BED. Another attempt might be to use 40 fractions to give the expected tolerance level of 100 $Gy_{[2]}$, which requires a dose per fraction of around 0.4 Gy, but then the tumour BED falls to be equivalent to 44.75 Gy in 2 Gy fractions.

So, the therapeutic window is not good and it would be reasonable not to proceed with particle therapy in this instance. In practice, a 'small amount' of tumour is sometimes given a reduced BED, sufficient to respect the tolerance of the chiasm.

6.4 The use of the linear quadratic model with large fraction sizes

It is known that deviations from the LQ model occur in some cellular (*in vitro*) systems at doses above 6–8 Gy. This is discussed in some detail in chapter 2. There is no evidence for such an effect *in vivo*. Some modellers apply linear models above a certain threshold dose and extrapolate the effect to higher doses. There is no entirely satisfactory method to overcome this, although alternative models are presented in chapter 2. However, it is important to realise that the increasing cell survival slope with dose provided by the LQ model can be considered to be an advantage when assessing normal tissue effects since the LQ inevitably provides the 'worst-case scenario' and is consequently protective on normal tissues. Deviations from the model matter less for tumours with high α/β and for very-high-LET radiations since the cell survival curves have reduced curvature compared with low-LET radiations.

6.5 Optimisation of fractionation using calculus methods

It is, in principle, possible to study tumour cell kill for an equivalent normal tissue toxicity grading or intensity level. A variety of mathematical techniques could be used such as numerical analysis or, most conveniently, graphical methods. However, relatively simple differential calculus (Jones & Dale 2000) can be used provided the discontinuous fraction number parameter n is replaced by a function of overall time, t, and the mean inter-fraction interval, f. The approximation

$$t = f(n - 1) \tag{6.17}$$

can be used to replace t and then n can be replaced by the normal tissue BED(NT), where

$$\mathrm{BED} = nd_H\left(\mathrm{RBE}_{\max} + \frac{\mathrm{RBE}^2_{\min}\, d_H}{k}\right), \tag{6.18}$$

where, for convenience, k is now the late-reacting normal tissue α/β ratio, so that

$$n = \frac{\mathrm{BED}}{d_H\left(\mathrm{RBE}_{\max} + \frac{\mathrm{RBE}^2_{\min}\, d_H}{\alpha/\beta}\right)}. \tag{6.19}$$

The dose per fraction d_H will be used as d from now.

With a repopulation correction factor included, we know that

$$\mathrm{BED} = nd\left(\mathrm{RBE}_{\max} + \frac{\mathrm{RBE}_{\min}{}^2\, d}{\left(\frac{\alpha}{\beta}\right)_{\mathrm{tum}}}\right) - Kt. \tag{6.20}$$

Then using the replacement given in equation (8.1), we obtain

$$\mathrm{BED} = nd\left(\mathrm{RBE}_{\max} + \frac{\mathrm{RBE}_{\min}{}^2\, d}{\left(\frac{\alpha}{\beta}\right)_{\mathrm{tum}}}\right) - Kf\,(n-1). \tag{6.21}$$

Then replacing n by equation (8.3), and defining z as the tumour dose and d the normal tissue dose (where $d = gz$) leads to

$$\mathrm{BED} = \frac{\mathrm{BED(NT)}}{(d(R\max_{NT} + R\min_{NT} d/k))}.\, z\left(\mathrm{RBE}\max + \frac{\mathrm{RBE}_{\min}{}^2 z}{\left(\frac{\alpha}{\beta}\right)_{\mathrm{tum}}}\right) - Kf\left(\frac{\mathrm{BED(NT)}}{(d(R\max_{NT} + R\min_{NT} d/k))} - 1\right). \tag{6.22}$$

Of course, if the normal tissues receive very-low-LET radiation, when the RBE factors will be close to unity, we can simplify as

$$\mathrm{BED} = \left(\frac{\mathrm{BED(NT)}}{(d(1 + d/k))} - 1\right).\, z\left(\mathrm{RBE}_{\max} + \frac{\mathrm{RBE}_{\min}{}^2 z}{\left(\frac{\alpha}{\beta}\right)_{\mathrm{tum}}}\right) - Kf\left(\frac{\mathrm{BED(NT)}}{(d(1 + d/k))} - 1\right). \tag{6.23}$$

The normal tissue dose per fraction symbol, d, can in all cases be replaced by $g \times z$ where z is the new tumour dose and g is the geometrical tissue sparing factor (i.e. if the organ at risk receives 80% of the prescribed tumour dose). Then, a maximum tumour BED (which is proportional to tumour cell kill) while preserving the same normal tissue response occurs only when

$$\frac{d(\mathrm{BED})}{dz} = 0. \tag{6.24}$$

This last equation can be solved easily using mathematical software and is, very interestingly, independent of the actual normal tissue BED constraint, but does include the normal tissue α/β (given the symbol k). Plots of the BED in this form show that optimum turnover points are found especially when the normal tissue sparing increases (i.e. with reduction of g values), as shown in figure 6.6(a). If the geometrical sparing (g factor) is further improved, as in figure 8(b), the tumour

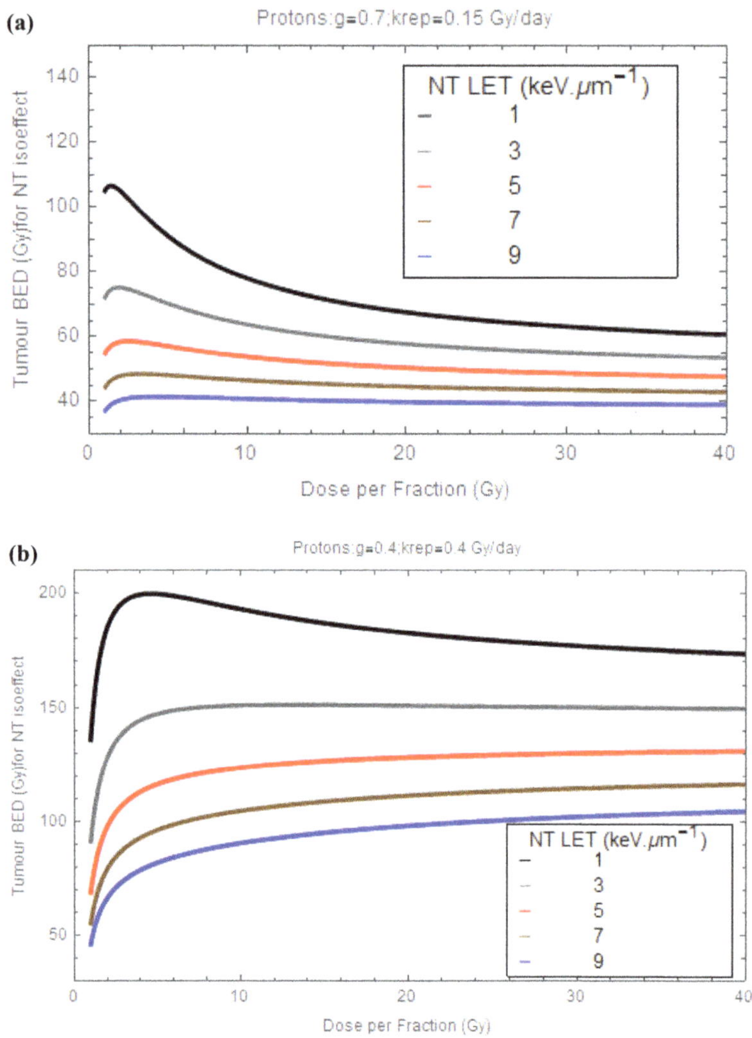

Figure 6.6. (a) and (b): Plots of tumour BED for an equal late normal tissue isoeffect against tumour dose per fraction using equations given above and in chapters 2 and 9. In (a) for a geometric sparing factor (g) of 0.7, the optimum dose per fraction is around 2 Gy day^{-1}, but in (b), where $g = 0.4$, much higher tumour BEDs are achievable, though there is only an optimum dose per fraction for one condition, when LET = 1 keV μm^{-1}. For higher values of LET there is no optimum dose per fraction. Both cases assumed a tumour $\alpha/\beta = 10$ Gy.

BEDs increase further, and in this case the tumour repopulation rate is lower. The flatness of the BED plateau in some cases show that there is no optimum dose per fraction (LET > 1 when $g = 0.4$) in the example given. Generally, the BED increases with improvement of treatment geometry (a lower g value), and also with low α/β ratios, although higher repopulation rates will also reduce the BEDs.

For this set of parameters and the other assumptions made, hypofractionation (to very high doses) is predicted to be a better option for conditions of good normal tissue sparing and for more rapidly growing tumours. Such calculations can only be a rough guide and it would be essential to take further measures to ensure excellent results: the aim should always be give the *lowest* possible normal tissue dose consistent with the highest tumour BED. As such, individual calculations will always be required. However, useful trends emerge such as the requirement of a higher dose per fraction for more rapidly growing tumours (with higher α/β ratios); the alternative would be to provide twice daily fractions using a lower dose per fraction (f is then shorter, around 0.78 d for, say, 10 fractions per week).

Further three-dimensional plots with inclusion of the optimum tumour dose per fraction (isoeffective for the normal tissue of concern) will be of interest. Two examples are given in figure 6.7. In figure 6.7(a), a broad front of optimal low dose per fraction (around 2 Gy) but which increases more sharply with increasing LET and with reducing g values, to high doses per fraction until there is no optimum value at lower values of g. The scope for an optimal dose per fraction is further reduced in figure 6.7(b), where the phase space occupied is far less due to the lower tumour α/β ratio (of 5 Gy) and repopulation equivalent (0.16 Gy day^{-1}).

A particular problem associated with the calculus method is that the parameters used must represent the average values during treatment and cannot easily be changed during the treatment. This creates a difficulty with accelerated repopulation, although this is only relevant perhaps to squamous cell cancers treated over durations longer than 28 days. Slower-growing tumours have less significant repopulation factors and, in any case, ion-beam therapy is normally completed well within this time frame. The present author considers it a mistake to assume that there is no repopulation up to 28 days even in squamous cell cancers, for there is always cellular turnover even if this is at a lower rate.

6.6 Other contributions to fractionation

No account of fractionation would be complete without mention of these other important mechanisms that influence FEs. Fractionation is often taught as being dependent on several factors beginning with 'R', including radiosensitivity, repopulation, reoxygenation, repair and reassortment (of the cell cycle). The α/β ratios used, if derived from clinical data, probably inherently include all these processes. We have already discussed repair and that α/β is the ratio of radiosensitivities, along with the different susceptibility of α and β to changes in LET.

Reoxygenation rates are thought to be rapid in most tumours, with perhaps sarcomas and high-grade gliomas being exceptions. Much will depend on tumour and vascular supply responsiveness, but there is insufficient knowledge of the rate of

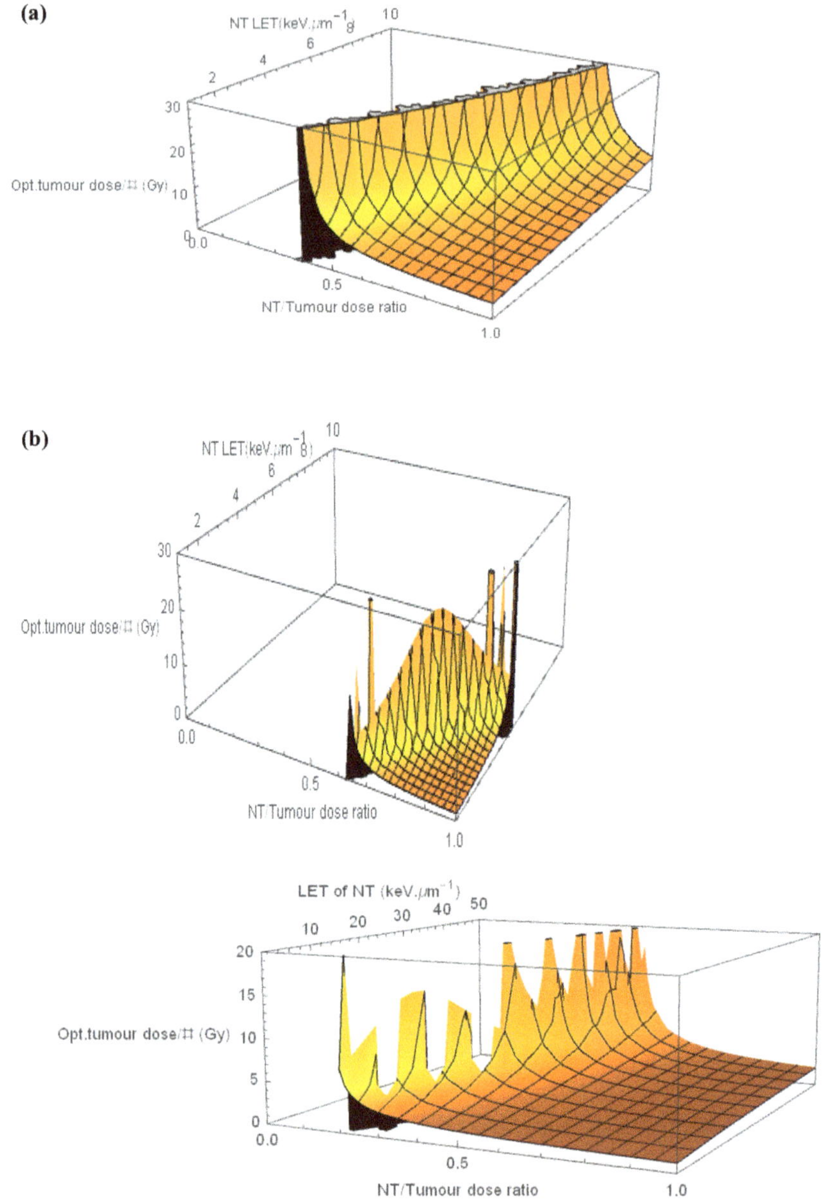

Figure 6.7. (a) and (b): Plots of optimum tumour dose per fraction for maximum cell kill, against tumour low-LET α/β ratio, for variations in normal tissue/tumour dose ratio, the sparing factor (g), for a constant BED of 100 $Gy_{[2]}$ in the normal tissue of interest, assuming five fractions per week are given. The tumour α/β ratios and repopulation equivalents were assumed to be (a) 10 Gy and 0.6 Gy day^{-1} and in (b) 5 Gy and 0.15 Gy day^{-1}, respectively.

reoxygenation in individual tumours at the present time. This key rate can in theory influence the potential outcomes of therapy even in the case of PCP. A single fraction offers no time for reoxygenation and even two fractions (given daily) will suffer from the fact that the second fraction will contain a greater fraction of hypoxic cells. The minimum time for significant although incomplete reoxygenation might be a week, consistent with four fractions given over 4–5 days. A greater number of fractions also might carry an advantage in the case of hypoxia caused by cyclical opening and closing of blood vessels in a tumour, since the volume of tumour treated during a hypoxic phase is expected to be less.

Reassortment of the cell cycle was thought to be important, since high-LET radiations exhibit less variation in radiosensitivity in the different phases of the cell cycle and so increasing fractionation would not be so important. This was established for neutron therapy but it is an effect which is mostly seen at low dose; higher doses which produce much lower surviving fractions appear to show less change with cell cycle position, presumably since the cell kill then follows the type B (β-related) cell-kill process, which has a lower RBE (the RBE_{min}). Such an effect will apply to both normal tissues and tumours.

The results obtained by Fowler and colleagues, in terms of an improvement in tumour control for x-rays by extending the number of fractions beyond a single fraction, were consistent with cell cycle reassortment and reoxygenation, in a tumour where reoxygenation was known to be almost complete in 3 days after a large single dose. The use of fast neutrons gave just as high a tumour control as the optimum dose per fraction and treatment time even if given in a single fraction because of their reduced dependency on hypoxia and perhaps to a lesser extent on cell cycle position.

Repopulation factors can be used for unintended treatment gap corrections, as discussed previously and included in overall BED calculations for longer treatment schedules. However, since most ion-beam treatments do not at present extend beyond a month, this is considered unnecessary in most tumour types. However, the use of ion beams as a boost after IMRT will usually cause treatment time to be more prolonged.

What if radiobiological parameters change during irradiation? We assume that the parameters used in fractionation calculation are the average values during radiotherapy. Where abrupt changes occur it may be necessary to use different forms of mathematics such as series expansions.

The effect of irradiated normal tissue volumes has only been considered briefly above: the precise location of the radiation relative to the three-dimensional vascular supply of organs may yield further useful data that will permit more selective hadrontherapy, with reduction in normal tissue complications.

Another 'contribution' to the effective BED values would be those of chemotherapy, age, surgery, etc., which can provide a further increment in cell kill or susceptibility to radiation effects. In principle, these can be represented by a variable BED increment, as shown elsewhere (Jones *et al* 2006).

One further important issue is *malignant induction*. It has been argued that the most protective effect of PCP therapy is a reduction in normal tissue cell numbers exposed to radiation, especially since RBE effects can increase the risk of malignant induction in individual cells. This effectively means that hadrontherapy should only use the lowest number of treatment fields which meet with the treatment aims and tissue constraints. In principle, fractionation may alter the yield of malignant cells in some hypofractionated cases if the 'turnover points' of malignant induction rates are exceeded and cell killing rather than malignant induction then dominates. Much further work is required in this area, although the changes are likely to be small and must be assessed together with any detriments in tumour control or normal tissue side effects that could occur.

6.7 Summary

Fractionation of high-LET PCP therapy imposes challenges and opportunities to improve and optimise therapeutic index and cost effectiveness, given that hypofractionation, even if applicable in only some clinical situations, will allow greater patient throughput. This can be achieved by further experimental RBE and fractionation programmes, eventually leading to carefully constructed and conducted clinical trials that will compare PCP fairly with low-LET radiotherapy alternatives.

References

Carabe-Fernandez A, Dale R G and Jones B 2007 The incorporation of the concept of minimum RBE (RBE_{min}) into the linear-quadratic model and the potential for improved radiobiological analysis of high-LET treatments *Int. J. Radiat. Biol.* **83** 27–39

Collins C D, Lloyd-Davies R W and Swan A V 1991 Radical external beam radiotherapy for localised carcinoma of the prostate using a hypofractionation technique *Clin. Oncol. (R. Coll. Radiol.).* **3** 127–32

Dale R G 1989 Time-dependent tumour repopulation factors in the linear quadratic equations—implications for treatment strategies *Radiot. Oncol.* **15** 371–82

Denekamp J 1973 Changes in the rate of repopulation during multifraction irradiation of mouse skin *Br. J. Radiol.* **46** 381–7

Douglas B G and Fowler J F 1976 The effect of multiple small doses of x-rays on skin reactions in the mouse and a basic interpretation *Radiat. Res.* **66** 401–26

Fowler J F 1984 The first James Kirk memorial lecture. What next in fractionated radiotherapy? *Br. J. Cancer. Suppl* **1984** 285–300 PMID: 6365141

Fowler J F 1989 The linear quadratic formula and progress in fractionated radiotherapy *Br. J. Radiol.* **62** 679–94

Fowler J F 2010 21 years of biologically effective dose *Br. J. Radiol.* **83** 554–68

Fowler J F, Denekamp J, Sheldon P W *et al* 1974 Optimum fractionation in x-ray treatment of C3H mouse mammary tumours *Brit. J. Radiol.* **47** 781–9

Haviland J S, Owen J RStart Trialists' Group *et al* 2013 The UK standardisation of breast radiotherapy (START) trials of radiotherapy hypofractionation for treatment of early breast cancer: 10-year follow-up results of two randomised controlled trials *Lancet Oncol.* **14** 1086–94

Hopewell J W, Millar W T and Lindquist C 2012 Radiobiological principles: their application to γ knife therapy *Prog. Neurol. Surg.* **25** 39–54

Joiner M C 2004 A simple alpha/beta-independent method to derive fully isoeffective schedules following changes in dose per fraction *Int. J. Radiat. Oncol. Biol. Phys.* **58** 871–5

Jones B, Carabe-Fernandez A and Dale R G 2006 Calculation of high-LET radiotherapy dose required for compensation of overall treatment time extensions *Br. J. Radiol.* **79** 254–7

Jones B and Dale R G 2000 Estimation of optimum dose per fraction for high LET radiations: implications for proton radiotherapy *Int. J. Radiat. Oncol. Biol. Phys.* **48** 1549–57

Jones B and Dale R G 2008 Radiobiological compensation of treatment errors in radiotherapy *Brit. J. Radiol.* **81** 323–6

Jones B, Dale R G, Deehan C, Hopkins K I and Morgan D A L 2001 The role of biologically effective dose (BED) in clinical oncology *Clin. Oncol.* **13** 71–81

Jones B, Dale R G and Kakhsar S J 2000 Biological equivalent dose assessment of the consequences of hypofractionated radiotherapy *Int. J. Radiat. Oncol. Biol. Phys.* **47** 1379–84

Jones B, Underwood T C, Carabe-Fernandez A and Dale R G 2011 Further analysis of fast neutron relative biological effects and implications for charged particle therapy *Br. J. Radiol.* **84** S11–8

Jones B, Wilson P, Nagano A, Fenwick J and Mckenna G 2012 Dilemmas concerning dose distribution and the influence of relative biological effect (RBE) in proton beam therapy of medulloblastoma *Brit. J. Radiol.* **85** 912–8

Kanai T, Furusawa Y, Fukutsu K *et al* 1997 Irradiation of mixed beam and design of spread-out Bragg peak for heavy-ion radiotherapy *Radiat. Res.* **147** 78–85

Karube M, Yamamoto N, Nakajima M *et al* 2016 Single-fraction carbon-ion radiation therapy for patients 80 years of age and older with stage I non-small cell lung cancer *Int. J. Radiat. Oncol. Biol. Phys.* **95** 542–8

Lea D E 1962 *Action of Radiation on Living Cells* (Cambridge: Cambridge University Press) 1st edn (1946) 2nd edn (1962)

Niemierko A 1997 Reporting and analyzing dose distributions: a concept of equivalent uniform dose *Med. Phys.* **24** 103–10

Pop L A, Millar W T, Van Der Plas M and Van Der Kogel A J 2000 Radiation tolerance of rat spinal cord to pulsed dose rate (PDR-) brachytherapy: the impact of differences in temporal dose distribution *Radiother. Oncol.* **55** 301–15

Thames H D and Hendry J H 1987 *Fractionation in Radiotherapy* (London: Taylor and Francis)

Tree A C, Ostler P, Van Der Voet H *et al* 2022 Intensity-modulated radiotherapy versus stereotactic body radiotherapy for prostate cancer (PACE-B): 2-year toxicity results from an open-label, randomised, phase 3, non-inferiority trial *Lancet Oncol.* **23** 1308–20

Withers H R 1985 Biological basis for altered fractionation schemes *Cancer* **55** 2086–95

Chapter 7

The scientific case for using a variable proton RBE rather than a constant RBE

The debate as to the most correct way of prescribing proton therapy continues, although it is changing. The conventional method of assuming that the relative biological effect (RBE) is 1.1 in all tissues and at all doses has been criticised on both theoretical and practical grounds. Further analysis of the well-known data set used to justify the use of a 1.1 RBE shows that this assumption is probably incorrect, but was an expedient decision taken in the early days of proton therapy and applies only to the mid spread-out Bragg peak regions. The critiques include the following:

(1) The lack of late-reacting tissue assays in the data, since in such tissues the RBE values are likely to be higher than 1.1, especially at low dose per fraction. The tissue assays were mostly acute intestinal reactions with high α/β vales of around 10 Gy, and where the RBE is 1.1 with little or no change with dose per fraction.

(2) The use of ortho- and low-voltage x-ray reference radiations in many of the experiments are criticised, since they provided a lower RBE (often less than 1) than would be obtained with more clinically relevant megavoltage photon beams; even allowing a 10% RBE effect for such reference radiations may not be sufficient.

(3) Most doses used to determine RBE were high (often 8–12 Gy), with few experiments based on lower doses.

(4) The data fitting was made by eye: no formal statistical method was used for either linear or non-linear possibilities.

A more flexible RBE which changes with dose per fraction and is related to tissue α/β in subtle ways is likely to be more realistic and safer for normal tissues during proton therapy.

doi:10.1088/978-0-7503-6209-2ch7

7.1 Introduction

In standard practice, the delivered proton tumour dose is the intended photon equivalent physical dose divided by the relative biological effect (RBE), so if RBE allocations to different tissues and tumours are incorrect, there will be inevitable under- or overdosage in the tumour and/or in the normal tissues. The clinical significance of this will vary due to a variety of reasons such as the physical dose, treatment volume, local anatomy, medical history and other factors that may change normal tissue tolerances or influence tumour control. The degree of dose variation caused by an incorrect RBE assignment not only can exceed those in the International Commission on Radiation Units and Measurements (ICRU) prescription guidelines (of −5% to +7% of the prescribed dose), but also those allowed by legal requirements for dose precision in most countries of around 2% (Dale *et al* 2009, ICRU 2010). This is a sensitive issue in the clinic, since there are implications that tissue doses may be inappropriately high if the proton RBE is assumed to be 1.1 but the actual tissue RBE exceeds this number. This is the presently accepted international standard of practice. This policy of using a constant RBE of 1.1 in all tissues, tumours and at all levels of dose and linear energy transfer (LET) has been endorsed in ICRU report 78, but has been questioned by radiobiologists and clinicians for some time (unexpected serious complications such as blindness were reported as long ago as 2000; see Jones and Errington (2000), with recent calls for its reassessment, for example by Blomquist *et al* (1993), Jones & Dale (2000), Paganetti (2014), Tommasino & Durante (2015), Dasu & Toma-Dasu (2013), Jones (2015, 2017) and Jones (2016). Such caveats unfortunately were not heeded, and the constant RBE was strongly defended for several decades without any substantive justification apart from statements to the effect that protons were a low-LET form of radiation where RBE was not important, and that the available experimental data provided a good working value of a constant RBE of 1.1. Opponents of this viewpoint were often suppressed at international meetings, as well as in grant applications and journal publications in some countries.

However, at the present time there is some degree of concern throughout Europe on this issue, supported by increasing clinical experience, as reflected in questionnaires by a European Society of Therapeutic Radiation Oncology (ESTRO) subgroup initiative on this important topic (Heuchel *et al* 2022).

This chapter is largely based on the Jones (2016) reference (where further details can be obtained) and provides the rationale for rejecting the present standard policy. Alternative approaches, which use a variable RBE based either on LET or on risk estimations, are presented in chapters 8 and 9. The work was stimulated by the author's personal experience of observing blindness and/or brain necrosis following treatment in four proton therapy patients referred from the UK, with personal communications of further such events that would not have been predicted from the treatment-planning dose distributions if the RBE of 1.1 was correct. Also, the finding of a 1.4 RBE with respect to the α radiosensitivity parameter at Clatterbridge was incorporated into some predictive modelling (Jones & Dale 2000), which was not well received elsewhere.

The decision to adopt this single value was made on the basis of some well-intended radiobiological experiments. It also followed the precedent of using a constant RBE in UK fast neutron therapy, despite extensive evidence that RBE varied with dose per fraction (Field 1976), although this was in the era before the linear quadratic (LQ) model was used extensively. Subsequent studies of these data sets in a LQ setting show that the extent of the variation in RBE with dose per fraction depends on control of the low-LET α/β ratio in a dose-dependent manner (Carabe-Fernandez *et al* 2007, 2010, Jones *et al* 2011a), with examples shown in chapter 5. When these decisions were taken, the treatment planning was not computerised and so could not have accommodated a variable RBE easily, and the easier alternative option of reallocating tissue tolerances based on higher RBE values was not adopted, which may in part have been due to the lack of three-dimensional dose distributions.

This chapter considers the reasons why proton RBE must be a variable rather than a constant, by referring to basic radiobiological principles within the overall framework of the LQ model. Increased clustering of ionisation events with increasing LET produces an inevitable higher proportion of unrepairable damage, conferring increased radiosensitivity and reduced fraction sensitivity compared with lower-LET radiations. It has been misleading to define a boundary between 'low' and 'high' LET, since protons produce increasing RBE occur at 'low' LET values (from 1 to 2 keV μm^{-1}, as encountered in most spread-out Bragg peaks, SOBPs), and more so at values of 2–10 keV μm^{-1} (Belli *et al* 2000, Britten *et al* 2013, Paganetti *et al* 2002). In the present chapter, 'high LET' will refer to any LET which exceeds the control megavoltage photon or electron low-LET value of around 0.22 keV μm^{-1}. The literature is littered with experiments using kilovoltage x-rays with LET values of 1 keV μm^{-1} or more: these result in lower RBE values (often less than 1.0, which implies that the control radiation LET used is higher than the test irradiation), a situation which does not arise if megavoltage control irradiations are used (see also chapter 1). There is a steep increase in RBE beyond this value, and more so in the case of protons (Belli *et al* 2000, Britten *et al* 2013) than all other ions, because the LET and RBE gradient is increased compared to other ions, resulting in a maximum RBE at a much lower value of LET, as shown in chapters 8 and 9.

7.1.1 Arguments to preserve the status quo or avoid using RBE

Many authorities have claimed that there is no motivation to change the present system, since the clinical results are satisfactory. But there are few, if any, publications that can justify this, whereas examples of 'unexpected' toxicities have been a cause of concern to referring physicians. It is relevant to mention the case in the UK where two radiotherapy centres under- and overdosed patients for a number of years (due to 60-Co dose-rate errors). In neither of these centres did the clinicians notice either lack of effectiveness or enhanced complications, which were found when formal retrospective analysis was made. It should be incumbent on proton centres, or indeed any centre using new technologies, to report their data annually. It is salutary to note that when the British government purchased a large stock of radium and established radium institutes in most major cities in the first half of the twentieth century, it was mandatory to report all results on an annual basis, a practice which persisted until the 1970s. This may seem excessive in present times, but it is in the public interest. Perhaps such a policy should be reinstated.

Other authorities, mainly medical physicists, have argued that RBE values other than 1.1 perhaps should not be used, because RBE is so 'complex', and that LET mapping may be sufficient, along with some form of dose reduction.

Another suggestion has been to use the product of dose and LET: this may be useful in situations where dose and LET are both increased, but since the RBE falls as dose increases, this index will be non-linear, and must vary considerably in the provision of effect thresholds for different tissues and tumours. It is self-evident that when the dose is slightly reduced to be just below the threshold for toxicity, but LET is raised (slightly), toxicity could occur despite the product being unchanged. This follows due to the increase in RBE with both LET and the fall of dose per fraction. In terms of physical dimensions, this product also does not seem to refer to any useful physical concept (for further information, see chapter 4). Although such an approach may be helpful in the short term, it should be applied with caution. This is because should any dose modification factor be used based directly on LET, it will need to be adjusted for the dose itself, and the factor will inevitably vary with the tissue or tumour being considered. Also, changing the dose per fraction, such as use of hypofractionation, would require quite different parameters. The overall system will turn out to be non-linear and a masquerade for RBE. RBE is a physical reality which cannot be ignored. The situation can be compared with, for example, using the constant acceleration due to gravity at the surface of the Earth with good results for falling bodies, but then applying this universally; on the Moon or Mars it will be quite different. Better by far would be to have a general system for establishing reasonable values of RBE in all likely biological/medical situations, based on reasonable understanding of the underlying science.

7.1.2 Justification of a variable RBE

The justification for a variable rather than constant proton RBE is considered from considerations of standard radiobiological principles, beginning with the definition of RBE and how the ratio changes for different cell/tissue types, which with other physical reasons contribute to the multifactorial nature of RBE, as presented in the *British Journal of Radiology* by Jones (2016). Then two proton data sets are analysed in further detail than in the original publications:

(a) A further analysis of the data of Britten *et al* (2013), to find the relationship between RBE and dose per fraction at various depths along a SOBP in the beam. The published radiosensitivities of the control and test cells were used to provide RBE_{max} and RBE_{min} values, which were then used in equation (2.19) (see chapter 2 for further details) to provide the RBE plots.

(b) A reanalysis of the data of Paganetti *et al* (2002). This data set influenced the decision to continue with the 1.1 RBE to the present time.

The above points are now considered below:

1. The definition of RBE refers to its measurement as the low-LET (reference) dose divided by the high-LET dose:

$$\mathrm{RBE} = \frac{\text{Dose of low LET radiation (as reference)}}{\text{Dose of high LET radiation}},$$

   when the same bioeffect is achieved by each quality of radiation (i.e. when both are isoeffective). The numerator dose depends on repair proficiency to a greater extent than the denominator, due to the greater proportion of unrepairable damage with increasing LET. To meet isoeffective conditions for a specified denominator high-LET dose, the required low-LET numerator dose per fraction will be much larger in the case of a more radioresistant cell/tissue (with high repair capacity) than in the case of a more radiosensitive cell/tissue system (with lower repair capacity). In this way, slower-growing/more radioresistant systems (which have large fraction sensitivities associated with low α/β ratios) will have the highest RBEs. Conversely, cells that are highly radiosensitive, with a high α/β ratio, will require a lower numerator dose and the high-LET dose will not differ by as much, since the absence of repair proficiency will not be so influential where there is a higher proportion of unrepairable damage. Consequently, the RBE will be lower and can approach 1.0 in highly radiosensitive, repair-deficient mutant cells. For example, the data of Weyrather *et al* (1999) show that the low-LET radiosensitivity correlates inversely with RBE. The RBE ratio consequently depends mostly on the intrinsic radiosensitivity/repair proficiency of the cell/tissue type, being scaled mostly by the numerator dose. It follows that in the more radiosensitive/rapidly growing cells/tissues, or with reduced DNA repair capacity, the changes in RBE with dose per fraction will be small. Since repair capacities and radiosensitivities are determined by a large number of genes, then RBE must vary. This is similar to population frequency distributions of height, body weight, blood pressure, etc., where multifactorial influences cause variation.
2. Another reason is provided by the mathematical boundary conditions for RBE. These extreme RBE limits are defined by radiosensitivity ratios, of the higher-LET radiosensitivity state divided by the control LET radiosensitivity. This is represented by the separate non-linear increments in α and β, which occur with increasing LET. Derivations are provided in the appendix as in the original publication (Jones 2016). Fast neutron experiments are appropriate for simulation of proton RBE in the Bragg peak region, since most ionisation occurs due to the formation of recoil protons. Examples are provided in the fast neutron data (see Warenius *et al* 1994 and Carabe-Fernandez *et al* 2007, 2010, with further examples in chapter 5), and the proton data of Britten *et al* (2013), where α increases with LET to a much greater extent than β. The maximum RBE is then given by α_H/α_L, found at very low dose since the α radiosensitivity parameter dominates cell kill at low

doses. The minimum RBE is given by $\sqrt{\beta_H}/\sqrt{\beta_L}$ at very high doses, where the β component of cell killing dominates. For all doses between these limits, the RBE must be of a variable intermediate value which depends on the dose itself (due to the changing contribution of α and β to cell kill with dose). Also, since the intrinsic variability of the low-LET α and β values, which increase nonlinearly with LET, will further contribute to RBE variations.

3. It is commonly assumed that because the measured proton RBE in experiments is so close to unity then further deviations are insignificant, especially if compared with ion beams having higher RBEs of around 3. This rationale is often used to support the use of a constant proton RBE on the grounds that small deviations either side of 1.1 might not be significant in clinical practice, especially since the megavoltage photon control radiation by definition has an RBE of 1. This simplistic argument can be counteracted by considering the effect of a change in dose on the biological effective dose (BED). For further details, see Jones (2016), where it is shown that any error is just as significant regardless of the RBE value chosen.
4. RBE will depend on the following physical factors:
   - Particle charge (z) and energy.
   - Depth/position within a SOBP (RBE increases with depth along a given SOBP).
   - Treatment volume (due to superimposition of low- and high-LET regions off and within Bragg peaks, respectively), so that larger volumes should have the lowest mean RBE, yet retain the same maximum RBE.
   - Beam contamination with neutrons and gamma radiation can increase and decrease RBE, respectively.
   - Length of the SOBP: smaller SOBPs will inevitably contain higher LET (and RBE) values since there is less 'mixing' of low- and high-LET regions.
   - Depth placement of the SOBP if passively scattered beams are used (this is discussed further in chapters 1 and 11), since there is evidence of substantial reductions in RBE for SOBP placed at the extreme depth range. This does not occur in pencil scanned beams.

For all these reasons, it follows that RBE can only be a continuous variable. There will be an infinite number of RBEs in any practical treatment plan, just as with dose, although for convenience dose and RBEs can be binned into ranges, and the RBE at critical tissue levels should be estimated if possible, or assumed to be within certain limits which ensure safety and efficacy (see chapter 9).

5. Two experimental data sets:
   (a) The Britten *et al* (2013) data set.
   Most proton RBE experiments measure RBE using single fraction experiments conducted in the mid-SOBP region of a single field. Higher LET and RBE values will inevitably occur towards the end of the SOBP range. In the exemplary study of Britten *et al* (2013), experiments were performed in SOBPs at different depth/ranges and

for different LET values. Changes in the α radiosensitivity parameter with LET in human Hep-2 cells are shown in figure 7.1(a), with values dependent on the initial incident energy. There are insufficient data points to determine the true position of the α radiosensitivity and LET

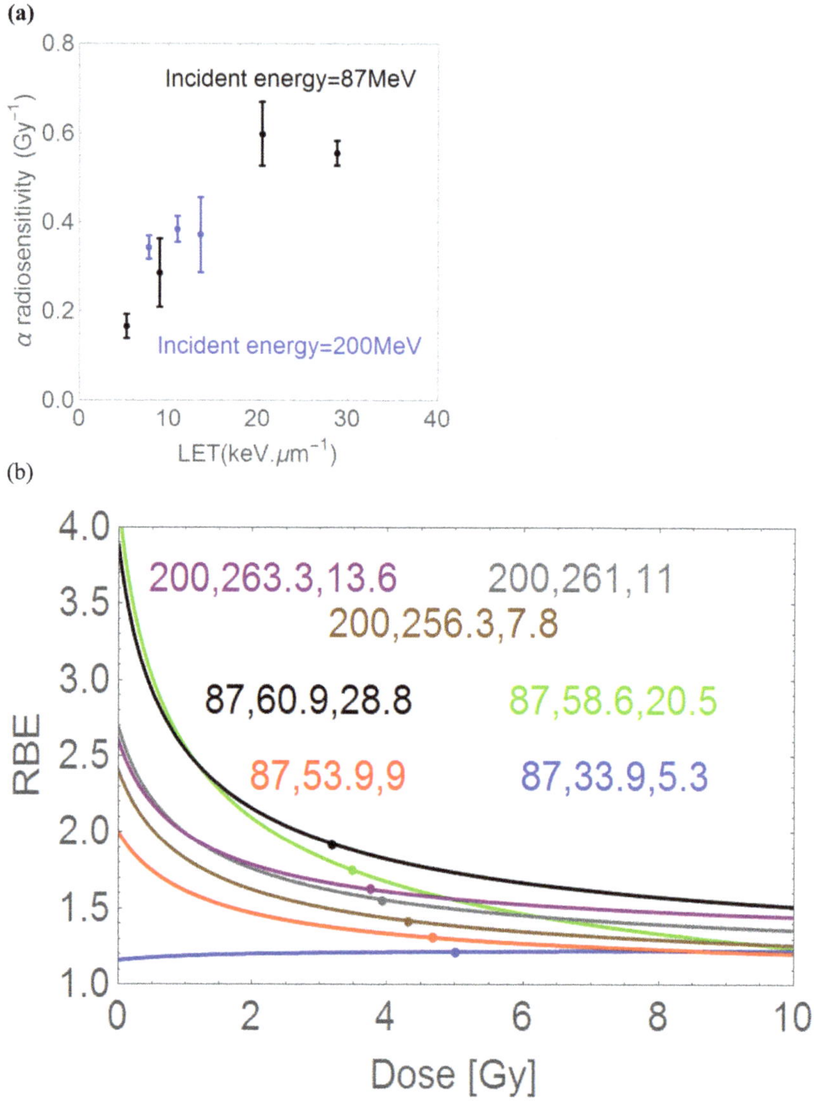

Figure 7.1. (a) and (b): Further analysis of the data of Britten *et al.* (a) For α radiosensitivity in Hep-2 cells with changes in LET, for two different values of the initial incident energy. (b) RBE plots with dose per fraction calculated using equation (2.19) (chapter 2), constructed from the α and β radiosensitivities reported in the data of Britten *et al* for Hep-2 human cells, at various positions in SOBPs and obtained using two different incident energies. For each colour, the set of three numbers, respectively, refer to incident energy (MeV), depth (mm) and LET (keV μm^{-1}). The superimposed points are the RBEs for a 0.1 surviving fraction.

turnover points, but the increase in α appears to be inversely related to the incident energy. Only the lower-incident-energy results appear to be similar to the data of Belli *et al* (2000), where turnover occurs at a LET value of around 30.5 keV μm^{-1}. The RBE variation with depth and dose per fraction in this study is shown in figure 7.1(b) for each incident energy. These curves show the large variation of RBE with dose per fraction and LET in different parts of a proton beam. The points shown in figure 7.1(b) are the published RBE values for a surviving fraction of 0.1: these fit on each curve almost exactly, although the curves were not fitted by their direct use, thus increasing the overall confidence in the high-LET LQ model when modified with RBE_{max} and RBE_{min} parameters. The Kolmogorov–Smirnov test statistic for goodness of fit of these points approaches 1, the prediction accuracy average being 0.998 ± 0.002.

(b) The Paganetti *et al* (2002) data set.

Linear regression models (with standard error weighting where possible) have been used to provide a linear fit of the form RBE = $m.dose + c$, where m is the slope and c the intercept. Also, the LQ model in its BED form (see the appendix of the original publication (Jones 2016)) was used to define isoeffective conditions for plots of RBE against dose per fraction, using least-squared non-linear fitting techniques. Statistical comparisons were made using absolute residual values comparing observed and expected data results, the summated chi-squared statistic and the distribution-free KS test. The data sets were analysed separately for (a) all data, and (b) data where RBE exceeds unity, which eliminates all experiments where low-keV photon controls were used, since the latter may have a higher LET than the proton LET in the SOBP, thus causing an 'inverted' RBE ratio with a value below 1. Although this may introduce a bias, there is a good scientific *a priori* reason for not using such data; indeed, the original data set includes a reverse bias by inclusion of these experiments. For pre-clinical experiments, the control irradiation should always be megavoltage photons or very-well-filtered 250 keV x-ray beams (see chapter 1). Data with equivocal or no standard error estimates were also excluded from the present analysis, unlike in Paganetti *et al* (2002).

Both *in vitro* and *in vivo* data sets show a modest increase in mean and median values of RBE when RBE values below unity are excluded, as shown in table 7.1. For this reason, the further analysis contains only the RBE results greater than unity, and excludes experiments where the control radiation used relatively low-keV photons in the photoelectric energy range. The *in vitro* data contains four such exclusions and the *in vivo* data 14 exclusions.

Table 7.1. Comparison of mean and median values of data characterised as having RBE > 0 and RBE > 1.

	In vitro RBE	Dose (Gy)	*In vivo* RBE	Dose (Gy)
Data RBE > 0				
Mean (SD)	1.21 (0.20)	4.8 (2.69)	1.08 (0.14)	12.2 (9.02)
Median	1.20	5.37	1.05	12.4
Data RBE > 1				
Mean (SD)	1.22 (0.18)	5.0 (2.68)	1.12 (0.07)	8.7 (8.04)
Median	1.23	5.6	1.12	10.07

(1) *In vitro* assays.
In the published series there are considerable variations in proton RBE. Some data points at low dose per fraction substantially exceed 1.1, with small error bars. However, a greater number of experiments were performed at high dose per fraction, where lower RBEs predominate. These experiments can be criticised from the radiotherapy standpoint since most of the cell lines tested are from Chinese hamster ovary cells, with lower chromosome numbers than in somatic human cells. *In vitro* cell growth conditions also favour proliferation, which confers increasing photon radiosensitivity, and which will drive down RBE. The range of cells used is very limited and based on low-cost assays, rather than using a pool of human cell lines with a wide spectrum of cell kinetics and intrinsic radiosensitivities. Even so, the data does show an inverse relationship with dose, which may be fitted by simple-linear or LQ model functions (figures 7.2(a) and (b)).

(2) *In vivo* assays.
In general, *in vivo* tissue assays can be divided into two types: acute and late tissue reactions. Each have different mechanisms. Acute reactions are due to cellular depopulation and acute inflammatory reactions in tissues. In contrast, late reactions depend on chronic inflammatory processes, with late-developing vascular insufficiency along with the development of progressive fibrosis resulting in tissue dysfunction, and which typically occur at intervals of at least 6 months to many years after treatment. Late reactions are important since they determine long-term quality of life in cured cancer patients; they are highly fraction sensitive, with low radiosensitivity and α/β values, and with a high repair capacity, so that RBE values are expected to be higher on the basis of statements made in section 7.1.

After exposures to fast neutrons (and so recoil protons), the late reactions show by far the greatest changes in RBE with dose per fraction, compared with very little change in RBE with dose per fraction in acute-reacting tissues with high α/β ratios (see chapter 5). For convenience, the acute upper intestinal crypt assay came to be used for neutron beam inter-comparisons,

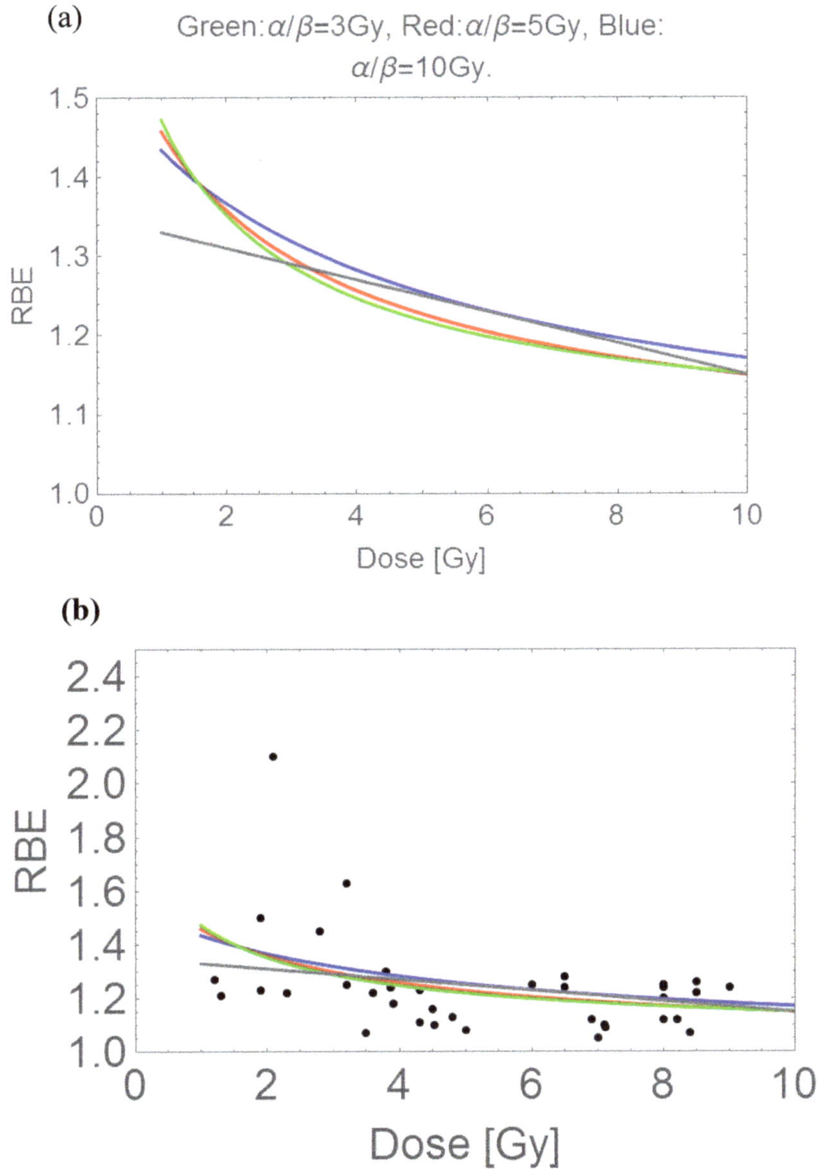

Figure 7.2. (a) and (b): *In vitro* data (RBEs > 1 only) of RBE and dose data derived from Paganetti *et al*, with modelled plots of dose per fraction and RBE plots using the weighted least-squares fitted 1.35–0.02d linear regression model (the straight line), and the LQ model, for varying α/β ratios (which provides curves): (a) magnified view of plotted models and (b) with superimposed data over a larger scale using the same colour codes. Due to frequent overlapping, error bars are omitted, but are in the original reference. The LQ RBE plots with dose per fraction are constructed using equation 17 in the appendix of the original publication (Jones 2016). Reprinted from Jones & Hopewell (2019), Copyright (2019), with permission from Elsevier.

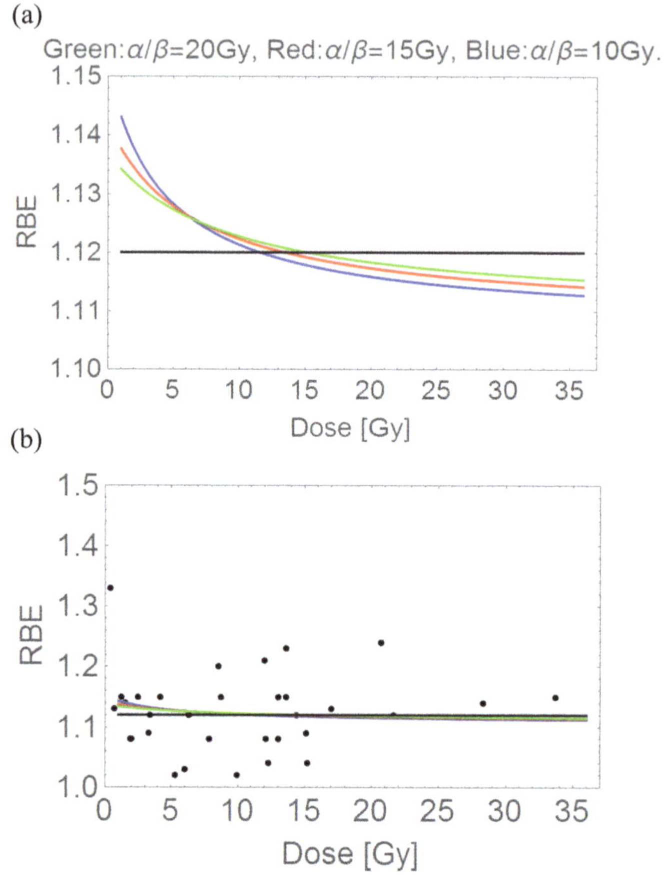

Figure 7.3. (a) and (b): *In vivo* data (RBE > 1) showing dose per fraction and RBE plots using parameters obtained from the linear fit of 1.12+d (shown as the grey coloured straight line), and the LQ model (for varying α/β ratios), which provides curves: (a) magnified view of plotted models, and (b) with superimposed data over a larger scale using the same colour codes. Error bars are omitted in order to improve visual inspection, but can be seen in the original reference.

as a beam quality assurance check in fast neutron and proton therapy: it is the most rapid animal tissue assay, with a low-LET α/β ratio of around 10 Gy (Gueulette *et al* 2004). Later onset and more clinically relevant effects, such as narrowing of the bowel lumen (stricture), ulceration and perforation, with a α/β of around 3 Gy, are not checked by this assay. It is the predominant assay used in the *in vivo* data in Paganetti *et al* (2002).

For the above reasons, this data set (seen in figures 7.3(a) and (b)), is unlikely to show significant changes in RBE with dose per fraction. Some tissues in the same data set did include later effects, such as the lens of the eye (which represents dose-related protein opacification and not a cellular clonogenic response associated with repair) and so is not a suitable assay to make any general conclusions. A few lung assays of early and later pneumonitis (but not the later development of lung fibrosis) were included, and there are some delayed skin reactions (these show consequential late effects in animals and so the overall RBE could reflect the severity of the acute reaction). These assays, when taken together, cannot adequately represent classical late tissue reactions in a variety of human tissues (e.g. kidney, heart, central nervous system, gut). Also, many of the experiments on these tissues were performed at between 9 and 12 Gy per fraction (because such large doses were in use for proton eye treatments). This is a dose range which should reveal low RBE values compared with those expected below 2.5 Gy per fraction. It is concluded that the most appropriate experiments for defining a range of clinically relevant RBEs remain to be done for late-reacting normal tissues.

Both of the Paganetti *et al* (2002) data sets with fitted lines and curves are shown in figure 7.2(a) and details of further analysis can be found in Jones (2016). However, due to the heterogeneity of the data, fitting exercises may be unreliable. Despite this, some broad conclusions emerge:

1. The modified *in vitro* data set can be fitted by a linear equation 1.35–0.02× dose; or by an averaged LQ model fit using $RBE_{max} = 1.67$, $RBE_{min} = 1.03$ with a α/β of 6 Gy.
2. The acute-reacting *in vivo* data set is reasonably fitted by either a constant RBE of 1.12 or by the LQ model with $RBE_{max} = 1.15$ and $RBE_{min} = 1.11$.

Interestingly, larger residual values were found for all attempted fits if RBE values >0 were used in the analysis.

7.2 Discussion

The existing data on proton RBEs refer to *in vitro* and acute-reacting *in vivo* experiments, which are likely to underestimate the RBE in late-reacting tissues, especially at lower doses per fraction. It is the latter class of tissues that contribute to long-term quality of life after all forms of radiotherapy, and their tolerances must be respected in the prescription process. Paganetti *et al* (2002) indicate how difficult it would be to detect deviations in RBE from an assumed value of 1.1: this would be especially true in experimental or clinical series where deviations in RBE may only produce clinically important changes in a small proportion of patients, depending on the degree of normal tissue sparing and the tumour dose achieved in each patient (Jones *et al* 2011b). For example, excess toxicity in the regions close to the planning target volume (PTV) would be expected if the RBE error were to override the degree of normal tissue sparing obtained. It is difficult to assess the true clinical significance, but the unexpected outcome results might occur in 5%–15% of all patients. Dasu & Toma-Dasu (2013) have performed interesting clinical simulations, with significant implications for patient safety. For tissues within the PTV, the RBE error may apply to all patients, but may not be clinically significant depending on the volume treated and the tissue functionality. For this to be detectable amid the large variation inherent in outcome studies, between 200 and 1000 patients might be required, even in the context of randomised studies (Bentzen 1994). An alternative and complimentary better approach might be to study all unexpected outcomes on an international basis and compare observed versus expected results, with a detailed analysis of LET, dose distributions, medical histories, etc., in order to identify if RBE uncertainties may be responsible. This is especially relevant to proton irradiations in the central nervous system (CNS), which have low α/β ratios of 2 Gy, with predicted RBE values >1.1 at low dose (as in chapter 9).

The new analysis also shows that further *in vitro* and *in vivo* work may be helpful to define to what extent the RBE changes with dose per fraction in many different cell and tissue types. This can be ascertained from cell-survival experiments which estimate α and β as accurately as possible, using large numbers of experiments to reduce the standard errors in a wide panel of cells with different radiobiological characteristics. This would involve the same overall experimental plan as in Britten *et al* (2013), but with greater numbers of LET variations in order to discern if the LET–radiosensitivity turnover point position varies with incident energy, as there are suggestions in figure 7.1(a) that this might be so. Such work would contribute to solving the remaining enigma about changes in RBE with depth in beams with different incident energies, and with different scattering or scanning modes (Calugaru *et al* 2011, Grassberger *et al* 2011). RBE–LET turnover points, where RBE is at a maximum, are important since these can be used as a reference to scale all other RBEs (see chapters 8, 9 and 11).

In future RBE experiments, it will be essential to pursue experiments across the same broad range of dose and LET for each cell/tissue type and to analyse them independently rather than in a combined analysis of all systems. This principle can be seen in the work of Sørensen *et al* (2011), where combined displays of data do not reveal what is most clearly shown for individual cell types and individual ions. Only then will the data provide useful parameters for each cell/tissue type, since the LET–RBE turnover points appear to be unique for each ion species and the RBE magnitude dependent on cell type (see chapter 8). Care must therefore be taken in analysis of large ion-beam data sets such as Friedrich *et al* (2013). The data analysis presented in this paper shows that analysing heterogenous systems will arguably provide results which do not well reflect what may be occurring in individual systems. When the LQ fits are so similar in a heterogenous population, it is inevitable that LQ-generated curves would show greater differences if derived from more individualised experiments.

There is now a greater appreciation that LET varies considerably in a complex treatment plan, for example when using multiple treatment field directions, or with intensity-modulated pencil beams. It follows that if a constant RBE is chosen, proton therapy will not completely achieve its intended promise. This can be assessed within the formal ICRU definitions of treatment volumes (examples given in chapter 4), with potential increases in effective dose in normal tissue volumes, as well as possibilities that radiosensitive tumours (with very low predicted RBE values less than 1.1) may be underdosed. In the absence of dose escalation, improved clinical outcomes will only be achieved if the tumour RBE exceeds that of the prescribed RBE (PRBE), and also if the PRBE is equal or less than the RBE assumed in each of the critical late-reacting normal tissues. These differences should also be compared to the potential advantages of the frequently large integral dose reduction, which must influence low-dose vascular and carcinogenic late effects over a much wider volume of interest. To make improvements possible, it will be necessary to allocate individual RBEs to different tissues and for different tumour types, from knowledge of the LET and dose per fraction they receive.

One suggestion is to display the most relevant tissue BED constraint (with allowances for individuals where tolerances may be reduced due to adverse histories), and to plot how these constraints might be breached with changes in LET for different degrees of normal tissue dose reduction (or sparing), expressed as the percentage of the prescribed tumour dose received by the normal tissue of concern, and where 100% represents the full dose and 40% is 40% of the full dose ('sparing' is highest when the percentage is lowest). The proton LET–RBE model described in chapter 9 is used to generate the BED by estimating RBE_{max} and RBE_{min}. This approach was designed to warn clinicians of potential risk and further details can be found in Jones & Hopewell (2019). A photon-only variant of this type of display where horizontal levels of normal tissue BED are used to alert clinicians and physicists has also been used recently in Jones *et al* (2023).

In comparison with the formal requirements for animal drug testing in the pharmaceutical industry, the past proton therapy experiments would be considered inadequate in terms of the range of tissues tested and the end points used. This is not necessarily a critique of particle therapy, since this also applies to other newer techniques in radiotherapy which are not subjected to an approved range of pre-clinical radiobiological experiments.

7.2.1 Inclusion of flexible RBEs in treatment plans

Nowadays it is possible to include a variable RBE within the treatment-planning process by incorporation of suitable radiobiological models within the software. An easier and short-term solution would be to use the existing 'in-built' 1.1, but further reduce the tolerance of late-reacting tissues. For very radiosensitive tumours, such as many forms of children's cancer, it might be preferable either not to include any RBE correction or to use a lesser correction of, say, 1.05, for the tumour itself. This is because the RBE may be significantly less than 1.1, which may result in tumour underdosage since the RBE is used to divide the photon equivalent dose to provide the physical dose of protons used. But care must be taken not to overdose important late-reacting normal tissues where a higher RBE should be applied. The eventual gold standard might be to use dose, LET and RBE three-dimensional maps to provide a more appropriately weighted dose, using agreed radiobiological input data. A more simple example of BED plotted against the available degree of normal tissue sparing for different LET conditions is given in figure 7.4 and has already been referred to above. Sharing of human data transnationally or internationally may provide greater statistical power to

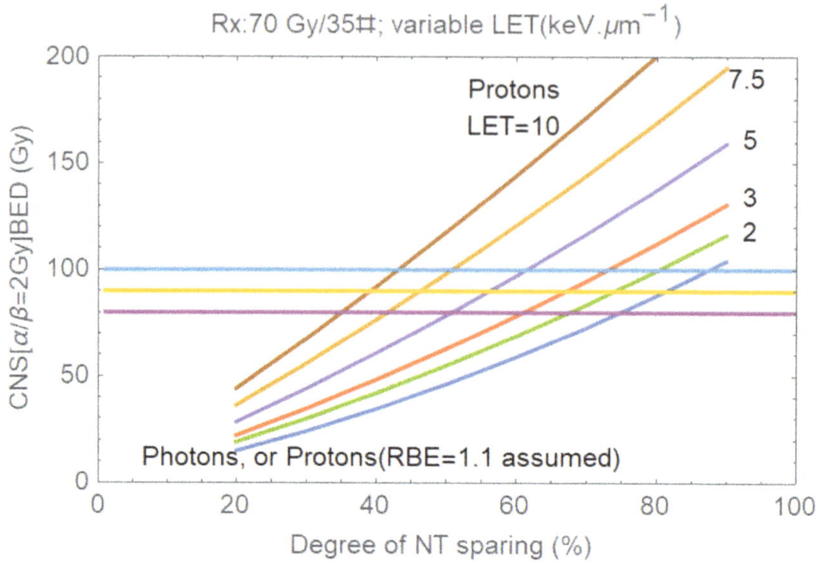

Figure 7.4. Graphical estimates of CNS BED (using $\alpha/\beta = 2$ Gy) against the percentage degree of achievable normal tissue dose sparing for variations in proton LET values between 2 and 10 keV μm^{-1}. The lowermost curve represents the reference megavoltage photon radiation, which would be identical to that for a proton treatment if RBE = 1.1 had been assumed to produce an isoeffect. The horizontal lines represent three possible CNS tolerance levels for spinal cord and other serially organised nervous tissues such as the brain stem and optic chiasm, which from above downwards are, namely, BED values of 100, 90 and 80 Gy_2, which, respectively, represent 0% conservatism (blue), 10% conservatism (yellow) and 20% conservatism (purple). All higher LET which exceeds 1 keV μm^{-1} have been linked to a RBE model that produces higher BEDs values for the CNS. For patient safety, the treatment conditions should fall below the relevant horizontal lines, which require a more favourable degree of normal tissue sparing if LET is increased. Reproduced with permission from Jones & Hopewell (2019), Copyright (2019), with permission from Elsevier.

detect subtle but important findings when using the above techniques, for example in the collection of unexpected outcomes and their detailed analysis. A suggested method would be to use graphical displays of CNS BED, as shown in figure 7.4, where the required safe degree of normal tissue sparing is seen to change with LET. Such an approach could be used where there is clinical concern. An interactive version of this graphic is given in chapter 9 (as figure 9.5).

There has been at least slow, if not steady, recognition that the RBE allocation requires modification in order to reduce severe and unnecessary proton-related side effects. The pleas made in 2000 in the UK for proton therapy prescription RBE reform, and subsequently reiterated by Jones & Errington (2000), Jones & Dale (2003), Jones (2015, 2016, 2017) and Jones *et al* (2018), went for many years unheeded, often being dismissed in a perfunctory manner and especially at international meetings. More recently, many research centres have been attempting to solve this fundamental error with combinations of pragmatic and theoretical approaches (McNamara *et al* 2020), or by summations of track ends in treatment-planning voxels (Henthorn *et al* 2023), and there is a growing consensus, at least in Europe and in some USA centres, that this problem must now be addressed (Sørensen *et al* 2021). ESTRO is presently forming a new initiative or task force in this respect.

In summary, there is an urgent need for coordinated *in vitro* and *in vivo* experiments that concentrate on a realistic dose range of 1.5–6 Gy per fraction in clinically relevant tissues such as the brain, spinal cord, lung, kidney and intestine for true late effects. Also, *in vitro* experiments must be used to test a wide range of human cancer cells in resting and growth conditions, to further investigate the relationship between LET, repair capacity, radiosensitivity and dose per fraction influences on RBE.

Some progress has been made with respect to neurological studies, but due to design economy within *in vivo* experiments and the use of large doses per fraction, the RBE of 1.1 seems to be exceeded in the CNS, although the experimental design cannot possibly provide the true RBE at the lower doses per fraction, which is essential for clinical use. It is possible that proton therapy fractionation policy will shift towards higher doses per fraction, thus competing with photon-based radiosurgical and stereotactic ablative radiotherapy (or SABR) techniques in some anatomical locations. These systems utilise arcing techniques and achieve sharp dose falloff outside target volumes with impressive conformity index statistics, although without the reduction in integral dose associated with proton therapy. Such techniques offer reasonable competition to proton therapy and have much lower treatment costs. The challenge will be to consider cost effectiveness comparisons in carefully conducted clinical trials where the proton (RBE-modified) dose must be known to a reasonable degree of accuracy by using the most appopriate (variable) RBE, otherwise such studies will not be regarded as reliable. Descriptions of these alternative techniques are available in standard textbooks of radiotherapy.

Ideally, there should be a randomised trial of a variable versus constant RBE, even if the degree of variability allowed is small. The present author suggests a trial of RBE = 1.18 versus RBE = 1.1 in neurological tissues, with RBE = 1.1 in tumours, with the exception of highly radiosensitive tumours such as lymphomas and childhood tumours where a tumour RBE of 1 or 1.05 (due to their high intrinsic radiosensitivity) would be reasonable. In this way, tumour dose would not be compromised and normal tissue protected as far as possible if the physical dose and LET distributions can be optimised.

References

Belli M, Bettega D, Calzolari P *et al* 2000 Inactivation of human normal and tumour cells irradiated with low energy protons *Int. J. Radiat. Biol.* **76** 831–9

Bentzen S M 1994 Radiobiological considerations in the design of clinical trials *Radiother. Oncol.* **32** 1–11

Britten R A, Nazaryan V, Davis L K *et al* 2013 Variations in the RBE for cell killing along the depth-dose profile of a modulated proton therapy beam *Radiat. Res.* **179** 21–8

Blomquist E, Russell K R, Stenerlöw B *et al* 1993 Relative biological effectiveness of intermediate energy protons. Comparisons with 60Co gamma-radiation using two cell lines *Radiother. Oncol.* **28** 44–51
Calugaru V, Nauraye C, Noël G *et al* 2011 Radiobiological characterization of two therapeutic proton beams with different initial energy spectra used at the institut curie proton therapy center in Orsay *Int. J. Radiat. Oncol. Biol. Phys.* **81** 1136–43
Carabe-Fernandez A, Dale R G and Jones B 2007 The incorporation of the concept of minimum RBE (RBE_{min}) into the linear-quadratic model and the potential for improved radio-biological analysis of high-LET treatments *Int. J. Radiat. Biol.* **83** 27–39
Carabe-Fernandez A, Dale R G, Hopewell J W, Jones B and Paganetti H 2010 Fractionation effects in particle radiotherapy: implications for hypo-fractionation regimes *Phys. Med. Biol.* **55** 5685–700
Dale R G, Jones B and Carabe-Fernandez A 2009 Why more needs to be known about RBE effects in modern radiotherapy *J. Appl. Radiat. Isot.* **67** 387–92
Dasu A and Toma-Dasu I 2013 Impact of variable RBE on proton therapy *Med. Phys.* **40** 01705
Field S B 1976 An historical survey of radiobiology and radiotherapy with fast neutrons *Curr. Top Radiat. Res.* Q **11** 1–86
Friedrich T, Scholz U, Elsässer T, Durante M and Scholz M 2013 Systematic analysis of RBE and related quantities using a database of cell survival experiments with ion beam irradiation *J. Radiat. Res. May* **54** 494–514
Gueulette J, Octave-Prignot M, De Costera B M, Wambersie A and Gregoire V 2004 Intestinal crypt regeneration in mice: a biological system for quality assurance in no-conventioanl radiation therapy *Radiother. Oncol.* **73** S148–54
Grassberger C, Trofimov A, Lomax A and Paganetti H 2011 Variations in linear energy transfer within clinical proton therapy fields and the potential for biological treatment planning *Int. J. Radiat. Oncol. Biol. Phys.* **80** 1559–66
Henthorn N T, Gardner L L, Aitkenhead A H *et al* 2023 Proposing a clinical model for RBE based on proton track-end counts *Int. J. Radiat. Oncol. Biol. Phys.* **116** 916–26
Heuchel L, Hahn C, Pawelke J, Sørensen B S, Dosanjh M and Lühr A 2022 Clinical use and future requirements of relative biological effectiveness: Survey among all European proton therapy centres *Radiother. Oncol.* **172** 134–9
ICRU 2010 *Prescribing, Recording, and Reporting Proton-Beam Therapy (Report 78)* (Bethesda, MD: International Commission on Radiation Units & Measurements)
Jones B and Errington R D 2000 Commentary: proton beam radiotherapy *Br. J. Radiol.* **73** 802–5
Jones B and Dale R G 2000 Estimation of optimum dose per fraction for high LET radiations: implications for proton radiotherapy *Int. J. Radiat. Oncol. Biol. Phys.* **48** 1549–57
Jones B, Underwood T C, Carabe-Fernandez A and Dale R G 2011a Further analysis of fast neutron relative biological effects and implications for charged particle therapy *Br. J. Radiol.* **84** S11–8
Jones B, Underwood T C and Dale R G 2011b The potential impact of RBE uncertainty on charged particle treatment prescriptions *Br. J. Radiol.* **84** S61–9
Jones B and Dale R G 2003 The clinical radiobiology of high linear energy transfer radiotherapy with particular reference to proton radiotherapy *Clin. Oncol. (R. Coll. Radiol. UK)* **15** S16–22
Jones B 2015 Towards achieving the full clinical potential of proton therapy by inclusion of LET and RBE models *Cancers (Basel).* **7** 460–80

Jones B 2016 Why RBE must be a variable and not a constant in proton therapy *Brit. J. Radiol.* **89** 20160116

Jones B 2017 Clinical radiobiology of proton therapy: modeling of RBE *Acta. Oncol.* **56** 1374–8

Jones B, McMahon S J and Prise K M 2018 The radiobiology of proton therapy: challenges and opportunities around relative biological effectiveness *Clin. Oncol.(R. Coll. Radiol.)* **30** 285–92

Jones B and Hopewell J W 2019 Spinal cord re-treatments using photon and proton based radiotherapy: LQ-derived tolerance doses *Phys. Med.* **64** 304–10

Jones M, Rogers J, Shrimali R K *et al* 2023 Feasibility and safety of shortened hypofractionated high-dose palliative lung radiotherapy—a retrospective planning study *Phys. Med.* **108** 102559

McNamara L A, Willers H and Paganetti H 2020 Modelling variable proton relative biological effectiveness for treatment planning *Br. J. Radiol.* **93** 20190334

Paganetti H, Niemierko A, Ancukiewicz M *et al* 2002 Relative biological effectiveness (RBE) values for proton beam therapy *Int. J. Radiat. Oncol. Biol. Phys.* **53** 407–21

Paganetti H 2014 Relative biological effectiveness (RBE) values for proton beam therapy. Variations as a function of biological endpoint, dose, and linear energy transfer *Phys. Med. Biol.* **59** R419–72

Sørensen B S, Overgaard J and Bassler N 2011 *In vitro* RBE-LET dependence for multiple particle types *Acta. Oncol.* **50** 757–62

Sørensen B S, Pawelke J, Bauer J *et al* 2021 Does the uncertainty in relative biological effectiveness affect patient treatment in proton therapy? *Radiother. Oncol.* **163** 177–84

Tommasino F and Durante M 2015 Proton radiobiology *Cancers* **7** 353–81

Warenius H M, Britten R A and Peacock J H 1994 The relative cellular radiosensitivity of 30 human *in vitro* cell lines of different histological type to high LET 62.5 MeV (p–>Be+) fast neutrons and 4 MeV photons *Radiother. Oncol.* **30** 83–9

Weyrather W K, Ritter S, Scholz M and Kraft G 1999 RBE for carbon track-segment irradiation in cell lines of differing repair capacity *Int. J. Radiat. Biol.* **75** 1357–64

IOP Publishing

Quantitative Radiobiology for Proton Therapy

Bleddyn Jones

Chapter 8

A general RBE linear energy-efficiency model for protons and light ions

There are many complex and often difficult to understand modelling systems for specific charged-ion relative biological effects (RBEs), as used in particle therapy, and which attempt to consider very fundamental aspects of biophysics with biological input data. These have their own limitations and specific assumptions, which have required successive modifications to produce more reliable data fitting.

As an alternative, this chapter provides a simple linear energy-efficiency model that is applicable to all ions based on their Z number and uses RBE values from many cell-survival data sets to provide the input parameters. The approach is semi-empirical, but involves exponential effect saturation equations, which provide realistic boundary conditions and appear more appropriate to the various data forms. Estimated values of α and β values at high linear energy transfer (LET) are scaled between those obtained using the reference (low-LET) radiation and their maximum possible (or ultimate) values α_U and β_U, which occur at the turnover point of the LET–RBE relationship, where energy efficiency is greatest at or around a LET value designated as LET_U. The model gives reasonable fits to several data sets that use a wide range of ion species, from protons to the heavier ions. In addition, because of its inherent use of linear quadratic radiosensitivity parameters, the model is also sensitive to dose per fraction changes. The physical kinematic properties of LET_U appear to show that it is determined by a combination of physical and biological factors (such as hypoxia) and that it occurs before the maximum LET value (LET_M) at the Bragg peak and may also be modified by extreme dose-rate intensification.

A graphical user interface is provided to allow rapid RBE estimations at any value of LET.

doi:10.1088/978-0-7503-6209-2ch8

8.1 Introduction

Positively charged particle therapy is associated with increased linear energy transfer (LET), creating clustered and complex DNA damage, which is less repairable and so causes enhanced biological effects. This changes normal tissue radiotolerances, as well as tumour control probabilities, with accompanying changes in fractionation sensitivity. LET can be expressed in different ways, either as the mean or the dose-averaged LET, but other variants exist (see chapter 1). Comparative changes in bioeffects are quantified by the relative biological effect (RBE) concept, defined and measured as the ratio of dose of a low-LET radiation divided by the control high-LET dose required for the same biological effect. RBE depends on the complexities of how radiation of different qualities interact with different biological systems due to the following:

(1) The LET depends on the particle energy, atomic charge, position along track (or tissue depth) and the mixture of Bragg-peak or non-Bragg-peak regions over a volume of interest (Newhauser & Zhang 2015), as in chapter 1.
(2) The increased local complexity, or clustering, of DNA damage with increasing LET (Anderson *et al* 2007), which consequently confers increased radiosensitivity due to repair mechanisms being overwhelmed.
(3) The latter results in reduced fractionation sensitivity and an increase in the α/β ratio (see chapter 2).

Some authors (e.g. Hall & Giaccia 2011, 2019) have stated that the LET–RBE turnover point is common for all ion species, at around 100–120 keV μm^{-1}, and that this value is determined by the average DNA strand thickness. This is not the case, upon detailed examination of data sets for each individual ion species. For example, those displayed by Sørensen *et al* (2011), which when combined appear to show a common turnover region, upon much closer inspection of each ion type shows an apparent unique value for the RBE turnover point. Furthermore, it can be seen that the turnover point LET value increases with the atomic number (Z), although the maximum RBE achieved by any ion is strikingly similar.

Some authors have developed relatively simple LET-RBE models for protons (Wilkens & Oelfke 2004, Carabe *et al* 2012, Jones 2015a). For ion beams, there are several complex formulations that tentatively describe the relationship between LET and RBE (Katz *et al* 1971, Hawkins *et al* 2003, Elsässer *et al* 2008, Kase *et al* 2008, Inaniwa *et al* 2013, Grün *et al* 2015), each with varying degrees of success, and which have been used for clinical applications. These ion-beam models are based on the fundamental interactions of particle physics with matter and contain multiple assumptions and input requirements, such as knowledge of particle trajectories relative to cells, cross-sectional probabilities, the relative proportion of cell nucleus to cell volume for each cell, critical biological sub-volumes, repair capacities, and extrapolations with dose, etc. Many of these parameters are continuously changing and will differ from cell to cell according to their position in the cell cycle, their relationship to blood vessels, and many biochemical variations. They all utilise long mathematical constructs that can be daunting to less mathematically gifted individuals.

Even though it is satisfying to build exploratory theoretical models in such a way, it is impossible to know these exact conditions within a real cancer and surrounding normal tissues. These various approaches have been used to predict ion-beam RBE values for variable LET values for the irradiation of specific cell types (usually the V-79 cell derived from Chinese hamster ovary, CHO, cells), but with mixed results, although they are used routinely in clinical practice for carbon-ion treatment planning. Only a few authors have attempted an approach for normalising the RBE differences between different ions, as in the work of Katz *et al* (1971), who developed the useful concept of the Katz radius of $Z^{*2}/(v/c)$, where v is the particle velocity and c the speed of light, the ratio usually expressed as β in physics although in the context of radiobiology it should not be confused with the second linear quadratic (LQ) model radiosensitivity coefficient. Since the radius is smallest for protons, with $Z = 1$, compared to all other ions, the ionisations are closer for protons and so capable of producing increases in RBE at relatively low LET values. As the Z values increase, the LET value of the maximum RBE occurs at increasingly higher LET values, as discussed below and with some further data analysis given in chapter 14.

What do we know with certainty about the LET and RBE? Measured relationships between LET and RBE generally show increases with LET until a maximum value is achieved, followed by a decrease to RBE values just above unity. Also, there are some important basic findings which models must incorporate in order to adequately describe how RBE changes with LET. These facts can be found in the reports of Barendsen (1968), Weyrather *et al* (1999) and Sørensen *et al* (2011). They are as follows:

- The initial slope of RBE with LET is linear when plotted on linear scales.
- The LET value (LET_U) which confers the maximum cell-killing efficiency (at the turnover point) increases non-linearly with the nuclear charge of a particle (the Z number), which denotes the electrostatic positive charge of the particle nucleus. LET_U values increase with Z, but smaller LET_U increments are apparent with increasing Z, which suggests a 'saturation' effect. Ions with the smallest Z values are consequently more efficient in increasing RBE per unit increase in LET, possibly because the energy released is more locally absorbed than is the case for higher Z ions with larger event sizes and more energetic gamma emissions.
- The magnitude of the RBE is not only dependent on the particle type (or Z), but also depends on LET, dose (and the surviving fraction of cells) and cell type (and its ability to repair radiation damage).
- The magnitude of the RBE for any ion also depends on cell type, with cells that are intrinsically more radiosensitive (to very-low-LET radiations) having lower RBEs than their more radioresistant counterparts.
- The RBE increases with dose reduction (when the cell surviving fraction is reduced), but the LET_U (turnover point position) remains constant. Thus the overall LET–RBE symmetry is preserved despite RBE decreasing with dose.

- In terms of the LQ model of radiation effect, the α value increases with LET to a far greater extent than β (Hawkins 2009, Jones 2010, Jones *et al* 2011, Jones 2015b). The relative increase in α with LET is greatest for cells/tissues which have the lowest, most radioresistant, low-LET α_L values, with smaller increases in α for systems which have the most radiosensitive, highest intrinsic α_L values, as will be shown later. A similar effect is assumed for β, and has been identified in some experiments (Weyrather *et al* 1999, Jones 2015b).
- These experimental findings apply to well-oxygenated cells, but are modified in radiologically hypoxic conditions (Furusawa *et al* 2000), probably since the α-parameter-related cell kill is not so influenced by oxygen as is the β-parameter-related cell kill (Jones *et al* 2007).

This chapter describes the development of a relatively simple linear energy-efficiency LET-based model using relatively simple linear mathematics to estimate RBE relationships and their modification with dose, Z, and the two low-LET reference intrinsic radiosensitivities, α_L and β_L. This model requires fewer input parameters and assumptions than do the far more complex models already referred to above. Such a model could be used to complement the other systems: in this sense, two predictions using different models are probably more reliable if they are in reasonably close agreement.

8.2 The available experimental data and its important limitations

There are relatively few published experiments that provide a reasonable estimate of LET turnover positions (LET_U) for clinically used particles. These include the data sets of Belli *et al* (2000), Barendsen (1968), Furusawa *et al* (2000) and Weyrather *et al* (1999). These experiments were not designed to accurately determine LET_U but to show overall phenomena and to determine the range of RBE values. Inevitably, overall accuracy is further undermined by biological variation, use of different cellular assays in various laboratories, use of different LET interpretations, and measurements over wide ranges with consequent use of a logarithmic scaled abscissa, which masks the uniform initial linear slope of the relationship. To obtain the best available estimate of LET_U, only the most unequivocal examples of maximum radiosensitivities, or RBE, over a small range of LET near to LET_U were used. Data where LET_U could not be determined to reasonable accuracy, as in some of the HRG cellular data of Furusawa *et al* (2000) and in some carbon-ion experiments, were excluded. The LET_U values (keV μm^{-1}) so obtained were 30.5 (protons), 103.4 (helium), 208 (carbon), and 233 (neon). Although data exist for heavier ions such as silicon and argon, these do not provide a sufficiently accurate estimate (23).

As a test of model fitting for each unique ion, the following experiments are used:

1. Todd (1967): deuterons, helium, lithium, boron, carbon, oxygen, nitrogen, neon and argon ions.
2. Barendsen (1968): deuterons and helium ions.
3. Weyrather *et al* (1999): carbon ions.

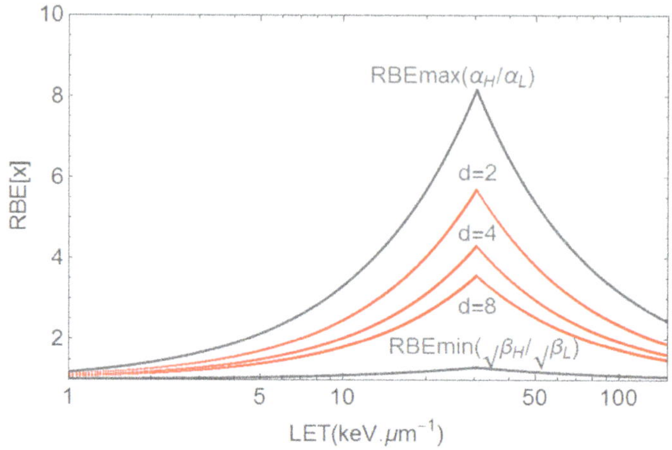

Figure 8.1. Theoretical plots of RBE_{max}, RBE_{min} and RBE values at doses of 2, 4 and 8 Gy with a low-LET α parameter of 0.1 Gy^{-1} and a α/β ratio of 3 Gy consistent with a normal tissue late effect. The overall symmetry can be seen for each plot. Thus the LET_U value here is typical of protons, around 30 keV μm^{-1}, for each of α, β and RBE, irrespective of dose.

The highest α radiosensitivity obtained (α_U), in the region of LET_U for each ion species was plotted against the low-LET (control) α_L value from the same data. These values are shown in later graphical plots, and include variation due to the LET_U position uncertainty. The accuracy of the β radiosensitivity parameter is less easy to determine for high-LET radiations (compared with low-LET radiations), for reasons discussed elsewhere (Jones 2015b). It is well established that β increases to a lesser extent than α with LET; but are their LET turnover points the same? In order to maintain the observed constant position of the maximum RBE occurring at LET_U, and this being constant at any dose (or surviving fraction), then in order to maintain the overall symmetry of the LET–RBE relationship, both α and β must follow symmetrical functions, each of which rises to a maximum value at LET_U. Otherwise, the overall symmetry of the LET–RBE curves with increasing dose would be broken. For instance, if the LET_U were different for α and β, the LET_U would be observed to change with dose, which is not the case. Figure 8.1 shows the overall symmetry of the LET–RBE relationship for different doses together with the phase-space limits given by the plots of RBE_{max} (or α_H/α_L) at near-zero dose and RBE_{min} (or $\sqrt{\beta H}/\sqrt{\beta L}$) at very high dose. The method for constructing these plots is described below, but it is useful to observe this effect here.

8.3 Description of the *Z*-specific model

8.3.1 The relationship between *Z* and LET_U

The position of the turnover point appears to be unique for each *Z* value. It is apparent from the publications quoted above that LET_U increases with *Z*, but the effect appears to saturate (i.e., further increases in LET have diminishing returns as far as the LET_U value is concerned). The Betha–Bloch equation for estimating the rate of energy loss with distance (x) traversed (dE/dx), which represents the LET, contains a Z^2 term in the numerator, usually reflecting the charge of a fully electron-stripped ion or proton. Larger Z values will also be associated with larger mass numbers and greater momentum with larger event volumes due to more complex nuclear collisions and energetic gamma-ray emissions. Beyond the necessary critical dimension (be this radial or linear as a surrogate), biological killing efficiency will not increase if the event size becomes too large and physically beyond the individual chromosome. So, a saturation effect is to be expected. The smallest values of $Z = 1$ for a proton effectively reduces dE/dx, but the proton LET_U is only 30.5 keV μm^{-1}, suggesting that lighter charged particles exert more localised effects (caused by short-range low-energy secondary electrons). In this respect, the proton is more efficient at causing an increment in RBE with LET, but proton LET values are quite small. For example, averaged LETs of only 1–8 keV μm^{-1} occur in radiological voxels during typical clinical exposures (Grassberger *et al* 2011), which when using scanned proton beams may cause RBEs as high as 1.8 or more (Jones 2015a).

The application of a simple differential equation can represent this process. Let us assume that Z is a continuous variable. If the initial rate of change in LET_U with Z is S, this value then decreases in proportion to LET_U itself, representing a saturation effect controlled by the constant k, so that

$$\frac{d\mathrm{LET}_U}{dZ} = S - k \cdot \mathrm{LET}_U, \tag{8.1}$$

which by integration of both sides and rearrangement leads to

$$\mathrm{LET}_U = S/k(1 - \mathrm{Exp}\,[-k(Z)]), \tag{8.2}$$

where S/k represents the maximum possible value of LET_U.

Equation (8.2) can be normalised to the proton ($Z = 1$) LET_U of around 30.5 keV μm^{-1} found by Belli *et al* (2000), so that for any Z a term $Z - 1$ is used such that

$$\mathrm{LET}_U = 30.5 + S/k(1 - \mathrm{Exp}[-k(Z - 1)]). \tag{8.3}$$

This equation is used for data-fitting purposes.

8.3.2 Changes in the radiosensitivities with LET

By increasing LET gradually, from a control low-LET value of, say, clinical 4–6 MeV photons (x-rays), we obtain small increases in the probability of additional lethal chromosomal breaks. The energy deposition becomes maximally efficient (let this be represented by 100% efficiency for normalisation purposes), and at higher LET values beyond LET_U the efficiency is reduced below 100% due to excess local energy deposition, which does not result in more effectiveness.

The separate relationship between α_L (the low-LET control α value) and α_U (the value of α at the turnover point where $LET = LET_U$) also exhibits saturation effects. In other words, increments in α with LET show diminishing returns, since the lowermost α_L values have the highest gain in α. This effect is found with fast neutrons and with charged-particle data, as shown in the results below (section 8.4).

For an initial slope of A and a rate constant j, the rate of change of α_U with α_L will fall in proportion to α_U, so that

$$\frac{d\alpha_U}{d\alpha_L} = A - j{\cdot}\alpha U, \tag{8.4}$$

which leads after integration to

$$\alpha U = A/j(1 - \mathrm{Exp}\,[-j\alpha L]). \tag{8.5}$$

The β parameter can either be modelled in a similar way, but with smaller overall changes, or to simplify matters for tentative modelling purposes it could be assumed to be invariant with LET, but only at low doses where β-related cell kill is small and where low-LET α/β ratios are high. It is preferable to use β modification for low-α/β value tumours and late-reacting normal tissues. The data of Weyrather *et al* (1999) show that β values rise from a control value of 0.026 Gy^{-2} to a maximum of 0.044 Gy^{-2} in V-79 cells, and likewise from 0.02 Gy^{-2} to 0.042 Gy^{-2} for CHO cells (one value of 0.192 Gy^{-2} in this data set must be erroneous due to the fitting programme or other assay-related issues). So, β appears to increase by up to a factor of around 2, which is small compared to the maximum increments in α with LET of around 10. There is more abundant data for 64 MeV fast neutrons, where β undoubtedly increases (22). However, such neutron experiments will probably underestimate the maximum possible rise in α and β, since the neutron LET spectrum (and its average value) may not necessarily be close to the LET_U for an ion beam. Nevertheless, further analysis of these data, which compare neutrons with megavoltage x-rays, shows fits of $\beta_{\mathrm{neu}} = 1.54\,\beta_x$-ray or $\beta_{\mathrm{neu}} = 0.097\,(1 - \mathrm{Exp}\,(23.6\,\beta_x$-ray), as will be shown below). The experimental variation in such data is considerable and the two fitted equations were obtained after elimination of repair-deficient cells (where $\alpha >$ 0.6 Gy^{-1}), or where neutron β values were close to zero, or if the increment in β exceeded that in α (suggesting an experimental artefact). It should be noted that α_U and β_U values will be higher than the maximum values obtained for fast (64 MeV) neutrons, and so the neutron data cannot be used directly to determine RBE changes for ion-beam data.

A similar saturation function is used to link β_L with β_U, as given elsewhere:

$$\beta_U = (R/u){\cdot}(1 - \exp[-u\beta_L]), \tag{8.6}$$

where $R = 2.5$ and $u = 25$, which provides a modest increase in b, and is compatible with the limited data discussed already, with a maximum ceiling value of 0.1 Gy^{-2} for β_U. It is possible that this maximum is underestimated since the available data cannot provide the true maximum RBE value from what is an inadequate number of data points in most experimental data sets.

8.3.3 Obtaining α_H and β_H values

In simple mathematical terms, a discontinuous or biphasic (efficiency followed by inefficiency) model can be used, where for LET values up to that of LET_U increasing efficiency is represented as a linear simple proportional relationship, as used by Wilkens & Oelfke (2004) for protons (equation (8.6)), and where the α value at any LET higher than the control and lower than the turnover value will be

$$\alpha_H = \alpha_L + \frac{\text{LET}x - \text{LET}_C}{\text{LET}_U - \text{LET}c}.(\alpha_U - \alpha_L), \tag{8.7}$$

where α_H is the α value at any particular LET value (LET_x) between the control and ultimate value of LET_x, which represents any LET value between the control value of LET_C (where α is α_L) and LET_U, where the maximum α of α_U occurs. To follow this reasoning a water tank analogy can be used (see figure 8.2), which accumulates water at a steady rate but overflows when its capacity is exceeded, causing inefficiency in terms of water collection. Water here represents energy deposition, and efficiency is the biological effectiveness.

For the initial linear portion of the relationship, there will be a uniform gradient of

$$\frac{\alpha_U - \alpha_L}{\text{LET}_U - \text{LET}_c} \tag{8.8}$$

between the values of LET_C and LET_U, which fulfils the requirement for linearity in this LET range.

It follows that, for example, if LET_C and LET_U are 1.2 and 120 KeV μm^{-1}, respectively, with a α_L and α_U of, say, 0.3 and 1.3 Gy^{-1}, then for a LET_x value of 60, the process is only (1.3 − 0.3)/(120 − 1.2) × (60 − 1.2), which is close to being 50% efficient, and for a LET_x of 90, the efficiency will be (1.3 − 0.3)/(120 − 1.2) × (90 − 1.2), which is close to 75% efficiency.

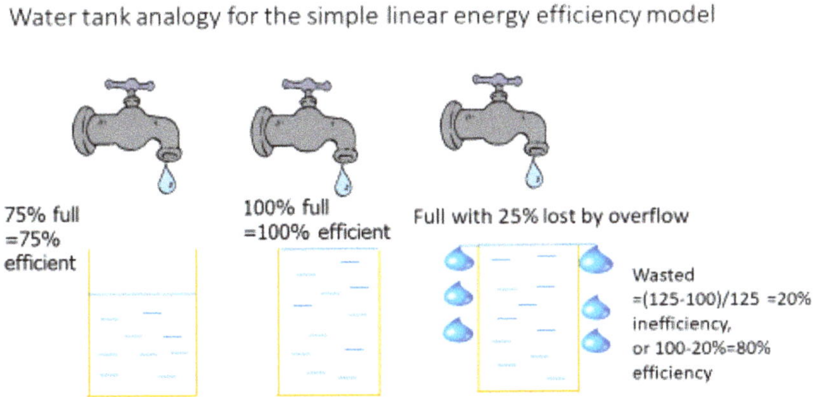

Figure 8.2. A water tank filling analogy for the simple linear energy efficiency model where the volume of water in the tank will increase linearly depending on the input rate, but after the tank is full the efficiency of the process must decline due to the proportion of wasted water.

In this way, the efficiency of cell kill per unit dose will increase linearly with LET, leading up to maximum efficiency (defined as 100%) at LET_U.

For values of LET beyond the turnover point (where LET > LET_U), the additional energy transferred does not contribute to extra lethality, but is wasted. That is, the excess energy (LET_x − LET_U) beyond the optimal released energy is wasted. Consequently, inefficiency, expressed in energy terms by energy wasted/energy released, or 1 − (LET_x − LET_U)/(LET_x − LET_C), increases with LET. To express this in terms of efficiency, the engineering relationship of % efficiency = 100 − % inefficiency is used, and the α_H value is then scaled between α_U and α_L.

Accordingly, the equation for α_H for LET > LET_U then changes to be

$$a_H = \alpha_L + \left(1 - \frac{LETx - LET_U}{LET_x - LET_C}\right) \cdot \left(\alpha_U - \alpha_L\right), \tag{8.9}$$

which effectively expresses a progressive reduction in α with further increasing LET. In this way, if LET_x is 180, $LET_C = 1$ and LET_U is 120, the value of α_U at the turnover point of 100% efficiency will fall to 1 − (180 − 120)/180, which provides around 67% efficiency. For a LET_x of 240, we obtain 1 − (240 − 120)/240, which is 50% efficient. These efficiencies are, of course, relative to a normalised value of 100% at the turnover point.

Similar equations are used to provide β_H, by proportionate scaling between β_L and β_U. These are obtained by simple replacement of α_L, α_H and α_U by β_L, β_H and β_U, respectively, in equations (8.7) and (8.9) and are not reproduced here.

The estimated RBE is then obtained using the isoeffect equations given below in section 8.3.5.

Whereas the above method can be used to tentatively estimate the RBE for any cellular system based on generic assumptions using only the input value of the low-LET radiosensitivity parameters. Alternatively, if there is available data sufficient to estimate the slope of the radiosensitivity parameters with LET then it is easy to estimate the RBE for any LET value within the range of the experiments, as described in the next section.

8.3.4 An alternative method which does not use LET_U but the slope of the radiosensitivity or measured RBE increments with increasing LET (up to the turnover point)

For RBE measurements at specified doses or bioeffects (such as surviving fraction), simple linear fitting should be sufficient, although in some instances a non-linear fit may be required if the relationship deviates from linearity. One cannot easily then predict the RBE at different dose or effect levels in the absence of radiosensitivity information.

Where detailed radiosensitivity measurements have been made, it is easy to estimate the slopes of α and β increasing with LET (noting that some cell lines show little or no increase in β). If the slopes are, respectively, S_α and S_β for each radiosensitivity parameter, then

$$\alpha_H = \alpha_L + S_\alpha.\ \mathrm{LET}_x - \mathrm{LET}_C,\ \mathrm{and}\beta_H = \beta_L + S_\beta.\ \mathrm{LET}_x - \mathrm{LET}_C, \tag{8.10}$$

then the RBEs can be estimated at any dose by applying the equations in the following section.

8.3.5 The RBE at any specified dose per fraction

The reduction in RBE with reduced surviving fraction and increasing dose is obtained by the solution of the following isoeffect equation for high- and low-LET radiations at a dose d_L and d_H, for low and high LET, respectively:

$$\alpha_L \quad d_L + \beta_L \quad d_L^2 = \alpha_H \quad d_H + \beta_H d_H^2. \tag{8.11}$$

The solution for d_L is then divided by d_H to provide the RBE, as shown elsewhere (Jones 2015a)

For clinical isoeffect calculations, the solution of the following biological effective dose (BED) equations are used for the low and high LET:

$$n \quad d_L\left(1 + \frac{d_L}{\left(\frac{\alpha}{\beta}\right)_L}\right) = m \quad d_H\left(\mathrm{RBE}_{\max} + \frac{\mathrm{RBE}_{\min}^2 \cdot d_H}{\left(\frac{\alpha}{\beta}\right)_L}\right), \tag{8.12}$$

where n and m are the respective number of fractions for the low and high LET.

The RBE parameters are replaced by LET (and the new parameters given in the sequence of equations described above) and then solved for d_H. Total doses to provide the same BED can then be calculated for different numbers of fractions.

8.4 The graphical results

8.4.1 Radiosensitivity data

In the previous edition, a different method for estimation of LET_U values for each ion was used (as described in Jones & Hill 2019), which used a linear function for the increase in RBE with LET and a reciprocal function for its later decrease, as is explained next.

For experiments where RBE results are available, a similar approach is used, with the reference RBE being 1 and by using simpler symbolism, with a linear relationship for LET values up to LET_U, and where x replaces $\mathrm{LET}_x - \mathrm{LET}_C$, U replaces $(\mathrm{LET}_U - \mathrm{LET}_C)$ and $\Delta\mathrm{RBE}$ is the increment in RBE. So that can be replaced as

$$\mathrm{RBE} = 1 + \frac{x}{U}\Delta\mathrm{RBE}. \tag{8.13}$$

$$\text{Or more simply as } \mathrm{RBE} = 1 + mx, \tag{8.14}$$

where m is the gradient.

The LET–RBE relationship beyond LET_U requires further replacements. These assume that since LET_x is then large compared to LET_C, that $\text{LET}_x - \text{LET}_C$ can be replaced by x and LET_U by u (since LET_C is small compared to LET_U). Then

$$\text{RBE} = 1 + \left(1 - \frac{(x - u)}{x}\right)\Delta\text{RBE}, \tag{8.15}$$

which can be simplified as

$$\text{RBE} = 1 + \frac{u}{x}\Delta\text{RBE}. \tag{8.16}$$

And more simply as

$$\text{RBE} = 1 + \frac{k}{x}, \tag{8.17}$$

where the coefficient k determines the displacement of the reciprocal function.

Equations (8.14) and (8.17) can be used to fit LET-RBE data sets and estimate m and k.

The intersection point where $\text{LET}_x = \text{LET}_U$ is then found from equating (8.13) and (8.17), so that

$$1 + m \quad \text{LET}_U = 1 + \frac{k}{\text{LET}_U}. \tag{8.18}$$

Then,

$$\text{LET}_U = \sqrt{\frac{k}{m}}. \tag{8.19}$$

Both k and m can be estimated by least-squares fitting of each of the LET-RBE data sets given in Jones & Hill (2019). Also, k/m should be related to Z in order for there to be a specific LET_U for each Z. Then

$$\text{LET}_U = f\left(\sqrt{Z}\right), \tag{8.20}$$

where $f(\surd Z)$ is some more complex function that contains $\surd Z$ or which might closely resemble such a function. The experimental relationship between Z and LET_U is shown in figure 8.3, using pooled data for helium and heavier ions, and this can be fitted by the equations given on each graphic below.

A range of potential fitted equations did not accommodate the practical LET_U value of the protons at 30.5 keV μm^{-1} with the results obtained with the heavier ions, but a good fit with the square-root function is obtained for helium and heavier ions (see figure 8.3) by excluding the protons due to the range issues described further below. Even if alternative equations such as $62.5 + 34\surd(Z - 1)$ are fitted, although the $R^2 = 0.995$ and parameter p values <0.01, this would be compatible with a proton LET_U value of 62.5 keV μm^{-1}, as estimated from fast neutron studies (Jones 2021), but the overall fitting is not as good as with $88.75 + 25.84\surd Z$ (as used

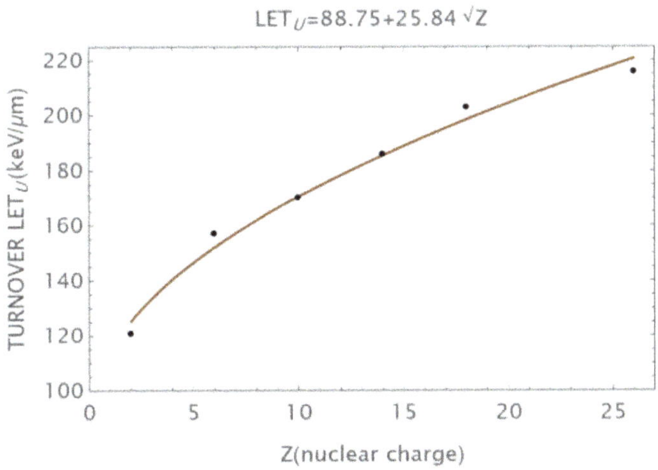

Figure 8.3. The experimental data relationships between Z and the LET_U value for different ions; the data are shown as black points. The black point at 30.5 keV μm^{-1} is the proton value found by Belli *et al*, which is thought to include cellular range limitations. The fitted equation is provided above the graphic with a statistical summary of $R^2 = 0.999$ and p values of <0.0002 for the numerical parameters.

in figure 8.3). If, alternatively, the experimental data includes the alternative value of 62.5 keV μm^{-1} for protons, the equation $79.7 + 29.4\sqrt{(Z - 1)}$ provides $R^2 = 0.995$ and parameter p values <0.0002, the suggested LET_U value for protons is then around 80 keV μm^{-1}, a value found in some experimental studies (but where the use of deuterons complicated the interpretation; Folkard *et al* 1996). It seems best to accept the practical value of 30.5 keV μm^{-1} for a pure proton beam due to the intracellular range limitations.

The relationships between α_L and α_U for various ions are shown in figure 8.4, fitted to data from the literature (with data where negative β values were obtained excluded).

The fitted equation is shown in the figure, but also with a least-squares fit for a linear no-intercept relationship of $\alpha_U = 6.47{\cdot}\alpha_L$ ($p < 0.001$, $R^2 = 0.899$) for α_L values less than 0.35 Gy^{-1}, the more radioresistant part of the radiosensitivity spectrum. These relationships, between α_L and α_U and β_L and β_U, can only be sought approximately due to data limitations (since there has been no formal study of these relationships), but from the existing data it is possible to make estimations from studies which include these parameters, especially if α_H and β_H are close to α_U and β_U. Also, if LET_U is known with reasonable accuracy, then

$$\alpha_U = \alpha_x - \alpha_C \frac{\text{LET}_U}{\text{LET}_x},$$

where α_x is the α parameter at LET_x, and α_C is the reference radiation α value (or α_{low}).

In the case of a non-monoenergetic fast neutron beam the LET is not known with precision since there is a LET spectrum to consider. However, the Clatterbridge fast

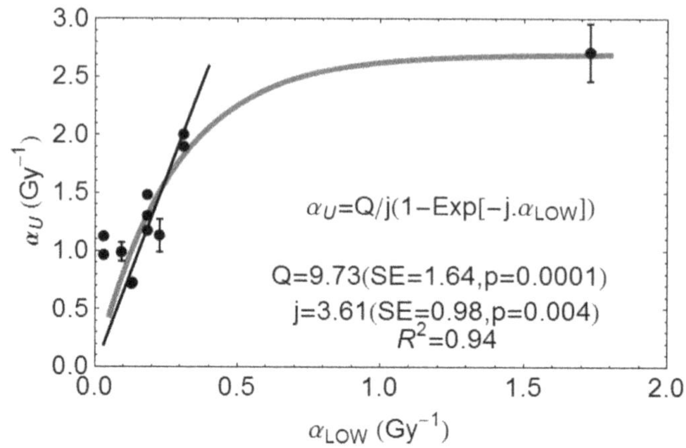

Figure 8.4. Ion-beam relationships between radiosensitivity parameters at low and high LET at the turnover point (α_H is here α_U) and fitted by the parameters shown, with α_{low} being the reference radiation α value. Error bars are not available for all data used.

neutron data (Warenius *et al* 1994), which show the relationship between α_L (for values up to 0.8 Gy^{-1}) and α_H and between β_L and β_H, are shown in figures 8.5(a) and (b), respectively. In each case, the linear and non-linear fits are not significantly different ($p > 0.05$), although the residuals are smallest for the non-linear equations, which also have the advantage of not extrapolating to infinitely high radiosensitivity values. Since these neutron RBE values are high relative to mid spread-out Bragg peak (SOBP) protons, and are mostly caused by recoiled protons, it is reasonable to assume that they will reflect the conditions near to the proton Bragg peak. For further discussion on this topic, see chapter 5.

8.4.2 Fits to experimental RBE data sets

The model is superimposed to the experimental data sets, using the different cell lines of Barendsen (figure 8.6), Weyrather *et al* (figures 8.7(a) and (b)) and Todd (figures 8.8(a) and (b)).

The data of Barendsen (1968) used monoenergetic deuterium or helium (alpha) particles in one human cell type, with highly symmetrical curves which turnover at around 110–120 keV μm^{-1}. In this case (see figure 8.6), the model fits the data reasonably well at all levels of surviving fraction. However, since this data set exists as plotted graphical surviving fraction results without access to the original data, there is inevitable uncertainty in assessing the low- and high-LET α and β values, which makes the RBE determination even more difficult. The plot was obtained by assessment using $\alpha_L = 0.16$, $\alpha_U = 1.31$, $\beta_L = 0.046$ and $\beta_U = 0.15$ obtained by crude measurements of survival curves and RBE plots, each on logarithmic and linear scales, drawn by artists, and which contain displacements of many data points for convenience of display, but the data set is better fitted by $\alpha_L = 0.15$, $\alpha_U = 1.35$, $\beta_L = 0.03$ and $\beta_U = 0.08$, as shown in figure 8.6. The Barendsen data set suffers from retrospective inaccuracies in estimating parameters from diagrams in publications

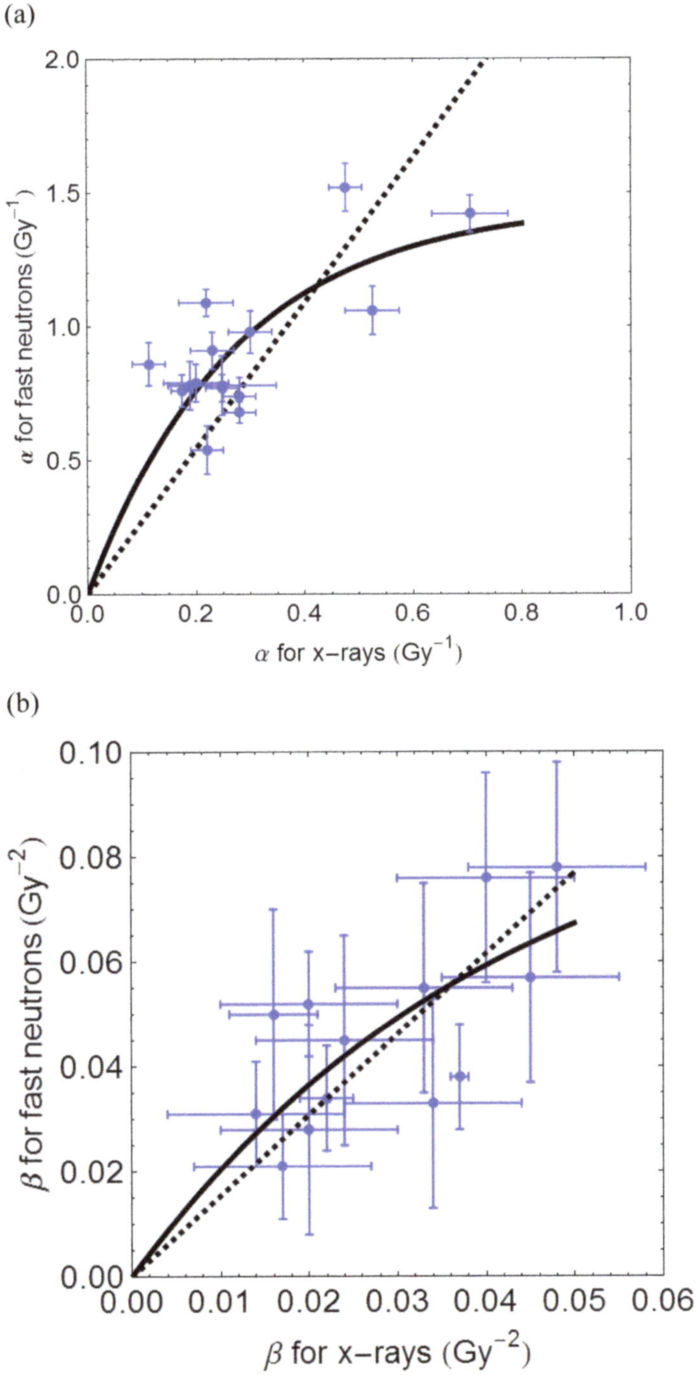

Figure 8.5. (a) and (b): 64 MeV fast neutron relationships between low- and high-LET radiosensitivity parameters. Linear no-intercept and non-linear least-squares fits are, respectively, (a) $\alpha_H = 2.72\alpha_{\text{low}}$ and $\alpha_H = 5.37/3.68(1 - \mathrm{e}^{-3.68.\ \alpha\text{low}})$, (b) $\alpha_H = 1.57{\cdot}\alpha_L$ and $2.29/23.57(1 - \mathrm{e}^{-23.57.\ \alpha\text{low}})$.

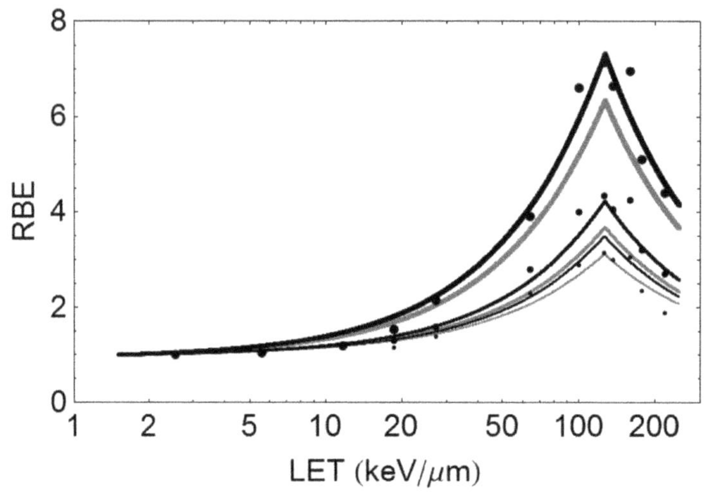

Figure 8.6. Monoenergetic alpha particle data of Barendsen (with large points indicating 50% survival, medium-sized points 10% survival and the smallest points 5% survival, using the proposed model to provide fit lines, with black indicating use of parameters $\alpha_L = 0.16$ Gy^{-1}, $\alpha_U = 1.31$ Gy^{-1}, $\beta_L = 0.046$ Gy^{-2} and $\beta_U = 0.15$ Gy^{-2}, and grey using parameters $\alpha_L = 0.15$ Gy^{-1}, $\alpha_U = 1.35$ Gy^{-1}, $\beta_L = 0.03$ Gy^{-2} and $\beta_U = 0.08$ Gy^{-2}. The thickest lines show the 5% survival.

rather than use of the raw data, but the graphic shows the sensitivity of the model to the input parameters.

The critical dependency of each RBE limit on the ratio of α and β at low and high LET, respectively, demonstrates the importance of obtaining the most accurate possible data, rather than depending on published material which does not contain precise surviving fraction outcomes. The Barendsen (1968) data set also suggests a higher value of LET_U for alpha particles than obtained above using the formula based on Z in pooled data, at around 127 instead of 103 keV μm^{-1}; also, the α_U is predicted to be 1.18 Gy^{-1} by equation (8.3). This illustrates the uniqueness of each data set and the distorting effect of pooling of data from different laboratories using different cell systems, etc.

The important carbon-ion data of Weyrather *et al* (1999), from GSI, which covers a broader range of LET values, shows an apparently constant turnover point for different cell types and surviving fractions (figure 8.7). The data are published with the LQ radiosensitivities, although the ions have a small variation in their LET spectrum (with a maximum spread of less than 5% for the highest LET values, which reduces further with decreasing LET). So, it is unlikely that energy and LET spread contribute to the deviations from the modelled curves seen at lower LET values. The RBE values found at low LET values seem higher than expected, possibly due to biological sample variation, especially since irradiations were performed using two different accelerator systems (for LET values above and below 100 keV μm^{-1}) in different laboratories and presumably at different times. These data, although very informative, inevitably contain greater heterogeneity than the data of Barendsen

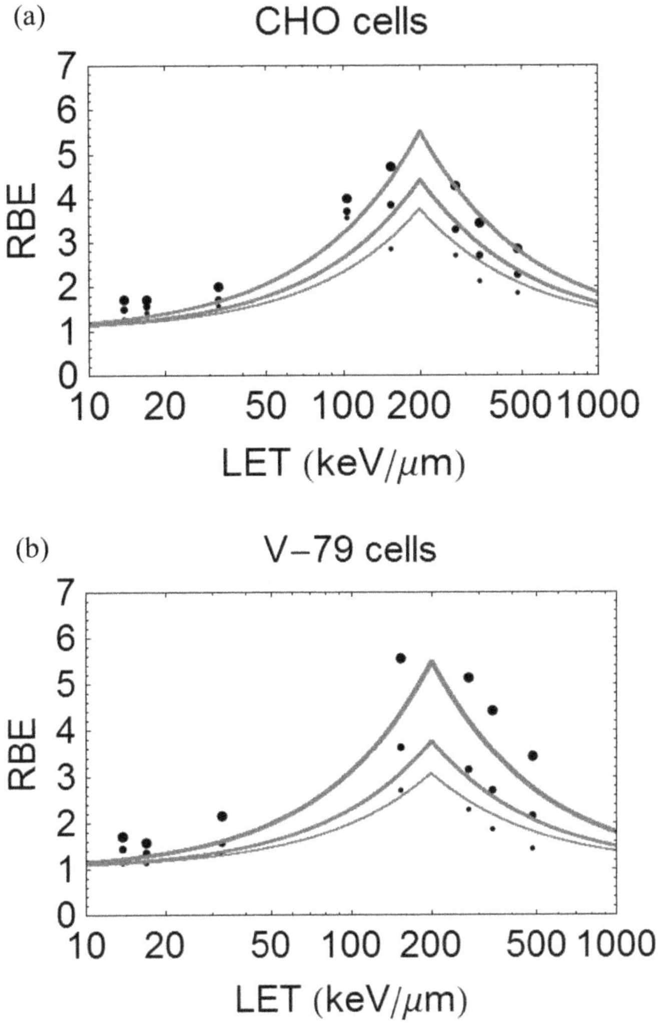

Figure 8.7. (a) and (b): Model-fitted data of Weyrether *et al* for carbon ions for three different cell lines and doses, coded in the same way as for figure 8.4 with respect to line thickness and surviving fraction, (a) for CHO cells and and (b) for V-79 cells.

(1968), and the data are less well fitted. Another more stochastic approach is to use a Poisson function, which will be presented in a further publication.

In the case of Todd's (1967) multi-ion data, a range of different monoenergetic ions were used (protons, deuterium, helium, lithium, boron, carbon, nitrogen, oxygen, neon and argon), which implies that there will be at least nine different curves, one for each Z value, and each with unique turnover points. Such heterogeneous data were fitted surprisingly well by allocating a unique turnover point for each ion species before estimation of the RBE, as shown in figure 8.8(a), followed by the RBE estimations for each ionic species, as shown in figure 8.8(b).

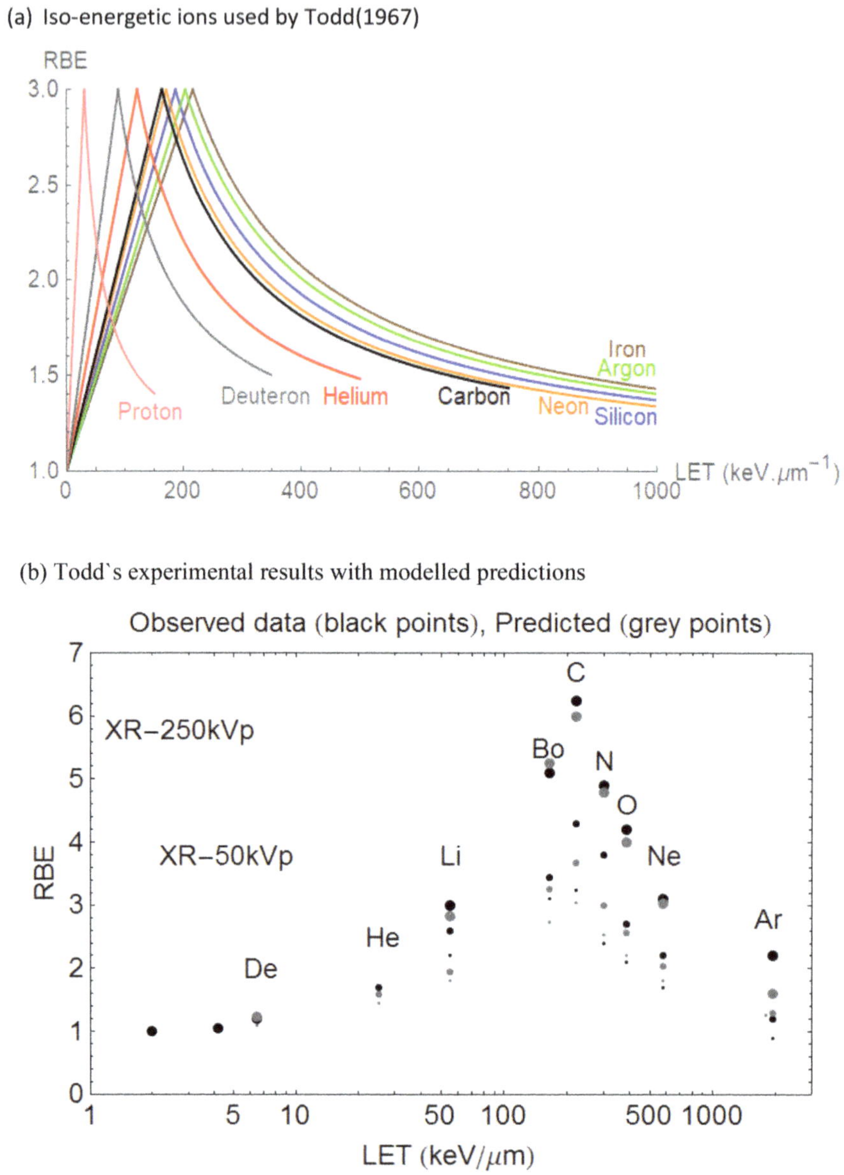

Figure 8.8. (a) and (b): In (a) the approximate LET–RBE relationships are plotted for the ions used by Todd and is useful to interpret figure (b), where the data points are displayed with the modelled estimations of the present Z-based model to determine LET_U and α_U and β_U, respectively, with LQ model correction for dose. The largest-sized points are for surviving fraction SF = 50%, the intermediate-sized points are for SF = 10% and the smallest-sized points are for SF = 1%. The ions used and their LET (keV μm^{-1}) values are given, respectively, in parentheses: deuterium (6.5), helium (25), lithium (55), boron (165), carbon (220), nitrogen (300), oxygen (385), neon (580) and argon (1940). Observed RBE data are printed as black points, with estimated RBE values as grey points. Starting on the left-hand side the first two black points are for 250 and 50 kVp x-rays, respectively, followed by deuterons, etc.

8.4.3 Applications of the model to clinical radiobiology

Not only is it possible to estimate RBE for any LET and dose, but also tentative assessments of changes in total dose required for different fractionation schedules using protons, helium and carbon ions become feasible, as shown in figures 8.9(a)–(c). The variations in LET are representative of the wide expected clinical ranges for non-Bragg-peak regions, SOBPs of different sizes, and for scanned beams. It should be noted that the changes in total dose required with number of fractions (and consequently dose per fraction) are remarkably similar for the respective LET ranges used. This indicates the importance of LET mapping as well as dose mapping in the clinic, since RBEs and consequently changes in total dose with fractionation can be the same for a wide range of ions, as determined by their Z value and LET.

Such graphics can be achieved by the interactive process as in figure 8.10.

8.5 Further investigations: properties of LET_U

The estimated kinematic results for the LET_U positions found in Jones & Hill (2019) are reproduced in table 8.1. These were acquired using the Stopping and Range of Ions in Matter (or SRIM) software (Ziegler *et al* 2008). They show unique features for each ion in terms of all parameters for each LET_U value obtained from experimental data sets, in terms of kinetic energies, relativistic velocity (β), velocity (v) and the various combinations of these studied where Z and atomic mass (A) were included. The index vA/Z^2 (nm fs^{-1}), appears to show the least variation, which suggests that each of its sub-parameters contributes to LET_U, and the presence of A may imply that mass is important (perhaps due to disruptive sonic effects on DNA in an aqueous medium).

Another interesting finding is that LET_U values have higher relativistic velocities than those for the LET values occurring at the Bragg peak (termed LET_M), as shown in figure 8.11, which indicates that the turnover of RBE occurs physically before the depth of a Bragg peak. This finding seems to be consistent with increasing Z, and remarkably the distance between LET_U and LET_M increases with Z number, as shown in table 8.2.

These results show that the physical separation differences between LET_U and LET_M are probably trivial for protons, and even for carbon ions the difference is not thought to be significant in treatment planning of therapy. Much larger differences occur with heavier ions and with iron in particular.

It has also been shown by plotting the data of Furusawa *et al* (2000) that LET_U values increase in hypoxic conditions (see chapter 2) and it has been suggested that LET_U values may reduce with intensification of dose rate (Jones 2022), as tentatively modelled for protons in chapter 9. Further work is required using carefully controlled dose rate and hypoxic experiments (see chapter 14).

The ranges of particles at specific energies is also of interest. Particle ranges for a range of Z values in comparison with cell thickness is shown in figure 8.12, where there is a significant limitation for protons. Range limitations probably contribute to the experimental LET_U value being as low as 30.5 keV $\mu\mathrm{m}^{-1}$ for monoenergetic protons (as discussed in chapter 9).

(a) Protons

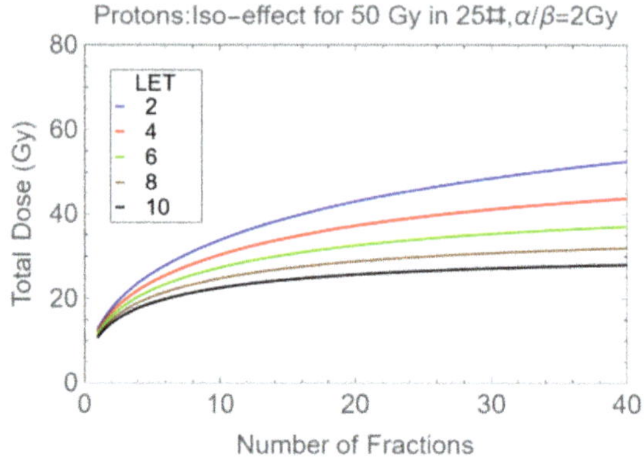

(b) Helium ions

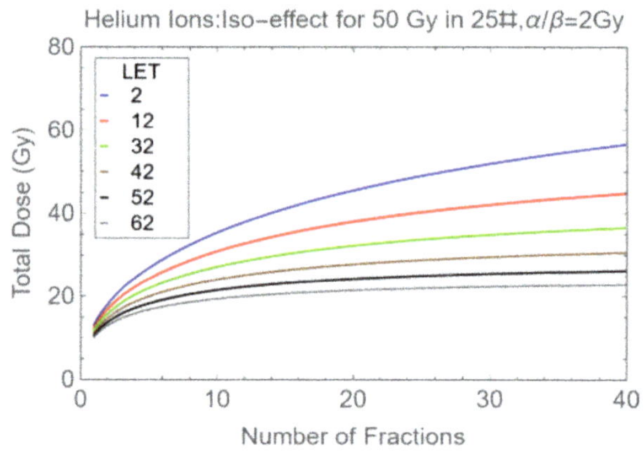

(c) Carbon ions

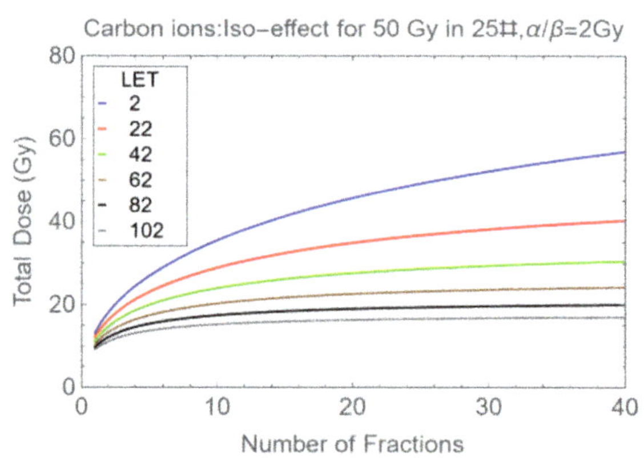

Figure 8.9. Plots of total isoeffective dose versus number of fractions for the given isoeffect and α/β ratio.

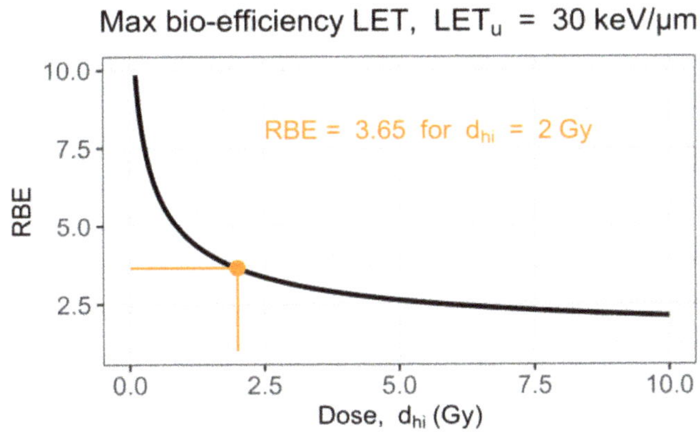

Figure 8.10. The RBE and dose relationship for variable LET_U values ranging from those of protons to argon ions for any LET value (LET_X). In the default graphic a dose of 2 Gy is shown by the orange point on the RBE–dose curve. A fully interactive version of this plot can be found at https://josh-will-moore.shinyapps.io/InteractivePlots_Jones_IOP/. Credit: Joshua Moore.

Table 8.1. Point estimates of kinematic parameters at the estimated mean LET_U positions.

	Proton $Z = 1$, $A = 1$	Helium $Z = 2$, $A = 4$	Carbon $Z = 6$, $A = 12$	Neon $Z = 10$, $A = 20$	Argon $Z = 18$, $A = 40$
LET_U (keV βm^{-1})	30.43	120.66	157.10	187.8	207.9
Kinetic energy (MeV)	0.74	3.25	135	685	5350
β ($=v/c$)	0.040	0.042	0.154	0.265	0.486
v (nm fs^{-1})	11.69	12.59	46.17	79.45	145.70
Z^*/Z	Not applicable	0.96	0.99	0.99	0.99
β/Z	0.040	0.021	0.027	0.027	0.027
v/Z (nm fs^{-1}per unit Z)	11.96	6.30	7.70	7.95	8.09
β/A	0.040	0.011	0.013	0.013	0.012
v/A (nm fs^{-1}/nucleon)	11.96	3.15	3.85	3.97	3.64
Index1 $= \beta A/Z^2$	0.040	0.042	0.051	0.053	0.060
Index2 $= vA/Z^2$(nm fs^{-1})	11.69	12.39	15.39	15.89	17.99
Katz ratio Z^{*2}/β^2	628	2111	1507	1421	1355

Comments: Z, A and β are dimensionless quantities. Statistics for (a) Index1: mean = 0.049, median = 0.051, $\sigma = 0.009$, $CV = 0.17$; (b) Index2: mean = 14.71, median = 15.39, $\sigma = 2.56$, $CV = 0.17$. Note that the speed of light is approximately 300 nm fs^{-1}. In comparison, the Katz ratio results from figure 3 have summary statistics of mean = 1410, median = 1421, $\sigma = 518$, $CV = 0.37$. Modified from Jones & Hill (2019).

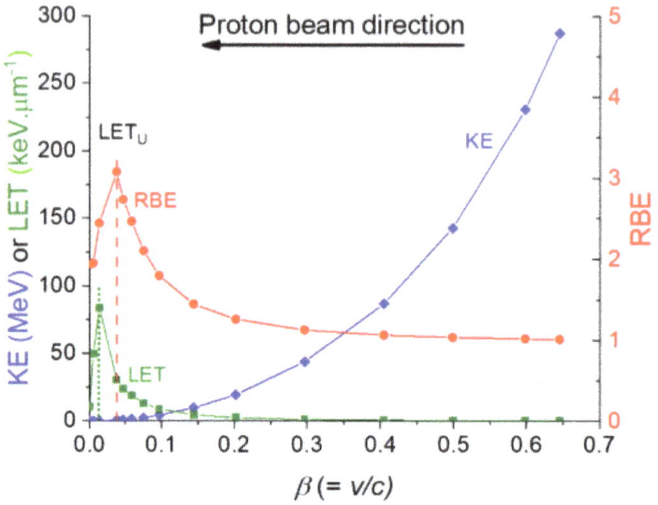

Figure 8.11. Plot of relativistic velocity (β) and changes in LET and RBE for protons. Similar changes are found for helium ions (see Jones & Hill 2020).

Table 8.2. LET, kinetic energy and particle ranges with the displacement distances between LET_U and LET_M (mm) for the ions under consideration (from Jones & Hill 2020).

	LET_U			LET_M			$\mathrm{LET}_M - \mathrm{LET}_U$
Particle	LET (keV μm^{-1})	K.E. (MeV)	Range (mm)	LET (keV μm^{-1})	K.E. (MeV)	Range (mm)	Displacement (mm)
Proton, $Z = 1$	30.4	0.68	0.014	85	0.08	0.0012	0.013
Helium, $Z = 2$	120.7	3.30	0.020	237	0.65	0.0040	0.016
Carbon, $Z = 6$	157.1	136	0.502	977	3.8	0.0061	0.496
Neon, $Z = 10$	170.1	685	2.26	1690	9	0.0086	2.17
Silicon, $Z = 14$	185.9	2020	6.15	2580	15	0.0094	6.14
Argon, $Z = 18$	202.8	5240	14.9	3320	25	0.0124	14.9
Iron, $Z = 26$	215.6	19 600	56.0	4750	45	0.0158	56.0

Further insights are gained by plotting relativistic velocity with LET_U energies per nucleon, which provides a smooth curve, as shown in figure 8.13.

This curve is useful when plotted together with the change in Z^* (the effective charge) which occurs with relativistic velocity (β), given by the empirically derived Barkas (1963) equation (which is shown in figure 8.14). This shows that LET_U occurs when β falls but remains within a plateau region where the fully electron-stripped charge is maintained and effective charge (Z^*) falls (by accepting electrons from the surrounding medium) with further slowing (by reductions in β) at around the LET_M value, where LET begins to fall beyond the Bragg peak. It can be seen

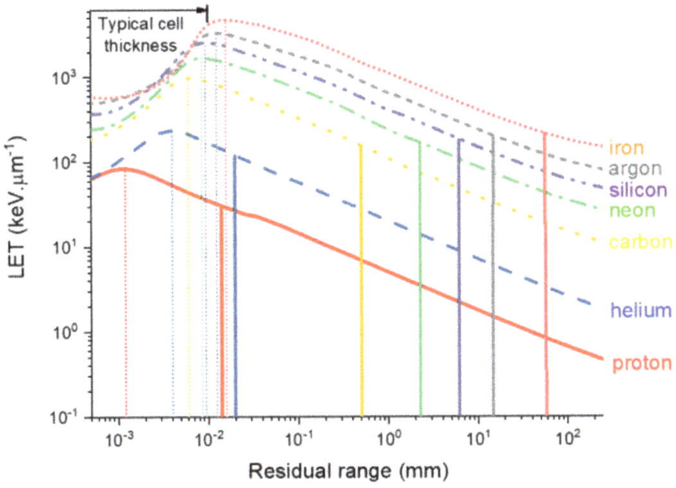

Figure 8.12. Plots of LET and residual range for the ion species under consideration. The typical cell thickness is shown. The colour-coded vertical dotted lines for each ionic species represent the LET_M position ranges and the vertical solid lines the LET_U values (see Jones & Hill (2020).

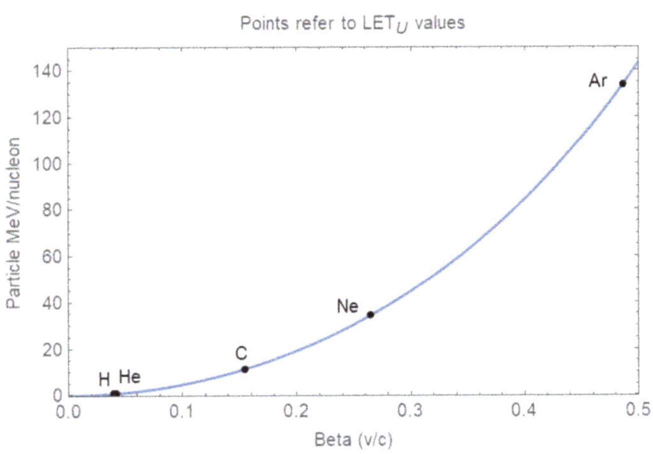

Figure 8.13. Plot of particle kinetic energies per nucleon with the relativistic velocity (β). The points indicate the values at the estimated LET_U turnover positions. Reproduced from Jones & Hill (2019).

that the separation between the LET_U value and the region where the plateau ends becomes larger with increasing Z.

This finding can be extended to all ions, as shown in figure 8.15, where the hatched curve provides the values at LET_U positions.

8.6 Conclusions and what remains to be done

Simple differential equations which model saturation effects are commonly used in the physical sciences and in biology, with notable examples in pharmacokinetics.

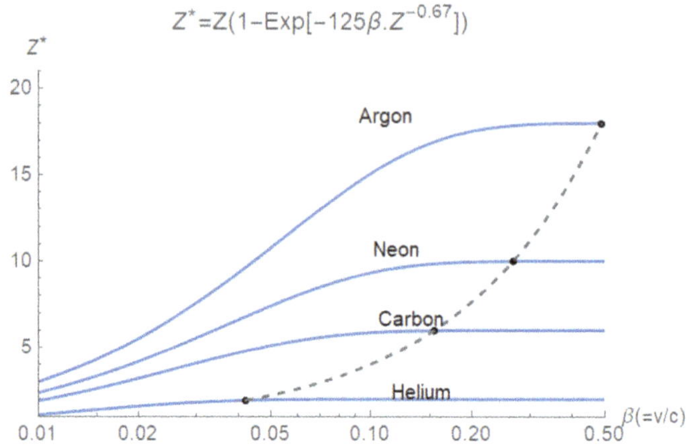

Figure 8.14. Plot of the relationship between effective value of Z, or (Z^*), and the relativistic velocity (β) for four ions. The black points are the estimated Z^* values at the LET_U turnover points. Protons cannot be included here because their own Z value cannot be reduced to a value <1. The fitted equation of the hatched curve was obtained by a non-linear equation least-squares fit yielding $Z^* = 0.41 + 36.16\beta$ at each LET–RBE turnover point. Reproduced from Jones & Hill (2019).

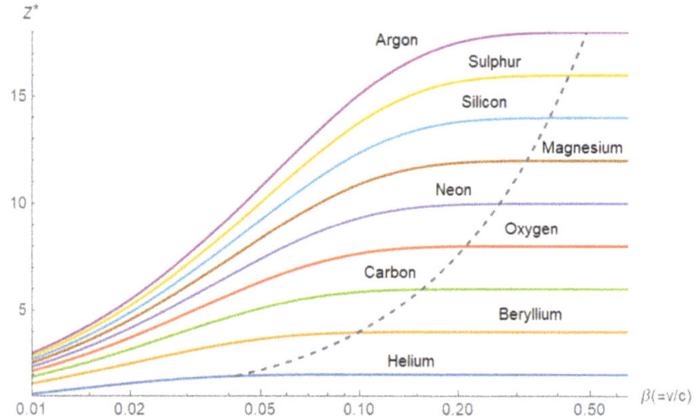

Figure 8.15. Further examples of the relationship between β and Z^*/Z for multiple further ions, where the hatched curve is the same function used in figure 8.3 and the crossing point for each curve provides the β parameter at the LET_U turnover points for each ion, and where the Z^*/Z value is around 0.99. Reproduced from Jones & Hill (2019).

Saturation in the radiation context applies to the relationship between the effective radiation event size and the biotarget. Maximum efficiency represents the maximum cell-killing effect caused by locally absorbed energy, which differs from the energy released, some of which may be wasted by causing more local damage than is necessary to cause lethality, or which is dissipated over a wider than necessary critical volume.

The new model offers a relatively more simple semi-empirical mathematical method for assessing changes in RBE with LET than has previously been available, and provides a second-order approximation. It can be more easily understood and used by clinicians, biologists and others without recourse to more complex mathematics. Also, the two saturation-based assumptions made, in comparison, are fewer than the assumptions required in other RBE models. For highly controlled and relatively homogenous data sets, this deterministic approach provides reasonable estimates of RBE by obtaining RBE_{max} and RBE_{min} from the incremental values of α and β at increasing LET. The model depends on the assumptions of the LQ model, where α and β are high-level parameters, being ultimate coefficients of radiation-induced cell death rather than basic components of radiation effect such as DNA strand breaks, etc.

The model is not intended to supplant existing models of RBE but to be complementary. It would be highly advantageous in clinical practice if more than one model could be used, with clinical decisions allowed to proceed if at least two are in reasonable agreement. Thus the local effect model (or LEM), micro-dosimetric kinetic model (or MKM) and their newest variants as well as the Katz model should continue to be used, and compared with the model described in this chapter.

Improved input data by further large-scale experiments would undoubtedly further improve the accuracy of the model (as discussed in chapter 14). Rather than attempt to fit historical data, which are limited in terms of accurate determination of 'maximum efficiency' turnover points, it would be better to conduct rigorous experiments to test hypotheses connected with the above models, such as the relationship of the initial slope to more precise estimates of the turnover point position (LET_U) in different ions. This also requires a further stochastic interpretation, necessary to match a range of LET values as would be encountered in many clinical beams. There is ample scope for research in this respect.

Some authors have emphasised the inverse association between low-LET α/β and the final RBE (Hawkins 2003, Elsässer *et al* 2008, Carabe *et al* 2012). This follows since α/β does represent cellular repair capacity and the intrinsic radiosensitivities, but is valid more at low doses. From the definitions of RBE_{max} and RBE_{min}, it is easy to show that the former will be inversely related to $(\alpha/\beta)_L$, but the latter directly proportional to the square root of $(\alpha/\beta)_L$ (Jones *et al* 2011), as shown in chapter 5. The former assumption can be used for low dose per fraction treatments, where RBE_{max} dominates the RBE. The need to include changes in β with LET is necessary for estimations of RBE at higher doses and where α/β is small, as in human late tissue effects. The new model also preserves the overall symmetry of the curves at increasing dose. Accurate estimation of β from cell-survival curves, especially when the α values are large, are notoriously difficult to achieve. Our knowledge of how β changes with increasing LET is less well documented than for the larger and easier to measure changes in α with increasing LET. Only by meticulously conducted large-scale experiments with greater than usual numbers of cell-survival experiments can these parameters be estimated to greater and sufficient accuracy.

Since neutrons are uncharged, they do not fall easily into this model, although the main products of neutron interactions such as recoil protons and other ions do, such that a spectrum of LET values will result, which in principle could be translated into RBE using the modelling described in this report. A crude estimate could be obtained from the specific or representative neutron LET (even if chosen from a spectrum) and applying $Z = 1$ in the model described.

There is considerable scope for the application of simpler RBE predictive models. Ideally, prospective experiments should be performed with specific attention to LET–RBE turnover point position for different ions, the initial slope of the increment in RBE, and the maximum value of α and β relative to their low LET values. These need to be determined for extensive *in vitro* libraries of human cell lines and, if confirmed, extended to more complex *in vivo* experiments, as discussed in chapter 14.

The next chapter will use the same model but for the specific application of protons.

Certain sections of text in this chapter have been reproduced from Jones (2015b).

References

Anderson R M, Stevens D L, Sumption N D *et al* 2007 Effect of linear energy transfer (LET) on the complexity of alpha-particle-induced chromosome aberrations in human CD34+ cells *Radiat. Res.* **167** 541–50

Barendsen G W 1968 Responses of cultured cells, tumours and normal tissues to radiations of different linear energy transfer *Curr. Topics Radiat. Res. Q.* **4** 293–356

Barkas H 1963 *Nuclear Research Emulsions* **vol 1** (New York: Academic) ch 9 p 371

Belli M, Bettega D, Calzolari P *et al* 2000 Inactivation of human normal and tumour cells irradiated with low energy protons *Int. J. Radiat. Biol.* **76** 831–9

Carabe A, Moteabbed M, Depauw N, Schuemann J and Paganetti H 2012 Range uncertainty in proton therapy due to variable biological effectiveness *Phys. Med. Biol.* **57** 1159–72

Elsässer T, Krämer M and Scholz M 2008 Accuracy of the local effect model for the prediction of biologic effects of carbon ion beams *in vitro* and *in vivo* *Int. J. Radiat. Oncol. Biol. Phys.* **71** 866–72

Folkard M, Prise K M, Voijnovic B *et al* 1996 Inactivation of V79 cells by low-energy protons, deuterons and helium-3 ions *Int. J. Radiat. Biol.* **69** 729–38

Furusawa Y, Fukutsu K, Aoki M *et al* 2000 Inactivation of aerobic and hypoxic cells from three different cell lines by accelerated (3)He-, (12)C- and (20)Ne-ion beams *Radiat. Res.* **154** 485–96
Erratum in: 2012 *Radiat. Res* **177** 129–31

Grassberger C, Trofimov A, Lomax A and Paganetti H 2011 Variations in linear energy transfer within clinical proton therapy fields and the potential for biological treatment planning *Int. J. Radiat. Oncol. Biol. Phys.* **80** 1559–66

Grün R, Friedrich T, Krämer M *et al* 2015 Assessment of potential advantages of relevant ions for particle therapy: a model based study *Med. Phys.* **42** 1037–47

Hall E J and Giaccia A 2011 *Radiobiology for the Radiologist* 7th edn (Lippincott) chs 6 and 7

Hall E J and Giaccia A J 2019 Linear energy transfer and relative biological effectiveness *Radiobiology for the Radiologist* ed E J Hall and A J Giaccia (Wolters Kluwer) ch 7 pp 105–6

Hawkins R B 2003 A microdosimetric-kinetic model for the effect of non-Poisson distribution of lethal lesions on the variation of RBE with LET *Radiat. Res.* **160** 61–9

Hawkins R B 2009 The relationship between the sensitivity of cells to high-energy photons and the RBE of particle radiation used in radiotherapy *Radiat. Res.* **172** 761–76

Inaniwa T, Suzuki M, Furukawa T *et al* 2013 Effects of dose-delivery time structure on biological effectiveness for therapeutic carbon-ion beams evaluated with microdosimetric kinetic model *Radiat. Res. Jul* **180** 44–59

Jones B, Carabe-Fernandez A and Dale R G 2007 Chapter: the oxygen effect *Radiobiological Modelling in Radiation Oncology* (London: British Institute of Radiology) pp 138–57

Jones B 2010 The apparent increase in the β-parameter of the linear quadratic model with increased linear energy transfer during particle irradiation *Br. J. Radiol.* **83** 433–6

Jones B, Underwood T C, Carabe-Fernandez A and Dale R G 2011 Further analysis of fast neutron relative biological effects and implications for charged particle therapy *Br. J. Radiol.* **84** S11–8

Jones B 2015a Towards achieving the full clinical potential of proton therapy by inclusion of LET and RBE models *Cancers (Basel).* **7** 460–80

Jones B 2015b A Simpler energy transfer efficiency model to predict relative biological effect (RBE) for protons and heavier ions *Front. Oncol.* **5** 184
Erratum in: 2016 *Front Oncol.* **6** 32

Jones B and Hill M A 2019 Physical characteristics at the turnover-points of relative biological effect (RBE) with linear energy transfer (LET) *Phys. Med. Biol.* **64** 225010

Jones B and Hill M A 2020 The physical separation between the LET associated with the ultimate relative biological effect (RBE) and the maximum LET in a proton or ion beam *Biomed. Phys. Eng. Express* **6** 055001

Jones B 2021 Fast neutron energy based modelling of biological effectiveness with implications for proton and ion beams *Phys. Med. Biol.* **14** 045028

Jones B 2022 The influence of hypoxia on LET and RBE relationships with implications for ultra-high dose rates and FLASH modelling *Phys. Med. Biol.* **67** 125011

Kase Y, Kanai T, Matsufuji N *et al* 2008 Biophysical calculation of cell survival probabilities using amorphous track structure models for heavy-ion irradiation *Phys. Med. Biol.* **53** 37–59

Katz R, Ackerson B, Homoyooufar M and Sharma S C 1971 Inactivation of cells by heavy ion bombardment *Radiat. Res.* **47** 402–25

Newhauser W D and Zhang R 2015 The physics of proton therapy *Phys. Med. Biol.* **60** R155–209

Sørensen B S, Overgaard J and Bassler N 2011 *In vitro* RBE-LET dependence for multiple particle types *Acta Oncol.* **50** 757–62

Todd P 1967 Heavy-ion irradiation of cultured human cells *Radiat. Res.* **7** 196–207

Warenius H M, Britten R A, Browning P G, Morton I E and Peacock J H 1994 Identification of human *in vitro* cell lines with greater intrinsic cellular radiosensitivity to 62.5 MeV (p-->Be+) neutrons than 4 MeV photons *Int. J. Radiat. Oncol. Biol. Phys.* **28** 913–20

Weyrather W K, Ritter S, Scholz M and Kraft G 1999 RBE for carbon track-segment irradiation in cell lines of differing repair capacity *Int. J. Radiat. Biol.* **75** 1357–64

Wilkens J J and Oelfke U 2004 A phenomenological model for the relative biological effectiveness in therapeutic proton beams *Phys. Med. Biol.* **49** 2811–25

Ziegler J F, Biersack J P and Ziegler M D 2008 *SRIM—The Stopping and Range of Ions in Matter* (Chester, MD: SRIM Co.) ch 3 and 4

IOP Publishing

Quantitative Radiobiology for Proton Therapy

Bleddyn Jones

Chapter 9

Inclusion of the energy-efficiency LET and RBE model in proton therapy

The energy-efficiency model presented in the previous chapter is used to estimate proton relative biological effect (RBE) values for a range of relevant linear energy transfer (LET) values which may occur within a spread-out Bragg peak (SOBP), with results presented as graphics of RBE with dose per fraction and as convenient tables with estimated statistical ranges of RBE values for different α/β values representing normal tissues and tumours. A graphical user interface for LET-RBE estimation is included. The isoeffective doses for different tissues may then be ascertained, and the values obtained may alert the physicist and clinician as to the need to change a treatment plan or reduce the proton dose weighting, or the prescribed dose itself. This approach is intended to make proton therapy safer and more effective by using a rational model for predicting RBE, rather than the untenable fixed RBE of 1.1 method which is error prone in late-reacting normal tissues if the actual RBE exceeds 1.1, but depending also on the degree of dose sparing advantage achieved. In situations where there is clinical concern, newer ways of presenting three-dimensional LET and RBE distributions need to be sought. The full potential of proton therapy will only be realised when this inherent RBE problem is eliminated as far as possible.

9.1 Introduction

Radiotherapy has evolved empirically, with most technical developments contributing to better clinical outcomes as either a better cure rate or reduced complication rate, or both. There are some exceptions to this, such as the increment in dose rate for brachytherapy purposes and fast neutron therapy, where clinical results were on the whole less than satisfactory.

The fundamental distinction between early and late tissue reactions, and their different fractionation sensitivities and dose ranges are important, and they provide limits to prescribed doses. Recent recognition that late vascular damage is responsible for many chronic effects of radiation and that the relative risk of

doi:10.1088/978-0-7503-6209-2ch9

radiation-induced coronary artery disease is estimated to be around 7.5% per Gy (Darby *et al* 2013), as well as the established cancer induction risks of at least 5% per Sv (Hall & Giaccia 2011), has led to a logical requirement for radiation beams that can markedly reduce the integral dose and so the amount of tissue traversed. This is achievable with positively charged particle beams such as protons and light ions, due to their reduced path length in tissues caused by the Bragg peak effect.

Technical developments in radiotherapy need careful assessment of their biological effects, since intended gains can occur along with subtle or even major disadvantages. In the case of proton-beam therapy (PBT), concerns remain about the lack of published evidence showing clear-cut improvements in outcomes. Many overviews point out the paucity of publications which show no obvious improvements in terms of tumour control and/or late normal tissue complications, as well as the lack of high-level medical evidence using randomised studies. Justification that proton therapy is safe, by using only paediatric data such as medulloblastoma (Yock *et al* 2016, Grosshans 2016) and some cases of ependymoma, should not be extrapolated to adult treatments. This is because lower prescribed doses of highly fractionated treatment (such as 30–35 Gy, which are well below the threshold for serious complications such as spinal myelitis and brain necrosis) are used in treating this tumour type in some regions, e.g. the whole brain and spinal cord. The present author is aware of considerable confusion amongst physicists who remember that doses of up to 60 Gy can be given for some of these conditions; but such doses are confined to the tumour itself, with a small additional margin only in order not to precipitate radionecrosis.

These concerns have received further support from some publications. There are reports of higher than expected radiological changes in ependymoma and meningioma patients after proton therapy (Peeler *et al* 2016, R. Mohan, personal communication), as well as markedly increased fibrosis occurring at the distal portions of proton spread-out Bragg peaks (SOBPs), compatible with RBE values of 3–4, which recalls the values found with fast neutrons (Underwood & Paganetti 2016). Also, there is some concern within the clinical community regarding results published from Switzerland's prestigious Paul Scherrer Institute laboratory, with serious neurological toxicity (blindness and cortical brain necrosis) as high as around 12.3% (Weber *et al* 2016), a result that would not be tolerated with photon-based therapy, where protocols are designed not to allow more than 1%–2% risks, and often aim for below this range, while being capable of delivering high tumour doses using modern photon techniques. In addition, the long-term results of children treated with protons in Japan show a significant rate of late complications: the grade 3 or higher late toxicities were 6%, 17% and 17% at 5, 10 and 20 years, respectively (Mizumoto *et al* 2016). As far as tumour control rates are concerned there is no clear-cut advantage from the use of protons for intracranial tumours, as reviewed by Combs (2017). Further clinical examples are given below.

Another barrier appears to be that Bragg peak placement issues seem to dominate discussions in physics-led meetings, with minimal attention to the radiobiological uncertainties, so that it becomes difficult to determine the cause of toxicity or failure to cure, even though both mechanisms may contribute in some particular cases. Realistic assessment of both is required, but it cannot be disputed that the range of known variation in RBE far exceeds that of Bragg peak positioning. This aspect must also be understood by the inevitable fact that displacement of Bragg peak position away from the International Commission on Radiation Units and Measurements (ICRU) target volumes might increase normal tissue toxicity outside the defined planning target volume (or PTV), but would be expected to be accompanied by reduced tumour control: there is no evidence that this has occurred, so it is reasonable to invoke RBE as being the main culprit.

RBE is of paramount importance since it determines the dose given to the patient in equivalent-Gy. Essentially, if the RBE is incorrect the proton dose may be too low or too high, with consequent effects in each patient.

RBE depends on multiple factors, as discussed in the previous chapter. This multi-factorial basis of RBE implies that it cannot be a constant value, but must be a continuous variable (as is height and weight in humans). Particularly relevant are the radiobiological properties of the control low LET of conventional megavoltage radiotherapy, which govern the numerator of the RBE definition. Report 16 of the ICRU (1970) states that the mean LET for megavoltage radiations (electrons and photons) is around 0.2–0.3 keV μm^{-1}. From the shapes of the cell-survival or bioeffect curves at low and high LET, it is inevitable that the numerator dose of the RBE ratio will increase to a greater extent than the denominator dose for a given isoeffect when dose per fraction is changed. An idealised example of cell survival isoeffects can be seen in figure 1.3 in chapter 1.

Proton therapy has two potential Achilles heels (unlike only one susceptible heel in the original Homeric poem). They are (1) physical dose placement uncertainty and (2) biological effect (RBE) uncertainties. First it is necessary to describe some of the physical uncertainties before considering the RBE issues in greater detail. The physical issues have already been discussed in chapter 1.

9.2 RBE uncertainties

The RBE concept is so often either misunderstood or underestimated in terms of complexity. It is vital to understand its multi-factorial dependency, already listed above. All clinicians should understand that if the RBE is incorrect, so also will be the dose given to the patient, sometimes by a percentage change that could exceed normally acceptable treatment plan dose variations, or the legally permitted range of dose due to errors in beam delivery (Dale *et al* 2009). RBE also has an impact on proton range uncertainties (Carabe *et al* 2012). A reported reduction in RBE at long range (Calugaru *et al* 2011) is possibly connected with the increasingly separating tracks, as discussed in chapter 1, and has important implications which need further experimentation (see chapters 11 and 14).

Proton RBEs have similarities with those for heavier ions than protons, but with some differences in scale. High proton RBEs have been found in various experiments, in high-LET parts of the beam (Belli *et al* 2000, Britten *et al* 2013, Marshall *et al* 2016). Also, the rise in RBE per unit increase in LET is larger at lower LET values for protons compared to all heavier ions (probably because of the smaller Katz radius of ionisation associated with each track; see chapter 1), which is directly proportional to the nuclear charge (Z), and protons have the lowest Z number of 1. So, protons are more efficient at increasing RBE at lower values of LET. This causes the turnover of RBE with LET at around 30.5 in Belli's experiments, rather than at between 100–120 and 180–220 keV μm^{-1} for protons, helium and carbon ions, respectively, as shown in the previous chapter. The potential for high RBE values occurring at deceptively low LET values consequently arises.

The essential clinical features of RBE are its inevitable dependency on LET, dose and tumour/tissue type. Changes in proton RBE with dose per fraction and tissue type have not been as extensively researched when compared with the range of experimental systems used for fast neutrons. In the latter case there was a clear dependency on tissue type: fast-proliferating, acute-reacting tissues (with high α/β ratios) had much smaller changes in RBE with dose than were the case for far more slowly proliferating, late-reacting tissues (with low α/β ratios) (Carabe-Fernandez *et al* 2007, 2010). The collected proton experiments, and the expedient decision to allocate an overall RBE of 1.1, representing a median value, to all tissues and tumours (regardless of their α/β ratio) is discussed in chapter 7; in order for proton therapy to improve, this must be reconsidered. This should be coupled with more detailed experimental studies and analysis of human clinical outcomes, including radiological changes in normal tissues for LET-RBE effects.

9.3 Description of the quantitative model

To determine the RBE, the same equations as in the preceding chapter 8 are used, but with a proton Z number of 1. Further details can be found in two publications (Jones 2015a, 2017) concerning the link between the low-LET reference values for α and β and their high-LET counterparts, and in the supplementary data in the most recent reference.

The efficiency of cell killing, in terms of the α and β parameters, are both assumed to rise linearly with LET to a maximum at around 30.5 keV μm^{-1}, as seen in figure 9.1, and to a maximum level which is related to the low-LET (reference, or control radiation) α and β parameters (respectively termed α_L and β_L, but where α/β is used it will refer to the low-LET state). The model considers increments in α and β that are proportional to LET, but using a saturation effect which limits the maximum possible increase in α and β, as given in the previous chapter. Some comments regarding the value of 30.5 keV μm^{-1} are given in Jones (2019) especially the comments of Dr P O'Neill regarding proton ranges, since at this and high LET values the particle range can become insufficient to reach the cellular nucleus in experimental conditions when using monoenergetic protons. Contrasting data using fast neutrons (see chapter 5) suggest that the proton LET_U should be round 62 keV μm^{-1}, but this would be in a beam where protons are being released stochastically along neutron tracks and so at any point within a cell such that range restrictions will not be as applicable.

Since the proton LET–RBE turnover point (defined as LET_U) is at 30.5 keV μm^{-1} (Belli *et al* 2000), and the increments in RBE (and consequently the radiosensitivity parameters) with LET appear to be linear (Belli *et al* 2000, Sørensen *et al* 2011), then with increasing dose the overall RBE will fall in proportion to the shift between the high-LET α and β parameters as shown in figure 9.2 (a more complete version of this graphic is given as figure 8.1 in chapter 8).

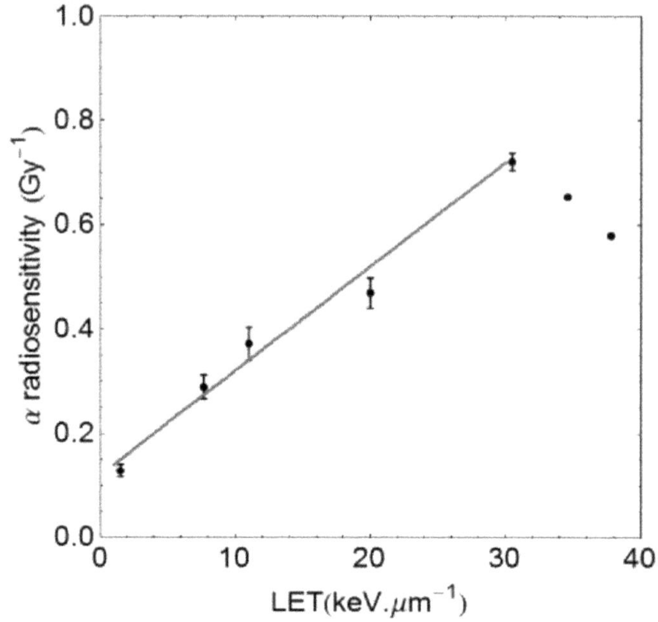

Figure 9.1. Data of Belli *et al* showing α rising linearly with linear energy transfer (LET). The least-squares fitted line is $\alpha_H = 0.12 + 0.02$ LET for data points below 31 keV μm^{-1}, which will only be the case for the strain of V-79 cells used, where 0.12 Gy^{-1} is the control low-LET α_L value.

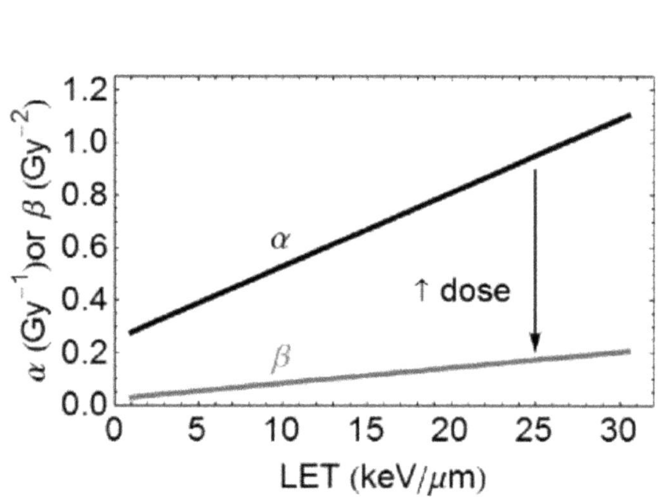

Figure 9.2. Schematic diagram of the linear increase change in α and β with LET. Increasing dose will increase the proportion of β-mediated cell kill and so cause a lower overall RBE (itself determined by the increments in α (changing RBE_{max}) and in β (changing RBE_{min}), and so the relative proportions of RBE_{max} and RBE_{min} which contribute to the overall RBE at any value of LET within this range. The increase in β with LET is always smaller than that in α. So, with increasing dose the overall RBE follows the direction of the arrow. The numbers used in this figure are not intended to represent any particular cell system.

The model outputs, using a baseline (control) LET of 0.22 keV μm^{-1} for megavoltage photons, are now displayed in the form of figures 9.3(a)–(e), where the fixed parameter was $\beta = 0.03$ Gy^{-2} (at the reference low LET), and tables 9.1–9.5, where stochastic estimates are obtained by assuming mean α values of 0.07 Gy^{-1} for a α/β of 2 and 3 Gy for late-reacting normal tissues, and reference radiation α values of 0.275, 0.375 and 0.55 Gy^{-1} for tumours with α/β ratios of, respectively, 4.5, 10 and 25 Gy. In all cases a standard deviation of 10% of the mean was used in Mathematica for random-sampling procedures using 1000 samples, from which the mean RBE and the 1% and 99% quantile ranges were found.

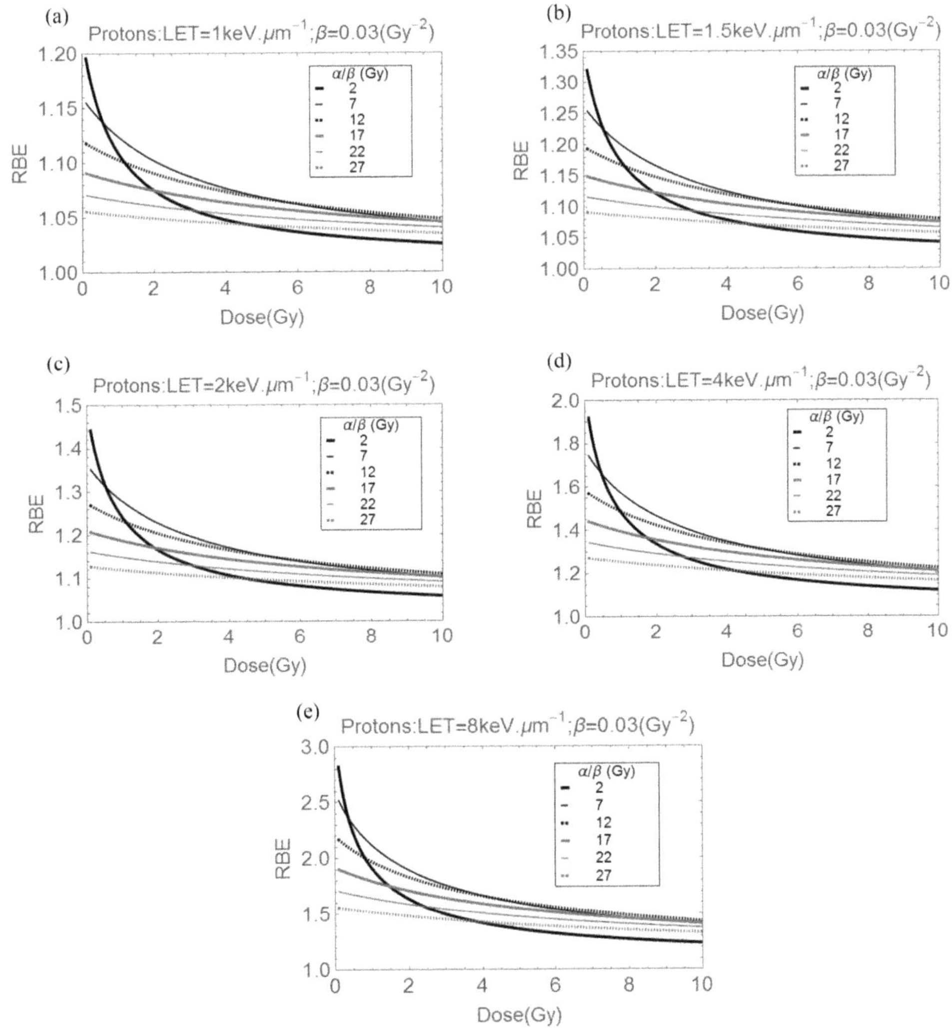

Figure 9.3. (a)–(e) Plots of proton RBE with dose per fraction at specified LET values.

Table 9.1. $\alpha/\beta = 2$ Gy: central nervous system late effects with mean $\alpha = 0.07$ Gy^{-1} (SD = 0.02).

Dose (Gy)	LET = 1	LET = 1.25	LET = 1.5	LET = 1.75	LET = 2.0	LET = 4.0	LET = 8.0
$d = 1.25$	1.10 (1.08, 1.11)	1.12 (1.08, 1.14)	1.15 (1.13, 1.18)	1.18 (1.16, 1.21)	1.21 (1.18, 1.24)	1.42 (1.37, 1.48)	1.80 (1.7, 1.9)
$d = 1.5$	1.09 (1.07, 1.10)	1.11 (1.10, 1.13)	1.14 (1.12, 1.16)	1.17 (1.14, 1.19)	1.19 (1.16,1.22)	1.38 (1.33,1.44)	1.72 (1.63, 1.82)
$d = 1.8$	1.08 (1.07, 1.09)	1.10 (1.09, 1.12)	1.13 (1.11, 1.15)	1.15 (1.13, 1.17)	1.17 (1.15, 1.20)	1.35 (1.30, 1.40)	1.66 (1.57, 1.75)
$d = 2$	1.07 (1.06, 1.09)	1.10 (1.08, 1.11)	1.12 (1.10, 1.14)	1.14 (1.12,1.16)	1.16 (1.14, 1.19)	1.33 (1.28, 1.38)	1.62 (1.53, 1.71)
$d = 2.5$	1.06 (1.05, 1.08)	1.08 (1.07, 1.10)	1.10 (1.09, 1.12)	1.12 (1.10, 1.15)	1.14 (1.12, 1.17)	1.29 (1.24, 1.34)	1.54 (1.46, 1.64)
$d = 3$	1.06 (1.05, 1.07)	1.07 (1.06, 1.09)	1.09 (1.07, 1.11)	1.11 (1.09, 1.13)	1.13 (1.10, 1.15)	1.25 (1.21, 1.31)	1.48 (1.41, 1.58)
$d = 5$	1.04 (1.03, 1.05)	1.05 (1.04, 1.07)	1.06 (1.05, 10.8)	1.08 (1.06, 1.10)	1.09 (1.07, 1.11)	1.18 (1.14, 1.23)	1.35 (1.28, 1.44)
$d = 10$	1.02 (1.01, 1.03)	1.03 (1.02, 10.5)	1.04 (1.03, 1.06)	1.05 (1.03, 1.07)	1.05 (1.04, 1.08)	1.11 (1.08, 1.12)	1.22 (1.15, 1.31)
$d = 12.5$	1.02 (1.01, 1.03)	1.03 (1.02, 1.04)	1.03 (1.02, 1.05)	1.04 (1.02, 1.06)	1.05 (1.03, 1.07)	1.10 (1.06, 1.15)	1.19 (1.12, 1.28)

SD = standard deviation, d = dose per fraction (Gy), LET= linear energy transfer (keV.μm^{-1}).

Table 9.2. $\alpha/\beta = 3$ Gy: general normal tissue late effects with mean $\alpha = 0.07$ Gy^{-1} (SD = 0.02).

Dose (Gy)	LET = 1	LET = 1.25	LET = 1.5	LET = 1.75	LET = 2.0	LET = 4.0	LET = 8.0
$d = 1.25$	1.12 (1.10, 1.13)	1.15 (1.13, 1.17)	1.19 (1.17, 1.21)	1.23 (1.20, 1.25)	1.26 (1.23, 1.29)	1.52 (1.46, 1.58)	1.98 (1.88, 2.09)
$d = 1.5$	1.11 (1.09, 1.12)	1.14 (1.12, 1.16)	1.18 (1.15, 1.20)	1.21 (1.18, 1.23)	1.24 (1.21, 1.27)	1.48 (1.42, 1.54)	1.91 (1.80, 2.01)
$d = 1.8$	1.10 (1.09, 1.11)	1.13 (1.11, 1.15)	1.16 (1.14, 1.18)	1.19 (1.17, 1.22)	1.22 (1.19, 1.25)	1.44 (1.39, 1.50)	1.83 (1.73, 1.93)
$d = 2$	1.09 (1.08, 1.11)	1.12 (1.11, 1.14)	1.15 (1.13, 1.17)	1.18 (1.16, 1.20)	1.21 (1.18, 1.24)	1.42, (1.37, 1.47)	1.79 (1.69, 1.88)

(Continued)

Table 9.2. (*Continued*)

Dose (Gy)	LET = 1	LET = 1.25	LET = 1.5	LET = 1.75	LET = 2.0	LET = 4.0	LET = 8.0
$d = 2.5$	1.08 (1.07, 1.10)	1.11 (1.09, 1.13)	1.14 (1.12, 1.16)	1.16 (1.14, 1.18)	1.19 (1.16, 1.21)	1.37 (1.32, 1.43)	1.70 (1.61, 1.79)
$d = 3$	1.08 (1.06, 1.09)	1.10 (1.08, 1.11)	1.12 (1.10, 1.14)	1.15 (1.12, 1.17)	1.17 (1.14, 1.19)	1.34 (1.29, 1.39)	1.64 (1.55, 1.73)
$d = 5$	1.06 (1.05, 1.07)	1.07 (1.06, 1.09)	1.09 (1.07, 1.10)	1.11 (1.09, 1.13)	1.13 (1.10, 1.50)	1.25 (1.21, 1.30)	1.48 (1.40, 1.56)
$d = 10$	1.04 (1.03, 1.05)	1.05 (1.04, 1.06)	1.06 (1.04, 1.07)	1.07 (1.05, 1.09)	1.08 (1.06, 1.10)	1.17 (1.13, 1.21)	1.32 (1.25, 1.40)
$d = 12.5$	1.03 (1.02, 1.04)	1.04 (1.03, 1.05)	1.05 (1.04, 1.07)	1.06 (1.04, 1.08)	1.07 (1.05, 1.09)	1.15 (1.11, 1.19)	1.28 (1.21, 1.36)

Table 9.3. $\alpha/\beta = 4.5$ Gy: tumours with mean $\alpha = 0.275$ Gy^{-1} (SD = 0.0275).

Dose (Gy)	LET = 1	LET = 1.25	LET = 1.5	LET = 1.75	LET = 2.0	LET = 4.0	LET = 8.0
$d = 1.25$	1.09 (1.08, 1.10)	1.12 (1.10, 1.13)	1.14 (1.12, 1.16)	1.17 (1.15, 1.20)	1.20 (1.17, 1.23)	1.41 (1.35, 1.46)	1.79 (1.69, 1.89)
$d = 1.5$	1.08 (1.07, 1.09)	1.11 (1.09, 1.12)	1.13 (1.11, 1.15)	1.16 (1.14, 1.18)	1.19 (1.16, 1.21)	1.38 (1.33, 1.43)	1.73 (1.64, 1.82)
$d = 1.8$	1.08 (1.07, 1.09)	1.10 (1.09, 1.11)	1.12 (1.11, 1.14)	1.15 (1.13, 1.17)	1.17 (1.15, 1.19)	1.35 (1.30, 1.40)	1.68 (1.59, 1.76)
$d = 2$	1.07 (1.06, 1.08)	1.10 (1.08, 1.11)	1.12 (1.10, 1.14)	1.14 (1.12. 1.16)	1.16 (1.14, 1.19)	1.33 (1.29, 1.38)	1.64 (1.56, 1.73)
$d = 2.5$	1.07 (1.06, 1.08)	1.09 (1.07, 1.11)	1.11 (1.09, 1.12)	1.13 (1.11, 1.14)	1.15 (1.12, 1.17)	1.30 (1.26, 1.34)	1.58 (1.50, 1.65)
$d = 3$	1.06 (1.05, 1.07)	1.08 (1.07, 1.09)	1.10 (1.08, 1.11)	1.11 (1.10, 1.13)	1.13 (1.11, 1.15)	1.27 (1,23, 1.31)	1.52 (1.49, 1.59)
$d = 5$	1.04 (1.03, 1.05)	1.06 (1.05, 1.07)	1.07 (1.06, 1.08)	1.08 (1.07, 1.10)	1.10 (1.08, 1.11)	1.20 (1.17, 1.23)	1.38 (1.33, 1.44)
$d = 10$	1.03 (1.02, 1.03)	1.03 (1.03, 1.04)	1.04 (1.03, 1.05)	1.05 (1.04, 1.06)	1.06 (1.04, 1.07)	1.12 (1.09, 1.14)	1.23 (1.19, 1.28)
$d = 12.5$	1.02 (1.02, 1.03)	1.03 (1.02, 1.03)	1.03 (1.03, 1.04)	1.04 (1.03, 1.05)	1.05 (1.04, 1.06)	1.10 (1.08, 1.12)	1.19 (1.15, 1.23)

Table 9.4. $\alpha/\beta = 10$ Gy: moderately radiosensitive tumours with mean $\alpha = 0.375$ Gy^{-1} (SD = 0.0375).

Dose (Gy)	LET = 1	LET = 1.25	LET = 1.5	LET = 1.75	LET = 2.0	LET = 4.0	LET = 8.0
$d = 1.25$	1.09 (1.8, 1.11)	1.12 (1.10, 1.14)	1.15 (1.13, 1.18)	1.18 (1.15, 1.21)	1.21 (1.18, 1.25)	1.44 (1.37, 1.51)	1.87 (1.73, 2.01)
$d = 1.5$	1.09 (1.07, 1.11)	1.12 (1.11, 1.14)	1.15 (1.12, 1.17)	1.18 (1.15, 1.21)	1.20 (1.17, 1.24)	1.42 (1.35, 1.49)	1.83 (1.70, 1.96)
$d = 1.8$	1.09 (1.07, 1.10)	1.11 (1.09, 1.13)	1.14 (1.12, 1.16)	1.17 (1.14, 1.20)	1.19 (1.16, 1.23)	1.40 (1.34, 1.47)	1.79 (1.66, 1.92)
$d = 2$	1.08 (1.07, 1.10)	1.11 (1.09, 1.13)	1.14 (1.11, 1.16)	1.16 (1.14, 1.19)	1.19 (1.16, 1.22)	1.39 (1.33, 1.45)	1.76 (1.64, 1.89)
$d = 2.5$	1.08 (1.07, 1.09)	1.09 (1.10, 1.12)	1.13 (1.11, 1.15)	1.15 (1.13, 1.18)	1.18 (1.15, 1.20)	1.36 (1.30, 1.42)	1.71 (1.60, 1.82)
$d = 3$	1.07 (1.06, 1.09)	1.10 (1.08, 1.11)	1.12 (1.10, 1.14)	1.14 (1.12, 1.17)	1.17 (1.14, 1.20)	1.34 (1.28, 1.40)	1.66 (1.55, 1.77)
$d = 5$	1.06 (1.05, 1.07)	1.08 (1.06, 1.09)	1.10 (1.08, 1.11)	1.12 (1.10, 1.14)	1.13 (1.11, 1.16)	1.28 (1.23, 1.32)	1.54 (1.45, 1.62)
$d = 10$	1.04 (1.03, 1.05)	1.05 (1.04, 1.07)	1.07 (1.05, 1.08)	1.08 (1.06, 1.10)	1.09 (1.08, 1.11)	1.19 (1.16, 1.23)	1.37 (1.30, 1.44)
$d = 12.5$	1.04 (1.03, 1.04)	1.05 (1.04, 1.06)	1.06 (1.05, 1.07)	1.07 (1.06, 1.08)	1.08 (1.06, 1.10)	1.17 (1.14, 1.20)	1.33 (1.27, 1.39)

Table 9.5. $\alpha/\beta = 25$ Gy: very radiosensitive tumours with mean $\alpha = 0.55$ Gy^{-1} (SD = 0.055).

Dose (Gy)	LET = 1	LET = 1.25	LET = 1.5	LET = 1.75	LET = 2.0	LET = 4.0	LET = 8.0
$d = 1.25$	1.08 (1.06, 1.10)	1.10 (1.08, 1.13)	1.13 (1.10, 1.16)	1.15 (1.12, 1.19)	1.18 (1.14, 1.22)	1.38 (1.30, 1.47)	1.77 (1.60–1.94)
$d = 1.5$	1.08 (1.06, 1.10)	1.10 (1.08, 1.13)	1.13 (1.10, 1.16)	1.15 (1.12, 1.19)	1.18 (1.14, 1.22)	1.37 (1.29, 1.46)	1.75 (1.59, 1.92)
$d = 1.8$	1.08 (1.06, 1.09)	1.10 (1.08, 1.12)	1.13 (1.10, 1.15)	1.15 (1.12, 1.18)	1.17 (1.14, 1.21)	1.37 (1.29, 1.45)	1.73 (1.58, 1.90)
$d = 2$	1.08 (1.06, 1.09)	1.10 (1.08, 1.12)	1.12 (1.10, 1.15)	1.15 (1.11, 1.18)	1.17 (1.13, 1.21)	1.36 (1.28, 1.44)	1.72 (1.57, 1.88)

(*Continued*)

Table 9.5. (*Continued*)

Dose (Gy)	LET = 1	LET = 1.25	LET = 1.5	LET = 1.75	LET = 2.0	LET = 4.0	LET = 8.0
$d = 2.5$	1.07 (1.06, 1.09)	1.10 (1.08, 1.12)	1.12 (1.09, 1.15)	1.14 (1.11, 1.18)	1.17 (1.13, 1.20)	1.35 (1.27, 1.43)	1.69 (1.55, 1.85)
$d = 3$	1.07 (1.06, 1.09)	1.09 (1.07, 1.12)	1.12 (1.09, 1.14)	1.14 (1.11, 1.17)	1.16 (1.13, 1.20)	1.34 (1.26, 1.41)	1.67 (1.53, 1.82)
$d = 5$	1.06 (1.05, 1.08)	1.08 (1.07, 1.10)	1.10 (1.08, 1.13)	1.12 (1.10, 1.15)	1.14 (1.11, 1.18)	1.30 (1.24, 1.37)	1.59 (1.47, 1.72)
$d = 10$	1.05 (1.04, 1.06)	1.07 (1.05, 1.08)	1.08 (1.07, 1.10)	1.10 (1.08, 1.12)	1.12 (1.09, 1.14)	1.24 (1.19, 1.30)	1.47 (1.38, 1.58)
$d = 12.5$	1.05 (1.04, 1.06)	1.06 (1.05, 1.08)	1.08 (1.06, 1.10)	1.09 (1.07, 1.11)	1.11 (1.08, 1.13)	1.22 (1.17, 1.27)	1.44 (1.35, 1.53)

The steps taken to estimate the RBE are as follows. The RBE calculation is based on the following scaling approach, an extension of the approach taken by Wilkens & Oelfke (2004) as in Jones (2015b, 2017), which includes the relevant parameters:

$$\alpha_H = \alpha_L + \frac{\text{LET}x - \text{LET}_C}{\text{LET}_U - \text{LET}c}.\ \alpha_U - \alpha_L,$$

$$\beta_H = \beta_L + \frac{\text{LET}x - \text{LET}_C}{\text{LET}_U - \text{LET}c}.\ \beta_U - \beta_L.$$

With LET_U, the slope of α and β with LET is found from the maximum radiosensitivity values:

$$\alpha_U = Q/j(1 - \exp[-j.\ \alpha L]),$$

and

$$\beta_U = (R/u).\ (1 - \exp[-u\ \beta L]).$$

If LET_U is not known, then use the highest available LET (let this be LET_S, and use this to replace LET_U, provided the radiosensitivity values at LET_S are known, which then replace α_U and β_U).

RBE is obtained by solving for d_L in the general isoeffect equation:
$\alpha_L\, d_L + \beta_L\, {d_L}^2 = \alpha_H\, d_H + \beta_H\, {d_H}^2$, and then dividing by the d_{H} to give

$$\text{RBE} = \frac{-\alpha_L + \sqrt{\alpha_L^2 + 4\alpha_H\beta_L d_H + 4\beta_H\beta_L d_H^2}}{(2\beta_L.\ d_H)}.$$

As an alternative to these tables, and with greater flexibility in terms of input parameter choices, as well as allowing LET and dose per fraction values on a continuous scale rather than discrete values, the graphical user interface used in the previous chapter 8 can be modified for estimating proton RBEs and for isoeffective dose calculations (figure 9.3 and tables 9.1–9.4).

These tabulated estimates and those in figures 9.3(a)–(e) all show increasing RBE with LET and an inverse relationship between RBE and dose per fraction. Greater complexity is introduced by varying the α/β ratios. It again can be seen that increases in LET above, say, 1.5 keV μm^{-1} can be accompanied by significant increments in RBE. The lowest α/β ratio systems give the largest RBE at near-zero dose, but then the values fall sharply, the rate of change depending on α/β. High-α/β systems have much flatter curves, showing less variation in RBE with dose per fraction. The curves cross over such that larger RBE values can exist for systems with high α/β ratios compared with low α/β ratios when dose per fraction is sufficiently large; it is important to note that the lowest RBE values then occur in the most fraction-sensitive tissues, suggesting that high dose per fraction can be relatively protective. This is because of enhanced repair capacity and fraction sensitivity in the case of low α/β ratios for the photon (numerator) part of the RBE definition and the converse for the high-LET denominator dose. Also, cells with low α/β, with the highest RBE_{max}, will asymptotically approach RBE_{min} with dose at a faster rate owing to the higher proportion of β-related cell killing than in cells where α/β is high.

Many of the RBE values shown exceed the conventional value of 1.1. Of particular concern is that for low-α/β systems such as brain spinal cord and late reactions, the RBE values are highest when dose per fraction is small. This finding represents a warning to clinicians, who should consider either using a suitably modified RBE or changing the tolerance of key organs at risk in such situations. Recognition of changes of RBE with tissue and tumour α/β ratios, and appropriate use of these ratios to the clinical setting will be important in PBT.

The method of estimation has assumed firm knowledge of the LET_U value for protons. The sensitivity of this value is considered in chapter 14. Should the slope of the radiosensitivities, or RBE, with increasing LET be known by experiment or clinical data, it would be possible to estimate the RBE more directly, as mentioned in chapter 8 (section 3.5). Without such data, the more generic method has to be pursued, or alternative approaches based on the low-LET α/β ratio, although such a method may incur some inaccuracies for high dose per fraction if β is assumed to be invariant with LET.

9.4 RBE graphical examples

Interactive graphics for respectively estimating proton RBE with dose per fraction and for estimating the degree of normal tissue sparing required for a defined BED isoeffect for different LET values are given in figures 9.4 and 9.5.

By solving for clinically relevant isoeffects (50 Gy in 25 fractions for spinal cord and optic chiasm, etc., and 60 Gy in 30 fractions for cortical brain) in the

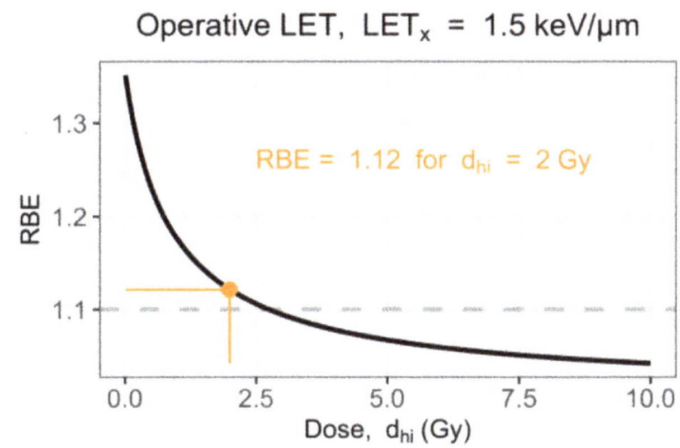

Figure 9.4. RBE as a function of proton physical dose, d_{hi}. The dashed line highlights a constant value of RBE = 1.1. The orange point on the RBE curve corresponds to the respective RBE value for a given dose, shown with a default d_{hi} = 2 Gy here. For a fully interactive version of this figure can be found at the link https://josh-will-moore.shinyapps.io/InteractivePlots_Jones_IOP/, where input variable may be changed on the relevant cursors. Credit: Joshua Moore.

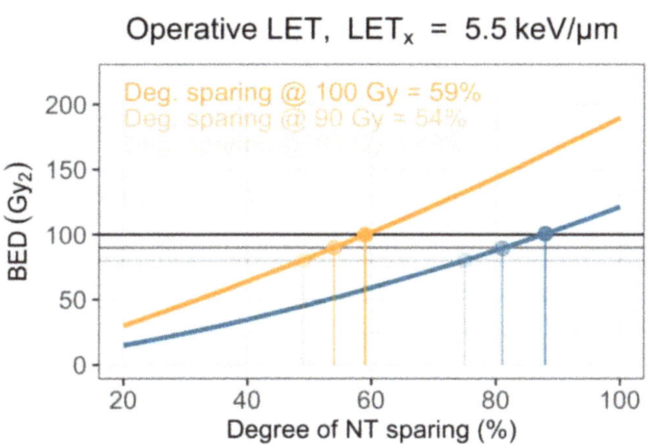

Figure 9.5. The relationship of the central nervous system biological effective dose (for BED values appropriate for spinal cord, optic chiasm and brain stem tolerances) and the degree of proton-beam normal tissue sparing with variable operative LET values. The three horizontal lines show BED levels of 100, 90 and 80 Gy[2], in order to represent different levels of CNS tissue radiotolerance according to medical histories. Higher tolerance levels are sometimes permitted for small irradiated volumes according to local protocols. For a fully interactive version of this figure, see https://josh-will-moore.shinyapps.io/InteractivePlots_Jones_IOP/. Credit: Joshua Moore.

biological effective dose (BED) equations with LET-RBE effects included (see chapter 6), the total doses required to maintain each isoeffect are given in figures 9.6(a) and (b), respectively.

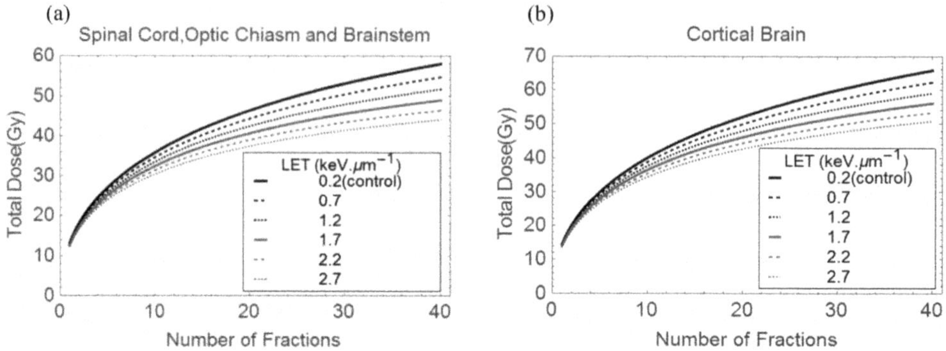

Figure 9.6. (a) and (b): Estimated total dose and number of fractions isoeffective with (a) 50 Gy in 25 fractions, and (b) 60 Gy in 30 fractions for the control megavoltage photon (x-ray) treatment with a LET of 0.2 keV μm^{-1}. The reduction of total dose to maintain these isoeffects are plotted for different LET values commonly encountered in proton therapy.

9.5 Some comparisons with experimental data sets

The data from Britten *et al* (2013) were used to compare experimentally determined RBE values with model predictions, with results shown in table 9.6 (where only the slope of the radiosenstivities is used, with β being extremely small) and table 9.7 (where the full LET_U and α_U assumptions are used). Because the RBE values were published as cobalt-equivalent RBE at 0.1 survival fraction using a simple 1.2 conversion from the 120 KeV x-rays control radiation data, the unmodified data were used since the 1.2 figure scould be erroneous. The problem then arises as to what was the most relevant value of LET in the control beam, there being no mention of filtration. The estimated RBE will depend on this value, and 1 keV μm^{-1} has been assumed, but which provides an accuracy of 22% due to systematic overestimation, though this reduces to 8.4% for LET values below 14 keV μm^{-1}. This raises the question as to the accuracy of the LET_U and α_U values used. Pragmatically, the α_U value could be reduced by the degree of inaccuracy to compensate for the systematic shift. If the LET_U value arrived at from simplistic consideration of the Belli *et al* (2000) data is incorrect, if higher turnover position values are used the error is reduced, as shown in figure 9.7, where the control irradiation LET is also varied. This approach would suggest that the LET_U may be between 45 and 55 keV μm^{-1}. Then, for example, the error falls to around 5% for a control LET of 1.25 and LET_U = 45 keV μm^{-1}. Further comprehensive experiments are indicated to determine a definitive value and are discussed further in chapter 14.

Such data, as well as many other examples in the literature, are hampered by the relatively few data points, imprecision about the actual position of LET_U and lack of standardisation to megavoltage radiation for control experiments. Further discussion of this problem and how research may better identify LET_U is given in the final chapter.

Table 9.6. Hep-2 cells (Britten *et al* 2013). The first four comparisons are for the 87 MeV incident energy and the final three for the 200 MeV data. The prediction is accurate to around ±3.5%.

LET (keV μm^{-1})	5.3	9	20.5	28.8	7.8	11	13.6
Predicted RBE[a]	1.17	1.32	1.81	2.18	1.27	1.40	1.51
Actual RBE[b]	1.22	1.31	1.75	1.92	1.42	1.55	1.63

[a] Using slope data and not the α_U concept.
[b] RBE values in publication are divided by 1.2 to avoid potential inaccurate values due to conversion to cobalt-equivalent RBE, and an assumed control LET of 1 keV μm^{-1} was used (120 keV x-rays).

Table 9.7. RBE estimations on Hep-2 cells (Britten *et al* 2013). The first four comparisons are for the 87 MeV incident energy and the final three for the 200 MeV data. These predictions are accurate to around 22%, but reduces to 7.5% for LET values below 14 keV μm^{-1}.

LET (keV μm^{-1})	5.3	9	20.5	28.8	7.8	11	13.6
Predicted RBE[a]	1.27	1.54	2.46	3.16	1.45	1.69	1.89
Actual RBE[b]	1.22	1.31	1.75	1.92	1.42	1.55	1.63

[a] Using the α_U concept and assumed LET_U at 30.5 keV μm^{-1}.
[b] RBE values in publication are divided by 1.2 to avoid potential inaccurate values due to conversion to cobalt-equivalent RBE, and an assumed control LET of 1 keV μm^{-1} was used (120 keV x-rays).

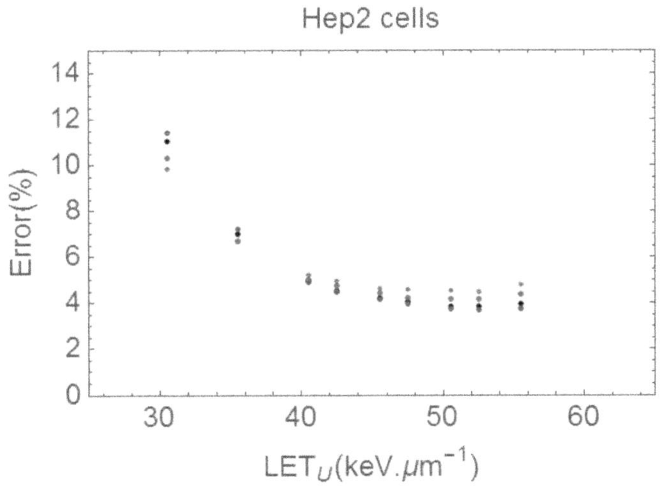

Figure 9.7. Estimation of error in predicting RBE with an assumed value of LET_U, with further variations in assumed control LET (coded as blue, black, red and grey for 0.75, 1, 1.5 and 2 keV μm^{-1}, respectively).

9.6 Two clinical examples where PBT could be sub-optimal

The following two clinical entities are relevant.

9.6.1 Prostate cancer

Most proton centres in the USA have based their business cases on treating high numbers of prostate cancer patients. There are some concerns about reports of enhanced side effects, but the outcomes are difficult to establish from small numbers in uncontrolled studies (Jones 2015b). The following list of techniques and assumptions could contribute to enhanced toxicity and have been used in some/all treatment centres:

a. To reduce gantry seep and repositioning time, one field per day treatments and use of only two field plans; both inevitably increase the dose per fraction outside the high-dose treatment volume.
b. Reduced beam shaping and conformity indices, especially with passive scattering, when compared to best photon techniques; this may be improved by scanned beams at the expense of closer inter-track distances (see chapter 1).
c. RBE values for late complications will probably exceed 1.1 in SOBPs, so the biological doses to relevant volumes of the small bowel and rectum will exceed those with photons.

It remains to be determined if better results emerge with scanned beams from all portals per day, with an emphasis of maximising LET in the gross tumour volume, and using a higher RBE allocation of, say, 1.2 for normal tissues.

9.6.2 Paediatric cancers and other radiosensitive tumours such as lymphomas

Here the tumour α radiosensitivity parameter is as high, resulting in an α/β ratio of 28 Gy (see chapter 2), leading to low RBEs, sometimes less than the 1.1 used for protons. In such cases, where RBEs may be as low as 1.03–1.07, the use of 1.05 or no RBE at all would, respectively, reduce or eliminate the chance of underdosage. Such an approach would require careful assessment of the normal tissues close to the tumours, since they might then be overdosed, but in many cases of radiosensitive tumours this should be acceptable, since the relatively low curative doses are within normal tissue tolerance for severe late effects. Random-sampling simulations of tumour control probabilities, including the numbers of patients required to reach significance, are given elsewhere (Jones 2014).

9.7 Prediction of tumour response from the RBE increment

It is always tempting to suggest that, at low dose per fraction, the reference low-LET α/β ratio will closely indicate the likely RBE, since this assumption is built into many proton RBE models. It is pertinent to mention some fast neutron data (Warenius & Britten 1994, Warenius *et al* 1994) in 30 human cell lines: the rank order of surviving fraction (SF) data after 2 Gy (photon) and 1.6 Gy (neutron) exposures, respectively,

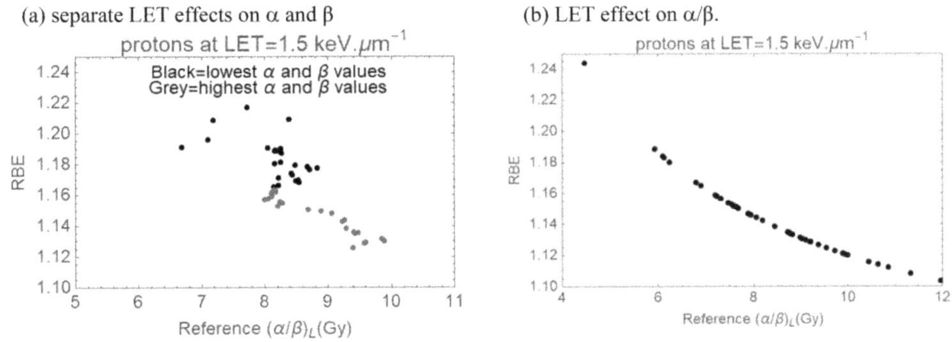

Figure 9.8. (a) and (b): Plot of estimated RBE against the low-LET reference radiation α/β using the assumptions given in the text (a) in the case where α and β are LET modified independently, and (b) where α/β is LET modified, for the LET value shown, which is typical of the mid-SOBP.

the SF_2 and $SF_{1.6}$, were not the same for photons and neutrons, but a trend was noted in that the most resistant cells seem to gain most in RBE. Since neutrons mainly ionise by forming recoil protons, these results are probably relevant to proton treatments.

A simulation of proton RBE for a typical range of human cancers is given in figure 9.8. Here two random samples are generated (mean $\alpha = 0.275$ Gy^{-1}, SD $= 0.07$; mean $\beta = 0.03$, SD $= 0.008$), and both parameters were ordered in lists from lowest to highest. In figure 9.8(a), the RBEs are then estimated for each pair of parameters, using the model used above with separate increments in α and β with LET. It can be seen that the rank order α/β ratios, although showing a general trend with RBE, will not determine the RBE ranking. This is because of the very different increments in α and β with increasing LET, which probably necessitates the independent estimation of these two radiosensitivity parameters. In comparison, the use of a variable α/β as the primary input to determine RBE, shown in figure 9.8(b), perfectly maintains the rank order from low to high α/β with the corresponding RBE, but this seems less realistic on consideration of the intrinsic biological variation which exists for α and β and consequently their ratio. For example, two cell types could have the same α/β ratio but have quite different α parameters which will dominate the increment in RBE at low dose per fraction. Further comparisons of the different published proton models has recently been published by Gardner, O'Connor and McMahon (2024), who find considerable variation in predicted RBEs. The model presented in the current chapter of this book give outputs which rank highly and especially for the important late reacting tissues.

9.8 Intensification of dose rates

The increasing interest in ultra-high dose rates, or FLASH radiotherapy, has inevitably attracted the attention of particle beam users, although considerable technical problems arise in providing accurate dosimetry and in controlling the effect. The overall mechanism is often disputed, but the best available explanation is that oxygen consumption occurs due to the enhanced dose rate, with consequent modifications to radiosensitivity. Any intensification of fluence rate will change the effective LET (the actual LET must remain the same) since the product of fluence and LET provides a micro-volumetric energy transfer (MVET), which itself should modify radiosensitivity. Increasing the fluence rate will increase MVET and in small regions such as 1 μm^3, typical of the cross-sectional area of a chromosome, the energy transfer, if sufficient, will exceed the mechanical integrity of the structure to cause a lethal and irreparable chromosomal break. At the same time, more rapid oxygen consumption due to free-radical production will also modify radiosensitivity. The combined effect will be a moderate increase in the α parameter (the increase being mitigated by the accompanying hypoxia), and a marked reduction in the β parameter (which normally increases with increasing energy transfer to a lesser extent than α, but is considerably more sensitive to severe hypoxia). Consequently, the α/β ratio is increased, and the β-parameter reduction ensures that for high doses per fraction the overall radiosensitivity is reduced, resulting in radioresistance.

The intensification of fluence rates to cause FLASH effects inevitably indicates that inter-track distances are reduced and in micro-volumes the mean inter-track distances (S) will be proportional to the inverse of the fluence rate cubed, which leads to a correction factor of $\sqrt[3]{\frac{R}{R_{\text{ref}}}}$, where R is a dose rate being compared with a reference rate R_{ref}. More extensive details can be found in Jones (2022).

Any LET_U changes, from LET_{u1} to LET_{u2} (relative to a reference experimental LET of LET_{ref}), are then expected to change in proportion to the cubed root of the exposure times T_1 and T_2 for the standard dose rate and a faster dose rate, respectively (where $T_2 < T_1$):

$$\text{LET}_{u2} = \text{LET}_{u1} - \text{LET}_{\text{ref}} \cdot \sqrt[3]{\frac{T_2}{T_1}} + \text{LET}_{\text{ref}}$$

Here time is used instead of dose rate when it is assumed that the same dose is delivered.

A similar function can be used for RBE, since there is direct proportionality between RBE and LET (below LET_U) (Sørensen *et al* 2011).

The adjusted RBE (RBE_2) is then

$$\text{RBE}_2 = \text{RBE}_1 - 1. \sqrt[3]{\frac{T_1}{T_2}} + 1.$$

The more rapid volumetric energy transfer was also reasoned to reduce LET_U values. Experimental evidence for increased LET_U in hypoxia is available in carbon- and neon-ion beams; see chapter 2 for graphical displays. These relationships were analysed and tentative modelling suggested that the proton LET–RBE relationship would change, as shown in figure 9.8. A method for estimating the oxygen enhancement ratio (OER) is given in the table 9.8.

The modelled effect of increasing dose-rate intensity on the LET and α-parameter relationship for protons is shown in figure 9.9. More substantial changes can be expected for the i parameter, but for which there is less available and reliable experimental data.

Table 9.8. Method for OER estimations.

From the data of Barendsen (1968), the cell-survival curve of the reference irradiation, with a LET of 1.3 keV μm^{-1}, provides $\alpha = 0.14$ Gy^{-1}, $\beta = 0.04$ Gy^{-2}, and the maximum helium α (α_u) given by $1.07e^{2.54\alpha}$, and the maximum $\beta(\beta_U)$ by 2β.

The LET_U value for oxic cells is 120.6 keV μm^{-1}, with the LET_U for hypoxic cells 158 keV μm^{-1}.

The Barendsen data set for OER is based on average OER values from multiple doses. To simplify, the input dose value here is for 3 Gy only for oxic cells.

For each LET value the α and β values are obtained using the scaling equations for the simple energy-efficiency model published elsewhere (Jones 2015a).

For values less than LET_U as

$$\alpha_H = \alpha_L + \frac{\mathrm{LET}_x - \mathrm{LET}_C}{\mathrm{LET}_U - \mathrm{LET}_C} \cdot \alpha_U - \alpha_L$$

and for values exceeding LET_U as

$$a_H = \alpha_L + \left(1 - \frac{\mathrm{LET}_x - \mathrm{LET}_U}{\mathrm{LET}_x - \mathrm{LET}_C}\right) \cdot \left(\alpha_U - \alpha_L\right).$$

The same equations are used for β.

Values of α and β can then be obtained for oxic and hypoxic cells by using the appropriate LET_U value (since α and β must share the same LET_U value to preserve symmetry when dose is increased).

The OER is then found for each LET value by solving for d_{hyp} in the equation, which contains suffixes to denote the oxic and hypoxic cells, in

$$\alpha_{\mathrm{ox}}\, d_{\mathrm{ox}} + \beta_{\mathrm{ox}}\, d_{\mathrm{ox}}^2 = \alpha_{\mathrm{hyp}}\, d_{\mathrm{hyp}} + \beta_{\mathrm{hyp}}\, d_{\mathrm{hyp}}^2.$$

The OER is then $d_{\mathrm{hyp}}/d_{\mathrm{ox}}$

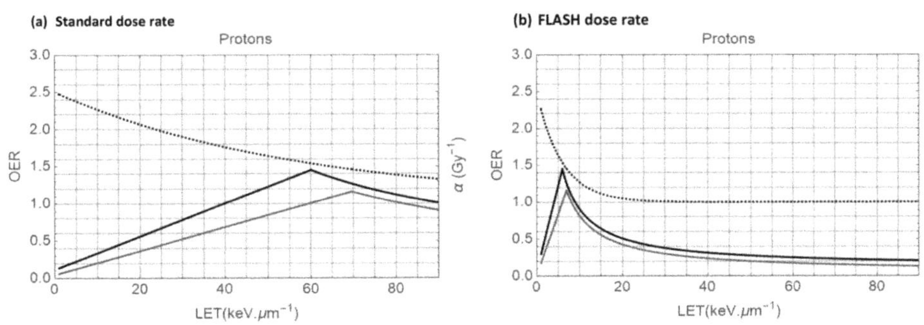

Figure 9.9. (a) and (b): Speculative graphic showing OER(α) and α parameters for protons in oxic (black) and hypoxic (grey) conditions. Graphic (a) is at a standard dose rate where the oxic and hypoxic LET_U is around 60 and 69 keV μm^{-1}, respectively. The OER(α) (dashed curve) is high in the standard LET range of 1–10 keV μm^{-1}, with a value of around 2.4 at a LET of 5 keV μm^{-1}. In (b) with a time-reduction factor of 10^{-2} the proton oxic and hypoxic LET_U are both below 10 keV μm^{-1}. The OER(α) is around 1.6 at the LET of 5 keV μm^{-1}.

For protons at 'high' fluence rates the LET_U positions, seen in figure 9.9(b), are predicted to shift to much lower values. Although the RBE will be expected to increase, it will be inversely depiendent on the dose per fraction, and so may not be apparent in high-dose *in vivo* experiments and will further reduce due to induced hypoxia when compared to the standard dose-rate condition.

9.9 Concluding discussion

Although proton therapy is the most promising external beam therapy method, it has its limitations. The obvious advantages of reduced or absent radiation exposure over wide tissue volumes will inevitably reduce many acute and late side effects. In the opinion of the present author, the physical and radiobiological uncertainties in tissues within and close to the target volumes could possibly be sufficient to cause unexpected late effects in some patients, by changing the delivered biological effective dose.

The above suggestions, along with more clinical research publications and molecular targeted approaches which might capitalise on the apparent reduction of RBE due to reduced repair capacity in some tumour types, as well as the better identification of RBE values in late-reacting tissues, together might further improve proton therapy results. There appears to be wider support for changing the RBE allocations within the proton therapy prescription process (Underwood & Paganetti 2016) and using LET maps (Grassberger *et al* 2011). Suggestions for the use of the product of LET and dose have been criticised because dose is inversely related to RBE while LET and RBE will in most instances be linearly related; there is also a wide variation in the product when plotted against SF (Jones 2017). The present writer is of the opinion that the treatment-planning process should include RBE effects, estimated from the LET and intended dose. Where important normal tissue structures exist along the distal ends of proton beams, then dose reduction should be applied if the RBE is found to indicate a potentially harmful dose (or BED). Some further approaches by other authors have been mentioned in chapter 7 and are not repeated here.

With respect to FLASH dose rates, a considerable body of experimental data is to be expected in this innovative area of research, although extreme caution is required regarding applications of FiLASH radiotherapy because of the requirement for extreme hypofractionation, dosimetry considerations and the potential for oxygen depletion causing radioresistance in tumour cells, although such lowering may be sufficient to cause enhanced cell killing providing diffusion of oxygen to depleted sites is limited. The capacity of tumour cells to exploit low oxygen tension should not be forgotten, and there is increasing interest in this topic, its molecular characterisation and exploitation (e.g. Warenius 2023).

Proton therapy clinicians and physicists must understand the full implications of a switch between photon and proton therapy. It is clear that the large capital investments in PBT equipment should be accompanied by further basic and applied research, with broader education of multi-disciplinary staff involved in its delivery.

References

Barendsen G W 1968 Responses of cultured cells, tumours and normal tissues to radiations of different linear energy transfer *Curr. Topics Radiat. Res.* Q. 4 293–356

Belli M, Bettega D, Calzolari P *et al* 2000 Inactivation of human normal and tumour cells irradiated with low energy protons *Int. J. Radiat. Biol.* **76** 831–9

Britten R A, Nazaryan V, Davis L K *et al* 2013 Variations in the RBE for cell killing along the depth-dose profile of a modulated proton therapy beam *Radiat. Res.* **179** 21–8

Calugaru V, Nauraye C, Noël G *et al* 2011 Radiobiological chariacterization of two therapeutic proton beams with different initial energy spectra used at the Institut Curie Proton Therapy Center in Orsay *Int. J. Radiat. Oncol. Biol. Phys.* **81** 1136–43

Carabe-Fernandez A, Dale R G and Jones B 2007 The incorporation of the concept of minimum RBE (RBE_{min}) into the linear-quadratic model and the potential for improved radiobiological analysis of high-LET treatments *Int. J. Radiat. Biol.* **83** 27–39

Carabe-Fernandez A, Dale R G, Hopewell J W, Jones B and Paganetti H 2010 Fractionation effects in particle radiotherapy: implications for hypo-fractionation regimes *Phys. Med. Biol.* **55** 5685–700

Carabe A, Moteabbed M, Depauw N, Schuemann J and Paganetti H 2012 Range uncertainty in proton therapy due to variable biological effectiveness *Phys Med. Biol.* **57** 1159–72

Combs S E 2017 Does proton therapy have a future in CNS tumors? *Curr. Treat. Options Neurol.* **19** 12

Dale R G, Jones B and Carabe-Fernandez A 2009 Why more needs to be known about RBE effects in modern radiotherapy *J. Appl. Radiat. Isot.* **67** 387–92

Darby S C, Ewertz M, McGale P *et al* 2013 Risk of ischemic heart disease in women after radiotherapy for breast cancer *N. Engl. J. Med.* **368** 987–98

Gardner L G, O'Connor J D and McMahon S J 2024 Benchmarking proton RBE models *Phys. Med. Biol.* **69** 085022

Grassberger C, Trofimov A, Lomax A and Paganetti H 2011 Variations in linear energy transfer within clinical proton therapy fields and the potential for biological treatment planning *Int. J. Radiat. Oncol. Biol. Phys.* **80** 1559–66

Grosshans D R 2016 Proton therapy for medulloblastoma *Lancet Oncol.* **29** 20i16

Hall E J and Giaccia A 2011 *Radiobiology for the Radiologist* (Philadelphia, PA: Lippincott Williams & Wilkins) 7th edn chs 6 and 7

ICRU 1970 *Linear Energy Transfer (Report 16)* (Bethesda, MD: International Commission on Radiation Units & Measurements)

Jones B 2014 Editorial: patterns of failure after proton therapy in Medulloblastoma *Int. J. Radiat. Oncol. Biol. Phys.* **90** 25–6

Jones B 2015a Towards achieving the full clinical potential of proton therapy by inclusion of LET and RBE models *Cancers (Basel)* **7** 460–80

Jones B 2015b A simpler energy transfer efficiency model to predict relative biological effect (RBE) for protons and Heavier ions *Front. Oncol.* **5** 184
Erratum in: 2016 *Front. Oncol.* **6** 32

Jones B 2017 Clinical radiobiology of proton therapy: modeling of RBE *Acta. Oncol.* **56** 1374–8

Jones B and Hill M A 2019 Physical characteristics at the turnover-points of relative biological effect (RBE) with linear energy transfer (LET) *Phys. Med. Biol.* **21** 225010

Jones B and Hopewell J W 2019 Spinal cord re-treatments using photon and proton based radiotherapy: LQ-derived tolerance doses *Phys. Med.* **64** 304–10

Marshall T I, Chaudhary P, Michaelidesová A *et al* 2016 Investigating the implications of a variable RBE on proton dose fractionation across a clinicali pencil beam scanned spread-out Bragg peak *Int. J. Radiat. Oncol. Biol. Phys.* **95** 70–7

Mizumoto M, Murayama S, Akimoto T *et al* 2016 Long-term follow-up after proton beam therapy for pediatric tumors: a Japanese national survey *Cancer Sci.* **108** 444–7

Peeler C R, Mirkovic D, Titt U *et al* 2016 Drinical evidence of variable proton biological effectiveness in pediatric patients treated for ependymoma *Radiother. Oncol.* **121** 395–401

Sørensen B S, Overgaard J and Bassler N 2011 In vitro RBE-LET dependence for multiple particle types *Acta. Oncol.* **50** 757–62

Warenius H M, Britten R A, Browning P G, Morton I E and Peacock J H 1994 Identification of human *in vitro* cell lines with greater intrinsic cellular radiosensitivity to 62.5 MeV (p->Be+) neutrons than 4 MeV phiotons *Int. J. Radiat. Oncol. Biol. Phys.* **28** 913–20

Warenius H M and Britten R A 1994 In vitro studies of intrinsic cellular radiosensitivity following 4 MeV photons or 62.5 MeV (p->Be+) neutrons. Potential implications for high LET therapy *Acta. Oncol.* **33** 241–9

Warenius H M 2023 The essential molecular requirements for the transformation of normal cells into established cancer cells, with implications for a novel anti-cancer agent *Cancer Rep.* **6** e1844

Weber D C, Malyapa R, Albertini F *et al* 2016 Long term outcomes of patients with skull-base low grade chondrosarcoma and chordoma patients treated with pencil beam scanning proton therapy *Radiother. Oncol.* **120** 169–74

Wilkens J J and Oelfke U 2004 A phenomenological model for the relative biological effectiveness in therapeutic proton beams *Phys. Med. Biol.* **49** 2811–25

Underwood T and Paganetti H 2016 Variable proton relative biological effectiveness: how do we move forward? *Int. J. Radiat. Oncol. Biol. Phys.* **95** 56–8

Yock T I, Yeap B Y, Ebb D H *et al* 2016 Long term toxic effects of proton radiotherapy for paediatric medulloblastoma: a phase 2 single arm study *Lancet Oncol.* **17** 287–98

Chapter 10

Proton therapy risk assessment using small increments in RBE in the central nervous system and estimation of remission times

The assumed constant proton relative biological effect (RBE) of 1.1 (Paganetti *et al* 2002) remains a controversial topic. Owing to its acceptance by international advisory bodies, clinicians have been reluctant to override this value. This chapter describes a method for the assessment of proton therapy dose prescriptions in clinical situations where little or no critical normal tissue dose reduction can be achieved. The routinely used RBE of 1.1 may not then be safe since higher values can be expected to occur, especially in neurological tissues.

The recommended method includes creating lists of biological effective dose (BED) and equivalent dose in 2 Gy fractions (EQD-2) in neurological tissues ($\alpha/\beta =$ 2 Gy), for small increments in RBE between 1.1 and 1.2 compatible with linear energy transfer (LET) values which occur in spread-out Bragg peaks. The method may be used where information on LET for RBE prediction is not available. It is also possible to include reductions in tissue tolerance due to adverse medical and surgical histories, age, etc., and is sufficiently simple for basic computer programming or pocket calculator estimates. It can also be used with formal tissue risk estimates based on human dose–response curves for spinal cord, brain stem and optic nerve tolerances.

The example of a brain stem low-grade glioma is followed, and there is no effective normal tissue dose sparing. Proton dose reductions to the normally prescribed photon dose must then be considered if accepted tissue tolerance levels are exceeded due to the assumed RBE increments above 1.1. This may then result in a decision to reduce the number of fractions and/or lower the total dose, while maintaining the same dose per fraction, since RBE is generally inversely related to dose per fraction (d), so it seems best not to change d. A reduction of total dose is not necessarily deleterious in this specific situation, since long-term cure cannot be

doi:10.1088/978-0-7503-6209-2ch10

achieved though long-term tumour control can be; but it is more likely to result in a better quality of life, although with a slightly shorter remission than would otherwise have occurred. BED-based methods for assessment of the remission-free durations are also provided.

This approach is considered to be feasible for use in routine clinical practice and, if followed, clinicians should find that this type of 'hands on' radiobiological information can should improve complication-free outcomes in proton therapy. Similar considerations apply to ion-beam treatments.

10.1 Introduction

It is essential to good medical practice that treatment-related toxicities should be minimised. The ancient advice of 'first do no harm' (*primum non nocere*) as well as 'To cure sometimes, to relieve often, to comfort always', attributed to Trudeau, should never be forgotten, and is not only restricted to palliative care situations, since long-term tumour control is sometimes the principal aim of treatment if complete cure is unachievable. In modern medical and surgical practice, including radiotherapy, it is necessary to accept a low risk probability in order to achieve long-term cancer control or cure, but in all situations avoidable risks should be eliminated. In daily practice, risk-related decisions are often made in the absence of complete predictive information, or with information which is not completely verifiable but regarded as the best available.

Physicians are accustomed to such situations more than physicists, although engineers often consider 'worst-case' limits in their designs and tend to use 'fail-safe' procedures where dangerous conditions are anticipated. There is a similar role for basic radiobiological modelling within radiotherapy, since clinically useful concepts such as biological effective dose (BED) can be used to guide therapeutic decisions in order to eliminate dangerous options (Jones *et al* 2001).

Proton therapy is used to treat various cancers, utilising the Bragg peak effect to achieve a reduction in radiation dose to unaffected volumes of normal tissues as well as critical tissues close to the cancer in many situations. Target volumes and their geometrical relationship to critical normal tissues are important.

There are two principal conditions for proton therapy:

1. Protons are mainly used to reduce radiation dose to critical organs situated outside the highest-dose region of the planning target volume (PTV). There will always be some normal tissue within the PTV and also within the smaller clinical target volume (CTV). In some clinical situations, for example if the normal tissue is liver (with regenerative capacity) or lung (which does not regenerate), some loss of function is usually accepted. When critical normal tissue sparing of tissues outside the PTV is sufficiently good, this advantage can override a disadvantage due small increments in relative biological effect (RBE) values beyond the standard 1.1 value (which effectively increases the dose).
2. In other situations, the CTV and PTV target volume itself includes a significant volume of important critical normal tissue, where a reduction of

> dose due to the Bragg peak effect is not possible. If this occurs in critical parts of the central nervous system (CNS) where radiation-induced loss of function is unacceptable (especially in serially organised structures and sometimes also in important parallel-organised areas), there is a potential serious problem if the RBE exceeds 1.1. Even in this situation, protons may be preferred because of the considerable reduction in dose to wider volumes of tissues (sometimes referred to as a reduced integral dose), but then the dose prescription requires closer scrutiny and possibly modification after very careful consideration of the potential impact of small increments in RBE.

Proton therapy contains two sources of uncertainty not present in standard megavoltage radiotherapy, namely errors of Bragg peak positioning and the RBE (Jones 2015, 2016, 2017, Jones *et al* 2018, Lühr *et al* 2018, Paganetti *et al* 2019, McNamara *et al* 2020, Sørensen *et al* 2021). Proton RBE has been a controversial but important topic since if the RBE is incorrect then the dose given to the patient may be incorrect, resulting in toxicity. Clinicians and physicists need to be increasingly aware of this.

Although RBE effects must be considered in all cases, it becomes even more important in the second case, or where there is inadequate critical normal tissue dose reduction, and especially within the CNS. This is because neurological tissue has a lower α/β ratio than for soft tissues outside the CNS, and is consequently at greater risk of higher RBE values due to the general inverse relationship between α/β ratio and RBE (Jones 2015, 2016, Jones *et al* 2018); this has been described in the earlier chapters 2, 7 and 9.

Consequently, the proton RBE of 1.1 can be exceeded in late-reacting tissues such as brain or spinal cord tissues, resulting in unintended overdosage. This can not only occur towards the distal end of the spread-out Bragg peak (SOBP, where the LET is highest), but also (although to a lesser extent) even in the mid-SOBP. The resulting amount of overdosage may be sufficiently small in some treatments to cause no damage in terms of functional losses, but in some instances it might be greater and become clinically significant, life-changing or even fatal. This places considerable responsibility on the treatment centre medical and supporting scientific staff.

A critique of the standard RBE value of 1.1 is given in chapter 7. There is presently a greater appreciation among the scientific community that the RBE can be higher than 1.1, with low doses per fraction in late-reacting tissues, even in regions of SOBPs (where LET values are normally between 1 and 2 keV μm^{-1}) and especially if the linear energy transfer (LET) exceeds 1.5 keV μm^{-1} (Jones 2016, 2017). It is then reasonable to assume increments in RBE of up to 1.2 when dose per fraction is low (2 Gy or less).

Until such a time arrives when there may be a fully validated method of predicting RBE from accurate LET and dose distributions, it is expedient to assume that small increases in RBE can occur in neurological tissues at low dose per fraction. This is because, on the balance of probabilities (which is the test level in medical judisprudence), it is more likely that the RBE exceeds 1.1 at low dose per fraction in this tissue. This is a prediction common to all radiobiological modelling systems based on LET and RBE. Some modelling systems predict a higher RBE than others (Rørvik *et al* 2018, Khachonkham *et al* 2020, Otterlei *et al* 2021), but in the present study only small increments are used, and in a very conservative manner.

10.2 Methods

The clinical dilemma is exemplified by choosing one difficult clinical site, although the advice can be applied in other intracranial or spinal situations.

For instance, a low-grade glioma is situated in the centre of the upper brain stem of a young adult. It is considered necessary to treat the entire cross section of the brain stem, as in condition (2) above. The standard photon (x-ray) dose would be 54 Gy in 30 fractions, so the chosen proton dose is 54 Gy(RBE) in 30 fractions, such that the proton physical dose is $1.8/1.1 = 1.64$ Gy. It is vital to make the distinction between physical Gy doses and the equivalent doses, designated as Gy(RBE) or Gy-equivalent (eq-Gy or Gy-eq) according to what form of units are in use. This dose-fractionation schedule is intended to deliver long-term tumour control, but will not eradicate the tumour, which will probably regrow at an extended time interval of many years. For example, the median survival after this dose schedule was 7.4 years in a randomised study (Van den Bent *et al* 2005), which inevitably includes many older patients.

The critical organ at risk (OAR, the brain stem in this case) receives the full prescribed dose, and which is slightly below radiotolerance levels. Then for the more likely CNS RBE values of between 1.12 and 1.2 (instead of 1.1) that will probably occur within a treatment volume, it is necessary to estimate the total equivalent photon doses, by using the BED and the equivalent dose in 2 Gy fraction (EQD-2) values for 30 fractions.

The simplest method of achieving this is to correct the proton dose per fraction with respect to potential small increments in RBE. BEDs and EQD-2 estimates for a photon equivalent treatment can then be obtained.

The steps are as follows (and the reader should remember that an RBE of 1.1 has already been used):

1. Multiply the intended equivalent photon dose per fraction (d) by the potential RBE divided by 1.1 (e.g. 1.12/1.1, 1.14/1.1, 1.16/1.1, 1.18/1.1 and 1.2/1.1) to give the estimated effective dose per fraction (d').
2. Then d' is used to estimate the respective BED values using

$$\mathrm{BED} = nd'\left(1 + \frac{d'}{\alpha/\beta}\right). \tag{10.1}$$

3. The EQD-2 is obtained by dividing each estimated BED by

$$\left(1 + \frac{2}{\alpha/\beta}\right). \tag{10.2}$$

4. These EQD-2 estimates must then be compared to that considered acceptable for the treatment volume under consideration.

This simple method avoids using RBE limits (RBE_{max} and RBE_{min}) and LET estimations, as would be required with some LET-based estimation methods, as described in chapter 9.

For risk determination, any locally preferred method can be used. In the present example, the estimated risks of overt radio-necrosis were obtained using the human dose–response curve for spinal cord and brain stem tolerance taken from the clinical data of K. Ang at the MD Anderson Hospital, and are embedded in software developed in the UK by Woolley *et al* (2018), which sets a tolerance of 50 Gy in 25 fractions, yielding a risk of around 0.11% for full-thickness irradiation of the spinal cord, though the risk level will increase with higher doses and larger numbers of fractions if d is kept constant. It can be used iteratively to obtain a risk for any dose-fractionation schedule. It is appreciated that in many proton treatments there may be partial irradiation of the OAR with a sharp dose falloff. This possibility is discussed further below.

It is important to consider what the effect of nervous tissue radiotolerance reduction might be due to previous cytotoxic chemotherapy, surgery or any other factor. The practical range of tolerance reduction used in radiotherapeutics for critical neural tissue is up to 20% (and sometimes more; see chapter 3). This range is exemplified by the typical clinical use of more cautious dose-fractionation schedules (with reductions in BED) where higher risks are anticipated, as from a normal prescribed dose of 50 Gy in 25 fractions to a serial structure such as spinal cord, to be safer at either 47.5 in 25 fractions, 45 Gy in 25 fractions or further to 40 Gy in 20 fractions (the CNS tolerance level BED then being progressively reduced by 20% from 100 $Gy_{[2]}$ to 80 $Gy_{[2]}$ for these changes in fractionation), and where the subscripts in parentheses denote the use of an α/β ratio of 2 Gy.

Where the estimated BED and EQD-2 values are considered by a clinician to be unacceptably high, a reduced dose, BED and EQD-2 must be considered. To achieve this, reductions in the number of fractions and/or total dose are probably safest, since lowering the proton dose per fraction (by further increasing the fraction number) will incur a further increase in RBE.

This can be achieved by iterative changes of n in the BED, where the α/β ratio is 2 Gy and the BED is divided by (1 + 2/2) in the subsequent EQD-2 equation, as in the following equation, where it has been assumed that the assumed RBE value of RBE is x. Thus if an RBE of 1.18 is assumed, $x = 1.18$ and the EQD-2 (in units of Gy delivered in 2 Gy fractions) is given by

$$\frac{1.8n\,\frac{x}{1.1}\left(1+\frac{x\quad\times 1.8}{1.1\times 2}\right)}{\left(1+\frac{2}{2}\right)}. \tag{10.3}$$

Each individual OAR must be considered according to their known radiotolerances. For example, cortical brain tissue will have a higher tolerance for radio-necrosis than brain stem, optic chiasm and spinal cord tissues, although some areas have a much lower tolerance for functional effects, such as the medial hippocampus. Clinicians will be aware of these. The general principles of how to proceed, given in the above examples, may then be used in each situation and similar percentage BED reductions can be applied.

In situations (category 1 above) where there is effective dose sparing (i.e. a reduction of dose in a critical tissue), the equations are modified by including the dose-sparing factor S (with range 0–1), where for example $S = 0.76$ for 76% of the prescribed dose or $S = 0.84$ for 84% of the prescribed dose, so that equation (10.1) becomes

$$\mathrm{BED} = nSd'\left(1 + \frac{Sd'}{\alpha/\beta}\right). \tag{10.4}$$

àAll the other steps can then be followed in the same way as outlined above. Essentially, the reduction in dose per fraction due to S must be sufficient to oppose any increase in dose per fraction caused by an RBE increment.

10.3 Results

Table 10.1 provides the estimated modifications in total doses, BED and EQD-2 due to sequential modest increases in RBE above 1.1. It can be seen that the BED and EQD-2 values become progressively larger. These estimates will cause concern to many clinicians when they realise that the EQD-2 changes from 51 Gy, if given by photons, to values of 54 Gy and above, to as high as 58 Gy.

The actual RBE values could be even higher in the presence of elevated LET regions within the treatment plan (especially at distal parts of SOBPs), but since the operative tissue LET may not be known outside research centres, these slightly elevated RBE estimates are reasonable for SOBPs with the LET values of 1–2 keV μm^{-1} obtained by scanning techniques in the first instance. It must also be recalled that there is evidence to suggest that, unlike the case of scattered beams, there is no appreciable fall in RBE with depth in scanned beams, so that clinicians must then be extra-vigilant on the RBE issues (this was introduced in chapters 1 and analysed further in chapter 11).

The clinician may decide to modify the prescription from the original 54 Gy (RBE) in 30 fractions, or to not proceed with proton therapy. If an RBE of around 1.18 is accepted as being reasonable instead of 1.1, with an EQD-2 of around 58 Gy

Table 10.1. Changes in total dose, BED and EQD-2 with assumed RBE for a prescription of 54 Gy in 30 fractions (using equations (10.1) and (10.2)).

Assumed RBE	1.10	1.12	1.14	1.16	1.18	1.20
Total dose (Gy)	54.0	55.0	56.0	56.9	57.9	58.9
BED ($Gy_{[2]}$)[a]	103	105	108	111	114	117
EQD-2 (Gy)[a]	51	52	54	55	57	58

[a] Rounded to nearest Gy.

Table 10.2. Number of fractions and EQD-2 values for an assumed RBE of 1.18 (using equation (10.3)).

n (number of fractions)	25	26	27	28	29
EQD-2 (Gy)[a]	47	49	51	53	55

[a] Rounded to nearest Gy.

Table 10.3. Changes in radiotolerance assumptions due to adverse histories and consequent estimated radio-necrosis risks within the PTV region, for an example of an unintended equivalent dose of 58 Gy in 29 fractions (an EQD-2 of 58 Gy) due to an RBE underestimation (taken from the final box in the EQD-2 results in table 10.1 under the assumption that the RBE is 1.2 rather than 1.1).

% BED tolerance change	0	−5	−10	−15	−20
% radio-necrosis risk	3	7	16	27	42

in 29 fractions, then further estimates of the number of fractions (of the same dose) should be obtained by modifying n in equation (10.3), giving the results shown in table 10.2.

Since the intended BED was $30 \times 1.8(1 + 1.8/2) = 102.6\ \text{Gy}_{[2]}$ with a EQD-2 of 51 Gy, the original intent is given by 27 fractions rather than 30 fractions (as seen in table 10.2). The prescription could then be modified as 48.6 Gy in 27 fractions.

Radio-necrosis risk estimates for assumed changes in tissue tolerance due to adverse clinical histories are given in table 10.3 by iteration of the re-treatment software systems (Woolley *et al* 2018, Moore *et al* 2021). It is self-evident that a considerably reduced radiation dose would be required to reduce the higher risk estimates, as can be expected if adverse clinical factors are present.

The same iterative procedure can be done using a different RBE assumption and with whatever method of normal tissue risk estimation is preferred at any treatment centre.

10.3.1 Remission duration considerations

In principle, it can be expected that the duration of remission is related to the cell kill achieved by therapy and so to its associated BED value. This duration will also be influenced by the expected growth rate of the tumour being treated. A series of publications have considered these issues (Jones *et al* 2003). Essentially, the remission duration ($T\text{rem}$) can be estimated from the BED and the repopulation equivalent BED term (K) as

$$T\text{rem} = \frac{\text{BED}}{K},$$

which is valid providing the duration of treatment is short when compared with the expected remission duration, as in the present example. Otherwise, subtractive corrections to the duration are required, as described by Jones & Sanghera (2007).

It follows that for any two different fractionation schedules (A and B), which provide BED_A and BED_B, respectively, then

$$T\mathrm{rem}_A = \frac{\mathrm{BED}_A}{K} \text{ and } T\mathrm{rem}_B = \frac{\mathrm{BED}_B}{K}.$$

So that $\frac{T\mathrm{rem}_B}{T\mathrm{rem}_A} = \frac{\mathrm{BED}_B}{\mathrm{BED}_A}$; then

$$T\mathrm{rem}_B = \frac{\mathrm{BED}_B}{\mathrm{BED}_A} \times T\mathrm{rem}_A.$$

If schedule A is the reference or standard schedule (with a known average remission duration) then the relative durations of remission can be expressed as the respective BED ratios without the need for inclusion of a repopulation factor.

Then by including the full BED terms as

$$T\mathrm{rem}_B = \frac{n_B d\left(1 + \frac{d}{\alpha/\beta}\right)}{n_A d\left(1 + \frac{d}{\alpha/\beta}\right)} \times T\mathrm{rem}_A,$$

where n_A and n_B are the number of fractions in schedules A and B, respectively, the simplified equation is then

$$T\mathrm{rem}_B = \frac{n_B d}{n_A d} \times T\mathrm{rem}_A,$$

which can be written as

$$T\mathrm{rem}_B = \frac{n_B}{n_A} \times T\mathrm{rem}_A,$$

and which no longer requires any assumptions about the α/β ratio.

This expression is only valid if schedules A and B have the same dose per fraction.

Estimated changes in remission durations for the changes in numbers of fractions are given in table 10.4 when based on an expected median survival of 7.4 years (where it is now assumed that recurrences were detectable around 1 year earlier), for the photon-based schedule of 54 Gy in 30 fractions.

For each fraction of treatment reduction there is a progressive reduction in Trem, although this may be considered acceptable provided that serious late complications are reduced. There is also a possibility of radiation re-treatments and other forms of treatment such as chemotherapy when recurrence is detected.

Table 10.4. The estimated median remission durations for different numbers of fractions in the altered dose-fractionation schedule (with dose per fraction kept constant). The standard photon-based treatment, given in 30 fractions, is expected to provide a remission duration of around 6.4 years.

Number of fractions (n_B)	25	26	27	28	29
Estimated Trem (years)	5.3	5.5	5.8	6.0	6.2

Table 10.5. The estimated median remission durations for different numbers of fractions in the altered dose-fractionation schedule (with dose per fraction kept constant). The standard photon-based treatment, given in 30 fractions, is expected to provide a remission duration of around 10 years.

Number of fractions (n_B)	25	26	27	28	29
Estimated *T*rem (years)	8.3	8.7	9.0	9.3	9.7

Table 10.6. The dose to the critical OAR is 90% of the prescribed dose and the operative RBE in the OAR is assumed to be 1.2.

Number of fractions (n_B)	25	26	27	28	29	30
BED ($Gy_{[2]}$)	83.2	86.6	89.9	93.2	96.5	99.9
EQD-2 (Gy)	41.6	43.3	44.9	46.6	48.3	49.9

Table 10.7. The dose to the critical OAR is 90% of the prescribed dose and the operative RBE in the OAR is assumed to be 1.25. The results in bold are above the chosen level of tolerance.

Number of fractions (n_B)	25	26	27	28	29	30
BED ($Gy_{[2]}$)	88.4	91.9	95.5	99.0	**102.5**	**106.1**
EQD-2 (Gy)	44.2	46.0	47.7	49.5	**51.3**	**53.0**

It is also instructive to consider a longer expected remission duration of, say, 10 years. Then the results shown in table 10.4 change to those given in table 10.5.

Also, it is necessary to consider the situation of a greater degree of critical OAR sparing in another location, where there might be physical separation between the OAR and the PTV. If, for example, the critical OAR receives 90% of the prescribed dose, then the BED and EQD-2 results are given in table 10.6 for an assumed RBE of 1.2 in the OAR. Here there is no need for total dose reduction since tolerance is not breached at 30 fractions.

If the RBE is assumed to be 1.25, then corrective action may be advisable, as can be seen in table 10.7, where the results in bold are above standard tolerance and a safe number of fractions would be 28.

In these examples, the results for the lower number of fractions may be relevant to individual patients who have reductions in radiotolerance due to other factors, as discussed above and in chapter 3.

10.4 Discussion

The above method involves no complex biophysical modelling and should be understandable to biologists and clinicians. These examples are at least important in an educative role, but serious consideration should be given to their implementation in routine practice, especially in situations where there is inadequate or no degree of critical OAR sparing, because of increasing concerns about higher than expected and anecdotal reports of a higher toxicity for proton therapy within the CNS. Predictions based on the use of a fixed RBE of 1.1 are probably inadequate in this region of the body. There is one report which shows that the grade 3 and 4 toxicities exceed 10%, a level which would be considered unacceptable following photon-based therapy (Weber *et al* 2018). A large German study has shown unacceptably high numbers of radio-necrotic brain lesions in magnetic resonance imaging studies following proton therapy (Eulitz *et al* 2023).

Critics of the above approach will usually claim that any reduction in prescribed dose will be detrimental to patients, although their quality of life may actually be enhanced (as discussed further below). They also demand that LET-based RBE estimations should be used, and that these should be fully validated: this standpoint represents an ideal situation which is probably many years from being fulfilled, and would require comprehensive ranges of *in vivo* studies at clinically relevant fractional doses and the use of randomised control trials to test the method in a large number of patients; functional radiology studies may find uncontrolled retrospective evidence but can contain substantial differences in irradiated volumes when comparing photons and protons, which may influence the outcomes. It may be possible that limited studies will be performed in some academic centres, but with insufficient standards of proof. Such attitudes will not help patients who need proton therapy in the immediate future. At the present time there is a real possibility that referrals for proton therapy will reduce with time if there is a perception amongst referring physicians and surgeons that there is an enhanced risk of toxicity in some clinical situations.

Returning to the clinical example described above, the key decision was what proton dose to prescribe. This is a clinical responsibility. A prescribed dose of 54 Gy in 30 fractions for conventional megavoltage radiotherapy would be tolerated in a patient without an adverse medical history, but if the RBE of 1.1 is exceeded the treatment delivered may be equivalent to the higher prescribed doses, as shown above. Severe adverse consequences of unintended overdosage in this situation might include major neurological deficits and possibly death. Also, if tolerance were to be further reduced by other factors (such as surgery, cytotoxic chemotherapy, other concomitant medical conditions or previous forms of neurological damage resulting in atrophic, or shrunken, brain appearances, such as after long-standing pressure effects on brain tissue in hydrocephalic conditions), then the treatment dose prescription should be further modified by reducing the BED by 5%–20% according to the clinical perception of risk, as would be done for photon-based treatments in order to be protective.

Consequently, the following is advised:

- An equivalence table for higher RBE values (as in table 10.1) should be considered on a routine basis by clinicians and physicists.
- If the BED and EQD-2 values seem unacceptably high, a choice of modified numbers of treatment fractions should be considered (as in table 10.2).
- Risk-based estimations may also be performed according to the clinical circumstances.

There will be clinical concerns about reducing total dose, but for many very radiosensitive childhood brain tumours the RBE is likely to be below 1.1, which implies slight tumour underdosage. It may be preferable to choose 28 rather than 27 fractions on this basis, since we do not know α/β for many tumor types. Also, the oncologist in charge must recognise that, in the example given of a low-grade glioma, the aim of treatment is to obtain reasonable long-term suppression of tumour growth, not complete tumour eradication, since low-grade gliomas are relatively radioresistant: cure would require a substantially higher dose, considerably above accepted radiotolerance. Thus a deliberate reduction in BED may lead to a shorter remission duration, but which may continue to amount to many years and would be regarded as a very successful treatment, especially if quality of life were to be maintained or improved rather than deteriorate at some time after treatment. The duration of remission is largely determined by the tumor growth rate after treatment in this type of situation (Jones *et al* 2003, Jones & Dale, 2007), which is likely to remain very slow in the case of a persisting low-grade glioma. In essence, the above quantitative techniques can be used only to a certain extent, after which qualitative considerations must be used to obtain the best overall outcomes. The success of proton therapy should be assessed not only by patient survival but also by quality-of-life assessments (Jones 2006). Furthermore, if careful primary treatment has been given to below radiotolerance, re-treatment to almost the same dose level may be possible many years later, thus further extending survival accompanied by a chosen low estimated risk of neurological deficit (Moore *et al* 2021).

The example given is appropriate to encourage clinicians and medical physicists to concentrate further on the RBE dilemmas that occur in some proton therapy patients. In other examples, the proton dose distribution across the spinal cord or brain stem will be non-uniform, with important consequences on tolerance, such that in some instances spinal cord doses of up to 63 Gy-eq or 63 Gy(RBE; or 57.3 Gy physical dose) could be delivered to a part of the spinal cord, even if given in 35 or more fractions (Chowdhry *et al* 2016) when the prescribed target doses could be as high as or exceed 70 Gy in 2 Gy fractions or equivalent (as in the treatment of some lung cancers). These authors also point out the importance of surgery, which can impair tissue vascularisation, in reducing radiotolerance. Such an effect can be accommodated in the tabulated estimations given above, although in their series there was negligible use of cytotoxic chemotherapy and other agents, which might also reduce tolerance.

Long-tract (serially arranged) CNS volume effects in animal models are insubstantial when assessed down to spinal cord lengths of 2.5 cm using photons in porcine experiments (Van den Aardweg *et al* 1995) but with uniform irradiation. It is also known that proton tolerances can be modified by the dose received by surrounding larger volumes of spinal cord tissues (Bijl *et al* 2006). There are some experimental *in vivo* assessments of proton RBE in the spinal cord, compatible with a value greater than 1.1, although what was observed may be limited by the large fraction sizes used in the experiments (Saager *et al* 2018), and some groups are preparing murine experiments (Howard *et al* 2021).

10.5 Conclusions

The above methods should be helpful to guide clinical decision-making in difficult treatment situations, in order for the full potential of proton therapy to be achieved by minimising adverse late-reacting tissue effects, leading to improved quality of life while maintaining reasonably long survival for patients who have tumours where the full advantages of proton- or ion-beam therapy may not be obtained because their anatomical location does not allow adequate neurological tissue dose sparing. The various disciplines within radiation oncology need to collaborate closely and understand the broad issues, which range from the clinical facts through medical physics and radiobiology, in order to achieve the best achievable outcomes.

Certain sections of text in this chapter have been reproduced from Jones (2022).

References

Bijl H P, van Luijk P, Coppes R P *et al* 2006 Influence of adjacent low-dose fields on tolerance to high doses of protons in rat cervical spinal cord *Int. J. Radiat. Oncol. Biol. Phys.* **64** 1204–10

Chowdhry V K, Liu L, Goldberg S *et al* 2016 Thoracolumbar spinal cord tolerance to high dose conformal proton-photon radiation therapy *Radiother Oncol.* **119** 35–9

Eulitz J, Troost E, Klünder L *et al* 2023 Increased relative biological effectiveness and periventricular radiosensitivity in proton therapy of glioma patients *Radiother. Oncol.* **178** 109422

Grassberger C, Trofimov A, Lomax A and Paganetti H 2011 Variations in linear energy transfer within clinical proton therapy fields and the potential for biological treatment planning *Int. J. Radiat. Oncol. Biol. Phys.* **80** 1559–66

Howard M E, Denbeigh J M, Debrot E K *et al* 2021 Dosimetric assessment of a high precision system for mouse proton irradiation to assess spinal cord toxicity *Radiat. Res.* **195** 541–8

Jones B, Dale R G, Deehan C, Hopkins K I and Morgan D A L 2001 The role of biologically effective dose (BED) in clinical oncology *Clin. Oncol. (R Coll. Radiol.)* **13** 71–81

Jones B, Cominos M and Dale R G 2003 Application of biological effective dose (BED) to estimate the duration of symptomatic relief and repopulation dose equivalent in palliative radiotherapy and chemotherapy *Int. J. Rad. Oncol. Biol. Phys.* **55** 736–42

Jones B, Cominos M and Dale R G 2003 Application of biological effective dose (BED) to estimate the duration of symptomatic relief and repopulation dose equivalent in palliative radiotherapy and chemotherapy *Int. J. Rad. Oncol. Biol. Phys.* **55** 736–42

Jones B 2006 Implications of quality adjusted survival for clinical trials in radiation oncology *Br. J. Radiol* **79** 353–5

Jones B and Dale R G 2007 Further radiobiological modelling of palliative radiotherapy: use of virtual trials *Int. J. Radiat. Oncol. Biol. Phys.* **69** 221–9

Jones B and Sanghera P 2007 Estimation of radiobiological parameters and equivalent radiation dose of cytotoxic chemotherapy in malignant glioma *Int. J. Radiat. Oncol. Biol Phys.* **68** 441–8

Jones B 2015 Towards achieving the full clinical potential of proton therapy by inclusion of LET and RBE models *Cancers (Basel)* **7** 460–80

Jones B 2016 Why RBE must be a variable and not a constant in proton therapy *Br. J. Radiol.* **89** 20160116

Jones B 2017 Clinical radiobiology of proton therapy: modelling of RBE *Acta Oncol.* **56** 1374–8

Jones B, McMahon S J and Prise K M 2018 The radiobiology of proton therapy: challenges and opportunities around relative biological effectiveness *Clin. Oncol. (R. Coll. Radiol.)* **30** 285–92

Khachonkham S, Mara E, Gruber S *et al* 2020 Investigating the impact of alpha/beta and LET_d on relative biological effectiveness in scanned proton beams: an *in vitro* study based on human cell lines *Med. Phys.* **47** 3691–702

Lühr A, von Neubeck C, Pawelke J *et al* 2018 Radiobiology of proton therapy: results of an international expert workshop *Radiother. Oncol.* **128** 56–67

McNamara A L, Willers H and Paganetti H 2020 Modelling variable proton relative biological effectiveness for treatment planning *Br. J. Radiol.* **93** 20190334

Moore J W, Woolley T E, Hopewell J H and Jones B 2021 Further development of spinal cord retreatment dose estimation: including radiotherapy with protons and light ions *Int. J. Radiat. Biol.* **97** 1657–66

Otterlei O M, Indelicato D J, Toussaint L *et al* 2021 Variation in relative biological effectiveness for cognitive structures in proton therapy of pediatric brain tumors *Acta Oncol.* **60** 267–74

Paganetti H, Niemierko A, Ancukiewicz M *et al* 2002 Relative biological effectiveness (RBE) values for proton beam therapy *Int. J. Radiat. Oncol. Biol. Phys.* **53** 407–21

Paganetti H, Eleanor Blakely E, Carabe-Fernandez A *et al* 2019 Report of the AAPM TG-256 on the relative biological effectiveness of proton beams in radiation therapy *Med. Phys.* **46** e53–78

Rørvik E, Fjæra L F, Dahle T J *et al* 2018 Exploration and application of phenomenological RBE models for proton therapy *Phys. Med. Biol.* **63** 185013

Saager M, Peschke P, Brons S, Debus J and Karger C P 2018 Determination of the proton RBE in the rat spinal cord: is there an increase towards the end of the spread-out Bragg peak? *Radiother. Oncol.* **128** 115–20

Sørensen B S, Pawelke J, Bauer J *et al* 2021 Does the uncertainty in relative biological effectiveness affect patient treatment in proton therapy? *Radiother. Oncol.* **163** 177–84

Van den Aardweg G J, Hopewell J W and Whitehouse E M 1995 The radiation response of the cervical spinal cord of the pig: effects of changing the irradiated volume *Int. J. Radiat. Oncol. Biol. Phys.* **31** 51–6

Van den Bent M J, Afra D, de Witte O *et al* 2005 Long-term efficacy of early versus delayed radiotherapy for low-grade astrocytoma and oligodendroglioma in adults: the EORTC 22845 randomised trial *Lancet* **366** 985–90

Weber D C, Murray F, Combescure C *et al* 2018 Long term outcome of skull-base chondrosarcoma patients treated with high-dose proton therapy with or without conventional radiation therapy *Radiother. Oncol.* **129** 520–6

Woolley T E, Belmonte-Beitia J, Calvo G F *et al* 2018 Changes in the retreatment radiation tolerance of the spinal cord with time after the initial treatment *Int. J. Radiat. Biol.* **94** 515–31

Chapter 11

Radiobiological interpretation of the finding of RBE changes within similar SOBPs placed at superficial and deep locations in passively scattered beams but not in scanned pencil beams

Marked differences in relative biological effect (RBE) were found in studies where spread-out Bragg peak (SOBP) placements were at (a) superficial depth and (b) at close to the maximum depth by varying the incident energy in each case. For pencil beam scanning, RBE did not change with SOBP placement depth (Britten *et al* 2013), but for passively scattered beams (PSBs), high RBE values (typically 1.2–1.3) in superficially placed SOBPs reduced to very low values (1–1.07) within SOBPs placed at an extreme depth (Calugaru *et al* 2011).

The physical parameters of dose, linear energy transfer (LET) distributions and kinetic energies along each SOBP were closely comparable regardless of SOBP depth placement. However, instantaneous changes in particle fluence, dose rate and inter-track distances must change substantially in the PSB beam with increasing SOBP depth placement, although the dose-rate changes that occurred in these experiments is insufficient to substantially increase sub-lethal damage DNA repair in the above experiments.

Equations are provided which allow α and β changes, resulting in reduced α/β ratios with falling dose rate (the converse to FLASH studies), and compatible with a reduction in micro-volumetric energy transfer (or MVET), with commensurate reductions in RBE. The published depth distances, the observed dose rates and the radiosensitivity ratios found in the experiments can be used to estimate the changes in RBE, which are compatible with the experimental PSB results of Calugaru *et al* (2011) to within a 5% tolerance limit, but with no significant RBE change for pencil beams, where high fluence rates and the same inter-track distances are maintained along the beam, compatible with the experimental results of Britten *et al* (2013).

doi:10.1088/978-0-7503-6209-2ch11

There are considerable clinical implications since excess proton therapy toxicity might occur with intense pencil spot beams when compared with PSBs when the SOBP is placed in a deep position. This poses a dilemma for scanned pencil beam users, who need to be vigilant about RBE allocations in proton therapy.

11.1 Introduction

It is crucial to appreciate that, although relative biological effect (RBE) always increases along a spread-out Bragg peak (SOBP), placement of the SOBP at a much greater depth (by means of an increase in incident beam energy) results in a marked reduction in RBE within the SOBP in the case of passively scattered beams (PSBs), although not in pencil scanned beams. This was found in comparative experimental studies. The last few pages of chapter 1 contain figures 1.4 and 1.5, which demonstrate the relevant experimental arrangements. It is essential to understand these, as confusion often occurs in readers who assume a more direct and simplistic interpretation of the meaning of depth in this context. The depth mainly being considered here is the placement depth of the SOBP and not the quite separate depth along the SOBP, a measurement which is carefully preserved in the experimental studies independently of the depth of the SOBP placement. The studies then go on to measure RBE at similar relative depths within the SOBPs themselves (these are referred to as point depths, called points 1, 2 and 3 at similar distances within the SOBP). Substantial comparative reductions in RBE were found between SOBPs placed at relatively superficial depths (with the highest RBE values) when compared with SOBPs placed at the deepest depths (the lowest RBE values) for scattered proton beams in the experiments of Calugaru *et al* (2011). These are in marked contrast with the remarkably constant ranges of RBE found in similarly designed experiments using scanned pencil beams by Britten *et al* (2013). For further details, see chapter 1, including the aforementioned figures 1.4 and 1.5, which illustrate the RBE findings for different SOBP placement depths; reading of the two experimental studies is also recommended in order to understand the experimental setups thoroughly.

These contrasting findings were noted from 2017 onwards and interpreted as being due to reduction in near-instantaneous beam fluence rate, dose rate and increased inter-track distances caused by scattered beam diversion that exceeds the more minimal diversion along pencil beams, which also maintain their higher dose-rate intensity in each pencil beam per unit time, as discussed in Jones (2017), Jones *et al* (2018) and Jones (2022). Such an effect on instantaneous dose rate is not found with scanned pencil beams, which maintain a fairly constant fluence rate and inter-track distances for SOBPs placed superficially or at the extreme depth.

This chapter considers how the PSB results in a reduced beam intensity per unit time if the SOBP is placed at a near end-of-range depth, which can then influence the radiosensitivity parameters that control RBE, probably caused by considerable reductions in the near-instantaneous dose rates and increased inter-track separations, but which do not have a substantial impact on enzymatic repair processes in the relevant short times.

11.2 Methods

The linear quadratic (LQ) model of radiation effect α and β radiosensitivity parameters are modified by linear energy transfer (LET) and dose rate. The SOBP depth positions and the three points of interest related to them, with the relevant dose rates as used by Calugaru *et al* (2011), are used to determine the most likely falloff in dose rate as an exponential function of depth. It is noted that the relationship with distance could be anywhere between an inverse square ($1/d^2$), where d is the depth, to a $1/d$ function, and this will vary with the type and functionality of scattering system used, which is often double rather than single. An exponential function linking dose rate and depth of SOBP is used in this chapter for minor changes in depth, but only to further refine the much larger reductions of dose rate found at the deepest SOBP placement.

The experimental designs included three designated points: P1 in the entrance region before the true SOBP, P2 in the mid-SOBP, and P3 towards the end of the SOBP for the 76 and 201 MeV beams in the Calugaru *et al* (2011) experiments. In this way, the three depths within each SOBP were kept constant and the only variable was the depth of SOBP placement. The Britten *et al* (2013) experiments followed a similar design, but used slightly different proton energies. These SOBP positions ensure comparable LET ranges for each energy used, since the dimensions of each SOBP were identical for each energy, ensuring that their LET distributions were comparable, the chief variable then being dose and fluence rates. The change in treatment times with beam energy change was insufficient to influence enzymatic DNA repair of sub-lethal damage, due to the much longer half-times of repair of 15–30 min occurring in cellular experiments: to give 2.86 Gy (the quoted D_{37} dose) would require $2.86/3 = 0.95$ min at 3 Gy hr^{-1} for the 201 MeV beam, but $2.86/7.5 = 0.38$ min at 7.5 Gy hr^{-1} for the 76 MeV beam.

11.2.1 Linear quadratic model base equations

The radiosensitivity parameters α and β and the α/β ratio will vary with dose or fluence rate due to changes in micro-volumetric energy transfer (or MVET, since the product of fluence rate and LET provides energy transfer per unit volume and time), and so influence radiosensitivity and RBE, using the equations derived by Jones (2022), where α/β changes with dose rate, in the context of FLASH radiotherapy, according to

$$J = \left(\frac{R}{R_{\text{ref}}}\right)^{0.3} = \frac{(\alpha/\beta)_R}{(\alpha/\beta)_{R\text{ref}}}, \tag{11.1}$$

where R is a dose rate, which can be greater or lesser than the reference dose rate R_{ref}, and where the same subscript symbols are used for their associated α/β ratio values.

These dose-rate changes are applied to the depth positions used for the two extreme SOBP positions used by Calugaru *et al* (2011), and for the reference radiation at the specified superficial and deep SOBP depth positions. No allowance for sub-lethal damage DNA repair is necessary.

11.2.2 The modelling method

1. The experimental reference photon dose rates reduce with depth (from 7.5 to 3 Gy min^{-1}) at each SOBP depth placement. The same dose rates were applied for 76 MeV protons (7.5 Gy min^{-1}) and 201 MeV protons (3 Gy min^{-1}), although with further changes for different locational points.
2. The field cross-sectional areas were 3 and 12 cm diameters at depths of 3 and 18 cm for 76 and 201 MeV beam energies, respectively. For exploratory modelling purposes, these areas are assumed to be changing exponentially as

$$\pi 1.5^2 = \pi 6^2 . \, e^{-a\Delta d}, \tag{11.2}$$

where the depth is Δd, since there is an inevitable component of scattering and attenuation as well as pure geometrical contributions, from which $a = 0.06\ \text{cm}^{-1}$.
3. α/β ratios can be influenced not only by high-LET effects but also by dose-rate effects when these fall into the domain where repair enzyme activity is low or insignificant (Jones 2022a). This is achieved by the operator J, where

$$J . \, (\alpha/\beta)_{R\text{ref}} = (\alpha/\beta)_R \text{ so that } J . = \frac{(\alpha/\beta)_R}{(\alpha/\beta)_{R\text{ref}}}, \tag{11.3}$$

and where the subscripts R and R' are, respectively, the reference dose rate and the altered dose rate for the same type of radiation. J is also a function of dose rate and consequently of beam divergence.
4. The LQ reference radiation BED is

$$\text{BED} = d_{\text{ref}}\left(1 + \frac{d_{\text{ref}}}{(\alpha/\beta)_{\text{ref}}}\right), \tag{11.4}$$

and for the 76 MeV proton beam must include RBE_{max} and $\text{RBE}^2_{\text{min}}$ (the ratio of α and β parameters obtained, respectively, divided by those of the reference radiation), with the subscripts 'pr' for proton dose:

$$\text{BED} = d_{\text{pr}}\left(\text{RBE}_{\text{max}} + d_{\text{pr}}\frac{\text{RBE}^2_{\text{min}}}{(\alpha/\beta)_{\text{ref}}}\right), \tag{11.5}$$

Equations (11.4) and (11.5) are then equated and solved for d_{ref}, then divided by d_{pr} to provide an estimated RBE using the RBE_{max} and $\text{RBE}^2_{\text{min}}$ values given for the caesium-137 (^{137}Cs) reference radiation and with 76 MeV protons in Calugaru *et al* (2011), given by the solution

$$\text{RBE} = \frac{0.5}{d_{\text{pr}}}\left(-(\alpha/\beta)_{\text{ref}} + \sqrt{(\alpha/\beta)^2_{\text{ref}} + 4 . \, d_{\text{pr}}\,(\alpha/\beta)_{\text{ref}}\text{RBE}_{\text{max}+}\,4d^2_{\text{pr}}\text{RBE}^2_{\text{min}}}\right). \tag{11.6}$$

For the higher energy, the J operator can be used with each of the RBE limit terms as a product with $\mathrm{RBE_{max}}$, but $\mathrm{RBE^2_{min}}$ is divided by J. J must also operate on the reference α/β ratio, since the reference dose rate also has changed in a time frame where DNA repair can be neglected. The partitioning of J between $\mathrm{RBE_{max}}$ and $\mathrm{RBE^2_{min}}$ (which determines the changes in α and β, respectively), using an index parameter m, ensures that the product of J^m and $J^{(1-m)}$ provides J. The partitioning should respect the unit of dose (which contributes to RBE although RBE is itself dimensionless) and also the units of α and β, namely $\mathrm{Gy^{-1}}$ and $\mathrm{Gy^{-2}}$, respectively, so that α and $\sqrt{\beta}$ should be used. Then the indices should follow the relationship

$$m + 0.5m = 1, \tag{11.7}$$

where $m = 0.667$ and $1 - m = 0.333$ approximately.

The BED for the 201 MeV protons is then given by

$$d_{\mathrm{pr}}\left(J^m \mathrm{RBE_{max}} + d_{pr}\frac{\mathrm{RBE^2_{min}}}{J^{(1-m)}.\ J(\alpha/\beta)_{\mathrm{ref}}}\right). \tag{11.8}$$

For isoeffective conditions, equation (11.8) can then be equated with the reference radiation BED given by

$$d_{\mathrm{ref}}\left(1 + \frac{d_{\mathrm{ref}}}{J(\alpha/\beta)_{\mathrm{ref}}}\right). \tag{11.9}$$

5. J is found from its original definition with respect to dose rates as in equation (11.1). The dose rates are incorporated in the J function by correction for depth based on the given dose rates at mid-SOBP positions: 7.5 and 3 Gy $\mathrm{min^{-1}}$ for points 2 in the SOBPs of the 76 and 2001 MeV beams, respectively. These dose rates are further corrected for positional changes relative to the mid-SOBP P2 positions in the case of points 1 and 3 by using equation (11.2), which results in P1: $J = 0.95$, P2: $J = 0.76$ and P3: $J = 0.74$ when the appropriate dose rates are divided and a 0.3 exponent applied to these ratios [5].
6. The isoeffect is then found by solving equation (11.8), equated with equation (11.9) for d_{ref}, and divided by the operative d_{pr} value to provide the RBE as

$$\mathrm{RBE} = \frac{0.5}{d_{pr}}\left(-J(\alpha/\beta)_{\mathrm{ref}} + \sqrt{\frac{J^3.\ (\alpha/\beta)^2_{\mathrm{ref}} + 4.\ d_{pr}\quad J^{m+2}(\alpha/\beta)_{\mathrm{ref}}\mathrm{RBE}_{\mathrm{max}+}\ 4d_{pr}{}^2J^m.\ \mathrm{RBE^2_{min}}}{\sqrt{J}}}\right). \tag{11.10}$$

7. When $J = 1$, as in the pencil scanned beams, equation (11.10) becomes equal to equation (11.6).

Table 11.1. Estimated RBEs for points of interest within the SOBPs. For the most superficial SOBP, α and β values were used to estimated RBE using equation (11.6); for the deep SOBP equation (11.10) was used. The RBE ranges in parentheses refer to 137Cs and 60Co as the reference radiation sources respectively[1].

Designated point in SOBP	76 MeV RBE	201 MeV RBE
P1 ($J = 0.95$)	1.00 (0.99, 1.07)	0.98 (1–1.07)
P2 ($J = 0.76$)	1.08 (1.07, 1.14)	0.97 (1–1.07)
P3 ($J = 0.74$)	1.21 (1.25, 1.33)	1.05 (1–1.07)

[1] From data of Calugaru *et al* (2011).

11.3 Results

Table 11.1 shows the close agreement between the predicted and experimental results obtained for the HeLa cells in the study by Calugaru *et al* (2011).

The HeLa cell analysis is consistent with LQ theory, with α increasing to a greater extent than β with increased LET, although the β values do reduce slightly which is probably due to β being more difficult to estimate.

The SQ20B cell line showed considerably more statistical variation and there is inconsistency in that the α and β values do not conform with their expected increases with distance along a SOBP (with β increasing by more than α with increasing LET, probably due to the imposed curve fitting due to the excessive surviving fraction variations) and so should not be taken further in terms of predicting RBE changes with depth of SOBP placement, since the input radiosensitivity α and β values would not be appropriate.

The 76 MeV energy resulting in a superficially placed SOBP shows consistent and supra-linear changes in RBE with depth along the SOBP as seen in figure 11.1.

Similarly, the Britten *et al* (2013) RBE values increase with depth along each of the two SOBPs, but in a linear placed at superficial and deep positions, as displayed in figure 11.2.

11.4 Discussion

From the above data, it can be appreciated that, although RBE increases along each SOBP, regardless of their depth placement, RBE can be reduced markedly in a scattered beam when the SOBP placement is near the extreme depth range compared with SOBP placement at a superficial depth. Such a change is not found with scanned pencil beams.

The modelled results in HeLa cells presented are compatible with the hypothesis that beam divergence of the entire beam in a scattered beam causes a marked reduction in RBE when a proton SOBP is repositioned from a superficial to a much deeper distance by increasing beam energy. Such changes were not found in closely comparable experiments using non-divergent (scanned) beams where particle tracks are near-parallel and no such change in dose and fluence rate occurs with increasing depth.

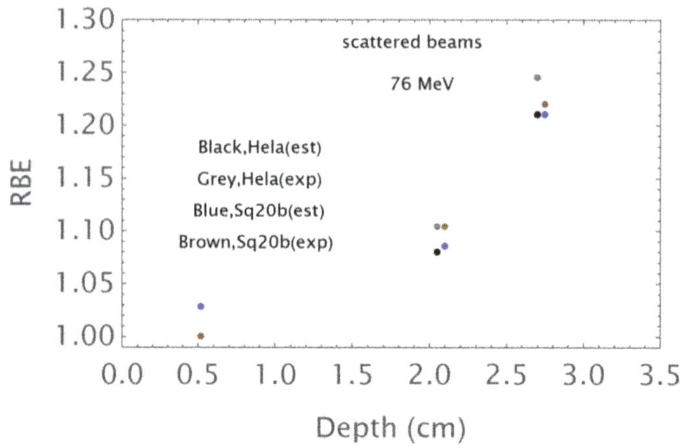

Figure 11.1. Results of Calugaru *et al* showing the experimental RBE results (exp) for each cell line compared with the estimated RBE results (est) obtained from the published α and β radiosensitivity values. The Hela cell line RBE at a depth of 0.5 cm were very close to 1, so are not shown.

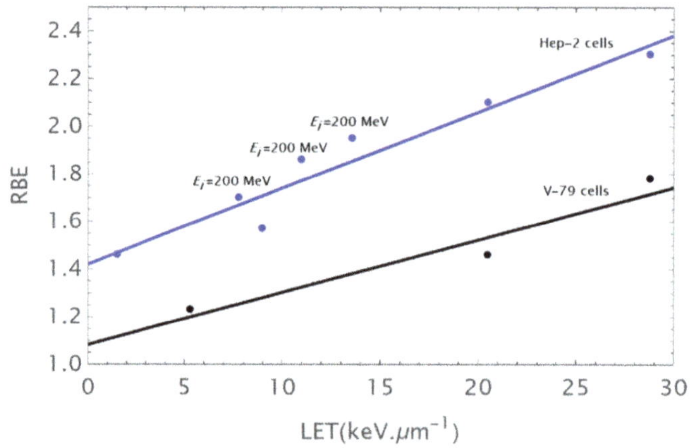

Figure 11.2. Plots of RBE with depth along SOBP obtained from the experiments of Britten *et al* using two different cell lines. The results obtained at energies at 200 MeV are marked; other points are results obtained using the 87 MeV beam energy.

These are important experiments, since the analysis of past proton therapy clinical results could be influenced similarly by the reduction in RBE: serious late normal tissue side effects might then be reduced in treatments where SOBP positions were at significant depths, e.g. in some CNS treatments with targets near midline where depths of around 7–10 cm may be used, but mostly in pelvic or thoracic treatments where greater skin-to-target distances occur. There could also be changes in tumour control if RBE falls to below the actual RBE used in the treatment prescription process.

At present, there has been a considerable shift in commercial accelerator beam delivery systems to produce only scanned beams for two reasons, namely some concern about low-dose fast neutron beam contamination from the scattering foils, and range shifters as published, respectively, by Polf & Newhauser (2005), Brenner & Hall (2008), Gerweck *et al* (2014) and Leite *et al* (2021). Pencil beam scanning techniques avoid much neutron generation before beam entry into the patient and can also achieve better dose–target 'conformity', as in the study by Brigitta *et al* (2004).

These two physical advantages could, in some critical clinical circumstances, be overridden by the higher RBE values maintained for SOBPs placed at increasing depths. A reliance on a fixed RBE of 1.1 would then incur greater susceptibility to produce unintended normal tissue damage if the RBE exceeds 1.1 and also if it is maintained with increasing depth. This is most likely to occur in anatomical sites such as the brain, where RBE values probably exceed 1.1, due to neural tissue having a low α/β ratio and the inevitable inclusion of brain tissue in the margin around a malignant tumour, as discussed in Jones (2016, 2022b) and covered in chapters 7 and 10 of this book.

A suggested method for immediate reduction of this risk has already been published (Jones 2022b), and the description forms chapter 10 in this book, whereas more complex methods involving LET and RBE considerations may take many years to be accepted depending on what level of rigorous proof is deemed necessary. It also remains to be seen whether some more scientifically informed clinicians will, in carefully selected patients, elect to use scattered beams for deeper tumour sites in order to deliberately reduce the risk of tissue damage caused by elevated RBE values. This may especially be required in re-treatment situations where enhanced RBE considerations can be especially important (Moore *et al* 2021).

There are reports containing higher than expected findings of neural radio-necrosis, or radiation-induced brain injuries, amounting to 64 events in 21 of 42 studied low-grade glioma patients (Eulitz *et al* 2023), and the above 10% risk of radio-necrotic changes in the treatment of skull-base tumours reported by Weber *et al* (2016) may be at least partly caused by non-divergent scanned beams and the inappropriate use of a 1.1 RBE.

Clinical commissioning of proton beams is at present limited mainly to physical depth–dose and reproducibility considerations. There needs to be greater attention to radiobiology along the beam for multiple SOBP depth placement positions. Users should ideally have a choice between the use of scattered and scanned beams in clinical circumstances where the correct choice may be advantageous. Analysis of clinical data sets should also take account of which beam scanning techniques and depth positions were used.

11.5 Conclusions

- The substantial fall of RBE in passively scattered beams in SOBPs placed at extreme depth ranges compared with superficially placed SOBP is compatible with a reduction with dispersion-related dose rates during such continuous exposures.
- Pencil beam scanning will not allow such an effect since the beam sweep, although covering the same area of dispersion, is delivered to separate small volumes at a much higher dose rate.

- Greater care is required for pencil beam scanning proton prescriptions since the average RBE for different SOBP placement depths will be higher than for passively scanned beams.

References

Brenner D J and Hall E J 2008 Secondary neutrons in clinical proton radiotherapy: a charged issue *Radiother. Oncol.* **86** 165–70

Brigitta G, Baumert B G, Norton I A, Lomax A J and Davis J B 2004 Dose conformation of intensity-modulated stereotactic photon beams, proton beams, and intensity-modulated proton beams for intracranial lesions *Int. J. Radiat. Oncol. Biol. Phys.* **60** 1314–24

Britten R A, Nazaryan V, Davis L K *et al* 2013 Variations in the RBE for cell killing along the depth-dose profile of a modulated proton therapy beam *Radiat. Res.* **179** 21–8

Calugaru V, Nauraye C, Noel G *et al* 2011 Radiobiological characterization of two therapeutic proton beams with different initial energy spectra used at the Institut Curie Proton Therapy Center in Orsay *Int. J. Radiat. Oncol. Biol. Phys.* **81** 1136–43

Eulitz J, Troost E G C, Klünder L *et al* 2023 Increased relative biological effectiveness and periventricular radiosensitivity in proton therapy of glioma patients *Radiother. Oncol.* **178** 109422

Gerweck L E, Huang P, Lu H-M, Paganetti H and Zhou Y 2014 Lifetime increased cancer risk in mice following exposure to clinical proton beam-generated neutrons *Int. J. Radiat. Oncol. Biol. Phys.* **89** 161–6

Jones B 2016 Why RBE must be a variable and not a constant in proton therapy *Br. J. Radiol.* **89** 20160116

Jones B 2017 Particle physics for biological interactions *Practical Radiobiology for Proton Therapy Treatment Planning* (Bristol: Institute of Physics Publishing) ch 1 (1.5–1.15)

Jones B, McMahon S J and Prise K M 2018 The radiobiology of proton therapy: challenges and opportunities around relative biological effectiveness *Clin. Oncol. (R. Coll. Radiol.)* **30** 285–92

Jones B 2022 The influence of hypoxia on LET and RBE relationships with implications for ultra-high dose rates and FLASH modelling *Phys. Med. Biol.* **67** 125011

Jones B 2022a The influence of hypoxia on LET and RBE relationships with implications for ultrahigh dose rates and FLASH modelling *Phys. Med. Biol.* **67** 125011

Jones B 2022b Risk assessment for proton therapy in the central nervous system by assuming small increments in RBE *Radiat. Phys. Chem.* **200** 110213

Leite A M M, Ronga M G, Giorgi M *et al* 2021 Secondary neutron dose contribution from pencil beam scanning, scattered and spatially fractionated proton therapy *Phys. Med. Biol.* **66** 225010

Polf J C and Newhauser W D 2005 Calculations of neutron dose equivalent exposures from range-modulated proton therapy beams *Phys. Med. Biol.* **50** 3859–73

Moore J W, Woolley T E, Hopewell J W and Jones B 2021 Further development of spinal cord retreatment dose estimation: including radiotherapy with protons and light ions *Int. J. Radiat. Biol.* **97** 1657–66

Weber D C, Malyapa R, Albertini F *et al* 2016 Long term outcomes of patients with skull-base low-grade chondrosarcoma and chordoma patients treated with pencil beam scanning proton therapy *Radiother. Oncol.: J. Eur. Soci. Ther. Radiol. Oncol.* **120** 169–74

Chapter 12

Particle therapy dose–time compensations in unintended interruptions and re-treatments

This chapter is concerned with the following:

(1) Numerical methods of how to compensate for unintended treatment interruptions by using biological effective dose (BED) and tumour cell repopulation considerations in the context of high-linear-energy-transfer (LET) therapy, which are more complex than in the case of conventional treatments since there must be associated RBE-related effects. Worked examples are presented.

(2) The difficult clinical problem of estimating changes in the recovery of normal tissue tolerance, which increases with time after an interval of around 90 days after previous radiation exposures in the central nervous system. The estimation process can be assisted by using carefully designed mathematical methods which have now been automated. These produce estimated re-treatment tissue tolerances in the central nervous system as a function of elapsed time following the initial treatment (expressed as the percentage BED of the accepted tissue tolerance BED). In the special context of particle therapy RBE factors must also be included in these formulations, since they will be sensitive to dose-per fraction changes, and which provide a final treatment BED obtained from the percentage tolerance BED given by the time-dependent equations.

12.1 Introduction

Two separate time-related issues are considered with respect to the estimation of the dose required to compensate for:

1. Continuing tumour cell repopulation during unintended treatment interruptions resulting in extension of the overall treatment time, usually by a few days or weeks, but may be longer.

doi:10.1088/978-0-7503-6209-2ch12

2. Recovery of normal tissue radiation tolerances at extended times between 3 and 6 months to many years after a treatment course, and which may allow further radiation therapy to be given.

To distinguish between these two different types of problems, it is important to recognise that interruptions of under 90 days should be considered as treatment interruptions (since normal tissue tolerance for late central nervous system (CNS) effects does not appear to change) but intervals of over 90 days should be classified as re-treatments (since normal tissue tolerance will then change after that time). This distinction was especially important during the COVID-19 pandemic when many treatment interruptions occurred, sometimes amounting to many months.

12.2 Unintended treatment interruptions

12.2.1 Background

A reduction in tumour control with extended overall treatment times was shown in classical experimental studies, such as Fowler *et al* (1974). The clinical problem of compensating for treatment interruptions was initially modelled using power-law equations, but which proved unreliable, since the parameters used were derived from acute-reacting tissue studies and inappropriately applied to late-reacting tissues; as a result, enhanced late toxicities occurred.

More realistic identification of the clinical problem was made by Withers *et al* (1988). Subsequent publications showed a reduction in tumour control by about 1%–2% per extended treatment day in the case of squamous cell cancers and transitional cell cancers. Rapid repopulation is now a better-understood cause of treatment failure (Kim & Tannock 2005). Ample references for the above facts can be obtained in the report of the UK Royal College of Radiologists (2008 and 2019). A longer time was required to identify a reduction in tumour control rates with treatment protraction in other forms of cancer, especially those associated with slower tumour cell kinetics such as prostate cancer (Thames *et al* 2010), which appear to manifest as around 0.25 Gy day^{-1} after 6–7 weeks (breast cancer probably behaves similarly). Further clinical data-set analysis is likely to produce new information about other classes of tumour in the future.

Modelling is used in these circumstances as the best guide to compensatory dose estimation, since clinical trials that allow deliberate treatment interruptions would not be ethical. The methods use equations given in chapter 2 (equations (2.6)–(2.10)). Especially important is the basic biological effective dose (BED) equation, which includes repopulation, but modified for high-linear-energy-transfer (LET) radiations as

$$\mathrm{BED} = nd\left(\mathrm{RBE}_{\max} + \mathrm{RBE}_{\min}^{2} \cdot \frac{d}{\left(\frac{\alpha}{\beta}\right)_L}\right) - K_L T - T_K, \tag{12.1}$$

where T is the overall time, K_L the low-LET daily BED repopulation equivalent and T_K a lag time until repopulation is active. This BED equation has been obtained from the basic equation given as equation (2.7) in chapter 2 by dividing throughout by α_L, so the BED units of K_L are the same as for any photon treatment, just as the α/β ratio used, with the RBE limits, is that of the low-LET condition. This last equation, with these specific parameters, will be the method used below. However, if $(\alpha/\beta)_H$ is used to compute BED without the necessity for using RBE values, then it is essential to use K_H and not K_L values. The alternative repopulation factor will be obtained by dividing by α_H rather than α_L, so that

$$K_H = \frac{0.693}{\alpha_H .\ T_{\mathrm{eff}}}, \tag{12.2}$$

and the relationship between K_L and K_H is given by

$$K_H = \frac{K_L}{\mathrm{RBE}_{\max}}. \tag{12.3}$$

Then the BED will be

$$\mathrm{BED} = nd\left(1 + \frac{d}{\left(\frac{\alpha}{\beta}\right)_H}\right) - K_H(T - T_K). \tag{12.4}$$

12.2.2 Treatment delays

The causes of treatment delays are numerous and include accelerator breakdown, patient illness, severe tissue reactions, chemotherapy complications, transport delays, etc. Particle therapy is especially vulnerable, since treatments normally depend on only one accelerator (rather than one per room for x-ray-based treatments). For long accelerator or gantry breakdowns, close liaison between the physicist and oncologist is required to discuss alternative treatment approaches such as x-ray intensity-modulated radiation therapy (or IMRT) or other focal x-ray-based techniques.

12.2.3 Calculations for compensation of treatment interruptions

The calculations are relatively simple but involve many steps and potential pitfalls (Dale *et al* 2002, Bese *et al* 2007). It must be appreciated that exact compensations for either a normal or a tumour tissue isoeffect will lead to a detriment in the other, so it is necessary to provide a range of solutions which can be chosen by the clinician in charge, and—where possible—the views of the patient.

Interruptions occurring early in the treatment course are easier to compensate, for example by working on weekends or by using two well-spaced treatments on some days close to the end of the week. The difficult cases are those interruptions which occur later during the treatment course. A model calculation for a delay in treatment when only part of the treatment was carbon ions has already been published (Jones *et al* 2006), and is more briefly given again below. In the case of hadrontherapy, great care is required, especially regarding the units of dose: if calculations involve the true physical dose (for example by conversion from the cobalt equivalent, or equivalent dose, or RBE-Gy) then the answer is in physical dose and any correction would need to be further adjusted to the original units such as RBE-Gy.

The following two worked examples are based on (1) pure proton and (2) pure carbon treatments. Protons are used to show how subtle differences in results are found from the two different calculation methods. The values used are not intended to be specific for any particular tumour, and the modelling examples are intended to demonstrate general principles. LET values have not been used in order to reduce the complexity, but the models described in other chapters 8 and 9 can be used to translate the working LET values to RBE_{max} and RBE_{min} values, which then allows the RBE to vary according to the specific dose per fraction under consideration. The results are compared with the use of a fixed (constant) RBE.

Worked example 1
A proton treatment of 46 Gy-eq in 23 fractions is prescribed for a paediatric sarcoma affecting the posterior orbit, treating daily five times per week over 31 days; the child does not require anaesthesia but mild sedation. The treatment is interrupted in the fourth week, on the day after 15 fractions had been given and for a duration of 7 days.

Assume that a simple 1.1 RBE factor has been applied to provide the Gy-eq dose, and that the tumour shows a constant low rate of repopulation equivalent to 0.3 Gy-eq day^{-1}. Then we use standard BED equations since it is assumed that there all doses are convertible by the 1.1 RBE factor. This assumption is used initially and will be compared with a more flexible RBE value using RBE_{max} and RBE_{min} later. For the sake of simplicity, equal doses to critical normal tissue and tumour are assumed; readers can calculate different BEDs for different isodose values using the following formula:

$$\mathrm{BED} = xnd\left(1 + \frac{xd}{\left(\frac{\alpha}{\beta}\right)}\right), \tag{12.5}$$

where x refers to the change in dose, n is the number of fractions and would be 0.6 for a 60% isodose line and 0.35 for a 35% isodose line, etc.

Calculations using a fixed RBE value for two different tissue types within the planning target volume (PTV).

Tissue A: Intended BED to PTV containing normal tissue late-reacting soft tissue using $\alpha/\beta = 3$ Gy; the BED is 46 (1 + 2/3) = 76.67 $\mathrm{Gy}_{[3]}$.

Tissue B: Intended BED to PTV containing normal tissue late-reacting brain/neural tissue using $\alpha/\beta = 2$ Gy; the BED is 46 (1 + 2/2) = 92 $Gy_{[2]}$.

Tumour: Intended tumour BED, using $\alpha/\beta = 10$ Gy, is 46(1 + 2/10) – 0.3 T = 45.90 $Gy_{[10]}$.

BEDs before interruptions:

Tissue A: 30 (1 + 2/3) = 50 $Gy_{[3]}$.

Tissue B: 30 (1 + 2/2) = 60 $Gy_{[2]}$.

Tumour: 30 (1+2/10) = 30.3 $Gy_{[10]}$.

The BED deficit is then

Tissue A: 26.67 $Gy_{[3]}$.

Tissue B: 32 $Gy_{[2]}$.

Tumour: 15.6 $Gy_{[10]}$.

If uncorrected, the tumour BED (over 31 + 7 days) would be

$= 46(1 + 2/10) - 0.3 \times 38 = 43.8$ $Gy_{[10]}$.

By treating with the same dose per fraction through one weekend, 2 days can be saved, so the tumour BED is then

$= 46(1 + 2/10) - 0.3 \times 36 = 44.4$ $Gy_{[10]}$.

By treating twice a day for all remaining weekday treatments (i.e. eight fractions in 4 days) the overall time is 32 days and the BED is then

$= 46(1 + 2/10) - 0.3 \times 32 = 45.6$ $Gy_{[10]}$.

This seems a good alternative and almost completely restores the BED, but may not be feasible if twice daily sedation is unacceptable.

Another way forward would be to give additional daily fractions, extending overall time further. If, for example, we try to give the remaining compensatory dose in one additional fraction of 2 Gy in one extra day after completing the prescribed dose, with all delays we obtain an overall treatment time of around 39 days.

For $d = 2$ Gy, the BED is

$= 46(1 + 2/10) + d(1 + d/10) - 0.3 \times 39 = 45.9$ Gy,

which is almost the same tumour BED as the original prescription, but the normal tissue BEDs will then be tissue A BED = 80 $Gy_{[3]}$ and tissue B BED = 96 $Gy_{[2]}$. These have increased. This additional normal tissue BED can be reduced by fractionating the final day of additional treatment into two treatments of 1.1 Gy, so that the BED is

$= 46(1 + 2/10) + 2 \times 1.1(1 + 1.1/10) - 0.3 \times 39.$

The tumour BED is then 45.94 $Gy_{[10]}$, tissue A = 79.67 $Gy_{[3]}$ and tissue B = 95.41 $Gy_{[2]}$. The normal tissue BEDs have reduced a little.

Consider what might happen if treatment is hypofractionated and given in only three remaining fractions in order to complete in the same overall treatment time but matched to give the same CNS effect in tissue B (a deficit BED of 32 $Gy_{[2]}$).

First, solve $32 = 3 \times d(1 + d/2)$; $d = 3.73$ Gy.

Then the tumour BED would then be lower:

BED = 30 (1 + 2/10) + 3 × 3.73(1 + 3.73/10) – 31 × 0.3 = 42.06 $Gy_{[10]}$.

This BED is probably unacceptable, so the alternative method given above would be preferred to maintain reasonable tumour control.

Another approach would be to give twice daily treatment for the entire remainder of treatment. In this way, 16 fractions could be given in 8 further days after the unintended gap, completing treatment in 36 days. For a dose per fraction of 1.15 Gy, we obtain the following.

The tumour BED would be

$15 \times 2(1 + 2/10) + 1.15 \times 16(1 + 1.15/10) - 36 \times 0.3 = 45.72\ \mathrm{Gy}_{[10]}$.

The tissue A BED is then

$$15 \times 2\left(1 + 2/3\right) + 1.15 \times 16\left(1 + 1.15/3\right) = 75.45\ \mathrm{Gy}_{[3]}.$$

And the tissue B BED is

$$15 \times 2\left(1 + 2/2\right) + 1.15 \times 16\left(1 + 1.15/2\right) = 88.98\ \mathrm{Gy}_{[3]}.$$

These BEDs all are slightly below the intended BEDs. It should be noted that these twice daily fractions have not taken into account the possibility of incomplete repair between fractions.

Since the above calculations have been done using a fixed RBE, it should be noted that dose units for the particle therapy are in equivalent Gy rather than Gy.

12.2.4 Calculations using a variable RBE value

In this case the actual physical dose of protons must be used along with the RBE_{max} and RBE_{min}. For the sake of simplicity, the repopulation equivalent remains 0.3 Gy day^{-1} as a physical dose.

The 2 Gy fraction was actually calculated from a 1.1 RBE so the actual dose given is 2/1.1 = 1.82 Gy. If we assume $\mathrm{RBE}_{max} = 1.15$, $\mathrm{RBE}_{min} = 1.05$ for tumour, and a higher value of $\mathrm{RBE}_{max} = 1.2$ for normal tissue and $\mathrm{RBE}_{max} = 1.3$ for brain tissue, but all have the same RBE_{min} (remember that RBE_{min} is mainly operative at high dose per fraction and will have little influence on the calculations below), we obtain the following.

Tissue A: Intended PTV containing normal soft tissue (late reacting) with $\alpha/\beta = 3$ Gy, the BED is then $23 \times 1.82\ (1.2 + 1.05^2 \times 1.82/3) = 78.23\ \mathrm{Gy}_{[3]}$.

Tissue B: Intended PTV containing late-reacting brain/neural tissue with $\alpha/\beta = 2$ Gy, the BED is then $23 \times 1.82\ (1.3 + 1.05^2 \times 1.82/2) = 96.42\ \mathrm{Gy}_{[2]}$.

Tumour: intended tumour BED, using $\alpha/\beta = 10$ Gy, is $23 \times 1.82(1.15 + 1.05^2 \times 1.82/2) - 0.3 \times 31 = 47.24\ \mathrm{Gy}_{[10]}$.

The BEDs given before interruptions are as follows:

Tissue A: $15 \times 1.82\ (1.2 + 1.05^2 \times 1.82/3) = 51.02\ \mathrm{Gy}_{[3]}$.

Tissue B: $15 \times 1.82\ (1.3 + 1.05^2 \times 1.82/2) = 62.88\ \mathrm{Gy}_{[2]}$.

Tumour: $15 \times 1.82\ (1.15 + 1.05^2 \times 1.82/10) - 0.3 \times 19 = 31.17\ \mathrm{Gy}_{[10]}$.

The BED deficit is then as follows:

Tissue A: 27.21 $\mathrm{Gy}_{[3]}$.

Tissue B: 33.54 $\mathrm{Gy}_{[2]}$.

Tumour: 16.07 $\mathrm{Gy}_{[10]}$.

If uncorrected, the tumour BED (over 31 + 7 days) would be $= 23 \times 1.82(1.15 + 1.05^2 \times 1.82/10) - 0.3 \times 38 = 45.14\ \mathrm{Gy}_{[10]}$.

By treating through one weekend 2 days can be saved, so the tumour BED is then

$$= 23 \times 1.82\left(1.15 + 1.05^2 \times 1.82/10\right) - 0.3 \times 36 = 45.74\ \mathrm{Gy}_{[10]}.$$

By treating twice a day for all remaining weekday treatments (i.e. eight fractions in 4 days), the overall time is 32 days and the BED is then

$$= 23 \times 1.82\left(1.15 + 1.05^2 \times 1.82/10\right) - 0.3 \times 32 = 46.94\ \mathrm{Gy}_{[10]}.$$

This seems a good alternative but may not be feasible if twice daily sedation is unacceptable.

Another possibility would be to give additional daily fractions, extending overall time further. If, for example, we try to give the remaining compensatory dose in one fraction in 1 extra day after completing the prescribed course (and the delay), we obtain an overall treatment time of around 39 days, then

$$\mathrm{BED} = 24 \times 1.82\left(1.15 + 1.05^2 \times 1.82/10\right)0.3 \times 39 = 47.30\ \mathrm{Gy}_{[10]},$$

which is almost the same tumour BED as the original prescription, but the normal tissue BEDs will then be tissue A BED = 81.63 $\mathrm{Gy}_{[3]}$ and tissue B BED = 100.61 $\mathrm{Gy}_{[2]}$. These have increased. This additional normal tissue BED can be reduced by fractionating the final days treatment into, say, two treatments of 1 Gy (physical dose).

The tumour BED is then 47.04 $\mathrm{Gy}_{[10]}$, the tissue A BED = 80.89$\mathrm{Gy}_{[3]}$ and the tissue B BED = 99.42 $\mathrm{Gy}_{[2]}$. This appears to be a reasonable compromise.

Consider what might happen if the remaining treatment is hypofractionated and given in only three fractions in order to complete in the same overall treatment time but matched to give the same CNS effect in tissue B (a deficit BED of 33.53 $\mathrm{Gy}_{[2]}$).

First, solve $33.53 = 3 \times d(1.3 + 1.05^2\ d/2)$; $d = 3.47$ Gy.

Then the tumour BED would be low at

$$\mathrm{BED} = 15 \times 1.82\left(1.15 + 1.05^2 \times 1.82/10\right) + 3 \times 3.47\left(1 + 3.47/10\right) - 31 \times 0.3 = 43.58\ \mathrm{Gy}_{[10]}.$$

This is probably not acceptable since the BED is less than the originally intended 47.24 $\mathrm{Gy}_{[10]}$. So, the alternative methods given above would be preferred to maintain reasonable tumour control.

Another possibility would be to use a dose such as 0.98 Gy (physical) twice daily for 8 days, completing treatment in 36 days.

The tumour BED would be

$$15 \times 1.82\left(1.15 + 1.05^2 \times 1.82/10\right) + 0.98 \times 16\left(1.15 + 1.05^2 \times 0.98/10\right) - 0.3 \times 36 = 45.80\mathrm{Gy}_{[10]}.$$

The tissue A BED is then

$$15 \times 1.82\left(1.2 + 1.05^2 \times 1.82/3\right) + 0.98 \times 16\left(1.2 + 1.05^2 \times 0.98/3\right) = 75.48\mathrm{Gy}_{[3]}.$$

And the tissue B BED is then

$$15 \times 1.82\ 1.3 + 1.05^2 \times 1.82/2 + 0.98 \times 16\ 1.3 + 1.05^2 \times 0.98/2 = 91.73\mathrm{Gy}_{[2]}.$$

Again, incomplete repair between fractions has not been used in the example, but could be used to further refine the BED.

12.2.5 Comparison of the two methods

The fixed and flexible RBE calculations give different answers when dose per fraction is changed. A comparison for one of the above alternatives is given in table 12.1. Also, in the case of giving three hypofractionated doses as compensation, we have BED values of 42.06 $Gy_{[10]}$ and 43.58 $Gy_{[10]}$ for the fixed and flexible RBE methods, respectively. These differences—due to the assumed changes in RBE with dose per fraction—provide a good reason why it might be best to deliver the remaining dose mostly using the same fraction size where possible and using altered fractionation on only a few days, especially those days preceding weekends if there is to be a further break in treatments, since over weekends accumulated incomplete repair will not occur. There is a difficulty in using 2 Gy twice daily for many treatments in acute-reacting tissues, since reactions can be made worse. General guidelines for limits of acute-reacting normal tissues have been given by Fowler *et al* (2003).

Worked example 2

An ion-beam schedule of 64 Gy-eq in 20 fractions over 26 days is interrupted after 15 fractions, for the entire fourth week and for a further 3 days into the following week (i.e. for 10 days). The tumour being treated is a squamous cell carcinoma of the peripheral bronchial tree. Here we assume a significant change in RBE with dose per fraction and only use the RBE_{max} and RBE_{min} concepts. There is no spinal cord dose. To simplify the calculations, we assume that the dose to lung tissue within the PTV will obliterate all lung function within the PTV; also that a surrounding volume (VLNT) for lung function receives approximately 50% of the prescribed dose and is relevant to the patients future wellbeing.

In this example the following assumptions are made:

RBE for dose conversion = 2.6, tumour RBE_{max} = 3.2, normal tissue RBE_{max} = 4, tumour and normal tissue RBE_{min} = 1.2, tumour α/β = 10 Gy and late-reacting normal

Table 12.1. BED calculations using two different modelling methods for twice daily fractions of 1.15 Gy-equivalent and 0.98 Gy (physical) on 8 treatment days, with treatment completion in 36 days.

	Fixed RBE	Flexible RBE
BED tumour ($Gy_{[10]}$)	45.72	45.80
BED tissue A ($Gy_{[3]}$)	75.45	75.48
BED tissue B ($Gy_{[2]}$)	88.98	91.73

tissue $\alpha/\beta = 3$ Gy. Tumour repopulation is modelled by no repopulation for 21 days followed by a repopulation rate equivalent to 0.9 Gy day^{-1}.

The 64 Gy-eq dose is a physical dose of 64/2.6 = 24.62 Gy and the physical dose per fraction consequently is 24.62/20 = 1.23 Gy.

Using the *flexible RBE* model we obtain the following.

The intended tumour BED is given by

$20 \times 1.23\left(3.2 + \frac{1.2^2 \times 1.23}{10}\right) - 0.9(T - T_K)$. The final repopulation term is zero since the intended T is less than T_K, so the BED is 83.08 $Gy_{[10]}$.

The intended normal tissue BED is

$20 \times 1.23 \times 0.5\left(4 + \frac{1.2^2 \times 1.23 \times 0.5}{3}\right) = 52.83\ Gy_{[3]}$.

The delivered tumour BED is

$15 \times 1.23\left(3.2 + \frac{1.2^2 \times 1.23}{10}\right) = 62.31\ Gy_{[10]}$.

The delivered normal tissue BED is

$15 \times 1.23 \times 0.5\left(4 + \frac{1.2^2 \times 1.23 \times 0.5}{3}\right) = 39.62\ Gy_{[3]}$.

The deficit BEDs are then as follows:

Tumour deficit: 83.08 – 62.31 = 20.77 $Gy_{[10]}$.

Normal tissue deficit: 52.83 – 39.62 = 13.21 $Gy_{[3]}$.

If it is intended to proceed by either

(1) giving the same fraction number (five) over 7 days (that is, 10 days longer than intended), but increasing the total dose; or

(2) giving six fractions of a lower dose in 3 days (that is, 6 days longer) by treating twice daily including on a Saturday.

Then for (1):

(a) If tumour control is to be maintained, we solve

$20.77 = 5d\,(3.2+1.2^2\,d/10) - (36 - 28)\,0.9$,

$d = 1.63$ Gy

The normal tissue BED will then have increased to be

$39.62 + 0.5 \times 5 \times 1.63\,(4 + 1.2^2 \times 1.63 \times 0.5/3) = 57.52\ Gy_{[3]}$, which has increased from 52.83 $Gy_{[3]}$. This could amount to 5%–10% additional complications in the volume of concern if complications increase at 1%–2% per Gy. If such a policy were to be followed, it might be appropriate to reduce the dose per fraction to, say, 1.5 Gy. This would then give a compromised tumour BED of

$62.31 + 5 \times 1.5\,(4 + 1.2^2 \times 1.5/3) - (36 - 28)\,0.9 = 80.73\ Gy_{[10]}$, instead of the intended 83.1 $Gy_{[10]}$.

Ultimately, it is the oncologist who has to decide which policy to pursue and alter the radiation prescription, but since the risks and benefits may have changed the patient should be informed as to the decision made and, ideally, they should be consulted when it comes to the choice of risks.

For method (2), where six fractions are given in 3 consecutive days (a total of 32 days), we can maintain the same tumour BED by solving for d in

$20.77 = 5d\,(3.2 + 1.2^2\, d/10) - (32 - 28)\,0.9,$
$d = 1.2$ Gy.
Then the normal tissue volume BED increases from the intended 52.83 $Gy_{[3]}$ to be $39.62 + 0.5 \times 5 \times 1.2\,(4 + 1.2^2 \times 1.2 \times 0.5/3) = 55.06$ $Gy_{[3]}$.

The latter option appears more acceptable than the former option (1), although we have not included a small increment for incomplete repair between fractions, which is considered to be small for inter-fraction intervals of 12 hr for only six fractions. This exercise has assumed that the RBE operative in the normal tissue is a worst-case scenario; at an increasing distance from the target the LET will fall, as will the RBE. However, with spread-out Bragg peaks (SOBPs) the LET remains quite high. Such details are more readily available using specially adapted treatment-planning systems, but which are beyond the scope of the present article. Again, as in the proton case discussed above, a lower dose per fraction could be chosen, e.g. 1.15 or 1.18 Gy. In all cases of a lower dose the tumour BED would fall below that intended originally.

A further example of an ion-beam boost following a first phase of x-ray-based treatment can be found in Jones *et al* (2006).

It must be remembered that there are three overall approaches to obtain a practical solution in these treatment interruption situations. These are as follows:

1. Treat with the same dose per fraction, but extend overall treatment time, possibly increasing the number of fractions. This at least has the potential advantage that the RBE will not change.
2. Treat with larger doses per fraction and complete in same overall treatment time. In this case the RBE will decrease since the fraction size has increased.
3. Treat with a larger number of fractions but with smaller dose per fraction over a slightly extended treatment time or the same treatment time. In this case the RBE will increase since the fraction size is smaller. This may have a larger effect in the normal tissues since the maximum RBE is greater in late-reacting tissues.

The above examples are meant to serve as a demonstration of how to approach treatment interruption corrections in charged-particle therapy (CPT) for treatments of curative (radical) intent. Similar approaches, with some modifications, can be applied to palliative treatments where the end point is the relief of symptoms for a reasonable duration.

It is essential to have close cooperation between all staff concerned, especially the input of clinicians to confirm the limits of normal tissue that might be acceptable as well as the medical and surgical histories of the patient, including cytotoxic chemotherapy exposures, which may influence the normal tissue tolerances. Also relevant is the detailed tumour histology, which may provide information on the rapidity of repopulation (the less well-differentiated tumours are expected to repopulate more rapidly, and possibly without a 'lag-time' effect). During the COVID-19 pandemic, the present author and Professor R. G. Dale advised many UK and some international treatment centres on extensions of photon-based treatments, and their combined experience has been published in two journals (see

Jones & Dale 2020, Dale & Jones 2022). This last reference provides the latest advice on compensatory techniques for photons (x-rays), which may be adapted for CPTs including protons. The authors also appeal for better overall standards, more specific education, and systems for ensuring good-quality assurance for such dose compensatory advice. So far, the national bodies have adopted a complacent attitude to these suggestions, and it remains to be seen if improvements might follow.

A further issue has arisen in that many European radiobiology textbooks have provided the EQD-2 (equivalent dose in 2 Gy) method for achieving these compensatory doses, with the result that many have been educated in this way and not using the simpler BED method. This appears to be satisfactory for normal tissue tolerances, but significant errors may occur with the repopulation factors. A method of overcoming this has recently been devised (Dale *et al* 2024). The method, essentially, finds a transitional BED below which simple methods of calculating tumour EQD-2 continue to be sufficient, but for higher BEDs the correct EQD-2 can be estimated from the reference schedule BED (BED_{ref}), using the relationship $\text{EQD-2} = A \times BED_{ref}\text{:}\ B$, where A and B are constants which contain the same radiobiological parameters as used in deriving BED method values. It also uses an approximate replacement of fraction number by time, depending on the number of fractions per week, as used in chapter 6. In principle, the same method could be used for CPTs by inclusion of RBE_{max} and RBE_{min}. Because of the inevitable increasing complexity, the present author recommends that the simpler BED method should be used instead, especially for proton- and ion-beam treatments.

12.2.6 Summary for unintended treatment gap corrections

- It can be appreciated that an individual approach should be used, although formulaic methods can also be devised for precise compensation for either the tumour or the normal tissue isoeffect. However, compromise solutions are inevitably required and individualisation is consequently essential.
- Ideally, such corrections should be done by persons who will practice and become used to these approaches, as there are many potential pitfalls.
- It has even been suggested that nation states should organise their own referral system for doing such calculations, although worldwide solutions and more global governance are feasible alternatives in an electronic data age.
- Data collection and sharing should be encouraged in order to study and gain further useful information.
- A BED-only method is suggested.

12.3 Re-treatments

12.3.1 Background

Radiotherapy re-treatment can be of benefit in carefully selected patients with recurrent local disease and where other salvage treatment options are inappropriate (Stewart 1999). It was traditional to assume there was no tissue recovery with time and that if several treatment courses were given over an extended time period (as is often the case in palliative treatment), their total BEDs should respect the standard tolerance BED.

Methods for estimating the change in spinal cord radiation tolerance with increasing time between the first and second radiotherapy courses have been published by Jones & Grant (2014) and Jones & Hopewell (2014). The mechanism of effect is late vascular damage, and although it is possible that the similar kinetics apply to late vascular damage in other organ systems, this is not necessarily the case: there may be anomalous tissues such as the kidney where late damage is amplified by hypertension caused by the initial renal damage itself, causing a vicious cycle of damage, and so the same relationships should not be applied. However, most late-reacting tissues, including the CNS, have similar time courses for late damage expression, although the α/β ratio used may differ. In this sense, we apply a more conservative approach to CNS sub-organs at risk than in many other anatomical sites by using $\alpha/\beta = 2$ Gy, rather than the 3 Gy elsewhere. There are also some unsatisfactory aspects to many of the classical small animal re-treatment experiments, where the beams also irradiated adjacent tissues or even the hemibody. Also, for example, bladder irradiations included the whole bladder rather than a part of it so the late effect studied was centripetal constriction, resulting in urinary frequency. Such a late effect be as severe after irradiating only a part of the organ.

These models rely on the basic linear quadratic concept of BED and some generic conclusions that after moderate to high doses of radiation there is around 50% recovery of tolerance in the spinal cord at around 6 months following radiotherapy. The study by Jones & Hopewell (2014) was based on the primate spinal cord study of Ang *et al* (2001), where an initial fixed dose was followed by re-treatment at time intervals of 1, 2 and 3 years. Essentially, if the first and second treatment courses are expressed as their BEDs as a percentage of their tolerance BED, i.e. (given BED/tolerance BED)%, then it is possible to apply a time-dependent function, $r(t)$, to estimate the final percentage tolerance BED from the first. It is important to carefully follow these definitions:

BED_{init} is the initial course BED; BED_{final} is the final course BED.
BED_1 is the % tolerance BED for the initial course (BED_{init}/tolerance BED)%.
BED_2 is the % tolerance BED for the final course (BED_{final}/tolerance BED)%.

From the shape of the experimental BED_1 versus BED_2 plots, a reasonable model which can be fitted to the animal data is

$$BED_2 = 100\left(1 - \frac{BED_1}{100}\right)^{\frac{1}{r(t)+1}}. \tag{12.6}$$

Further refinements were introduced to the model including the important 90 day lag time, which is necessary before the onset of vascular recovery processes in the CNS, and which is well established in animal models and is consistent with clinical experience, where examples of giving the full intended dose after a partial dose had been given but being interrupted by 4–6 weeks produced serious spinal cord damage. Also, it was necessary to include the human dose–response curve for spinal cord damage (which links increasing risk level with increasing BED) and relate this to the known animal dose–response curves from which the time factors were derived. Another essential feature was the allowance of a reduced normal tissue tolerance BED due to adverse medical histories, including significant surgery, age, chemotherapy exposure and other conditions. Such changes were complex to estimate by hand methods, so automation was introduced by a team of mathematicians, experimental and clinical radiobiologists, which resulted in a graphical user interface (GUI) that was later adapted to include particle therapies and RBE effects (Woolley *et al* 2018, Moore *et al* 2021).

It cannot be overemphasised that dose per fraction effects can be critical in standard forms of radiotherapy but also in proton therapy, but are probably even more important in re-treatments, so it was necessary to introduce predictive risk-based modelling with RBE values linked to LET in the second publication. To view some of the manually based explanatory estimations that were used with the GUI method, the separate publication by Jones & Hopewell (2019) should be consulted.

For charged particles, it is necessary to use the same BED approach where the particle BEDs are expressed as a function of α/β, dose, number of fractions, RBE_{max} and RBE_{min}. The latter two parameters can be estimated from the LET.

It could be the case that the initial treatment has used megavoltage photons and the second treatment charged particles. The appropriate form of the BEDs must be used in each case, for the prescription and the chosen tolerance level. Note that the chosen tolerance level should be the same in the first and second treatment courses, as this was the case in the experimental data analysis. Care is required after BED_2 has been estimated, not only to convert BED_2 to BED_{final} but also to determine the charged-particle physical dose.

To avoid manually based estimations, which can be long and tedious, a further GUI has been developed by Moore *et al* (2021); the article contains information on how to download the GUI. It allows re-treatment dose estimations for different risk levels for any combination of protons, light ions and photons (megavoltage x-rays) by using the models already described in chapters 8 and 9. Detailed worked examples are given of various initial and re-treatment permutations using these radiation modalities, with GUI screenshots. Again, the overall intention was to produce a safe re-treatment dose fractionation with an emphasis on tissue tolerance BED reductions due to adverse medical histories (as described in chapter 3). Readers are recommended to consult this publication in detail in order to obtain the necessary 'training', and no attempt has been made here to repeat the examples already published. However, the scope for re-treatment dose estimation using different modalities for initial and re-treatment can be appreciated in the form of a summary of the five worked examples (with particle doses being physical doses) in the above publication:

1. Photon–photon: Initial photon spinal cord dose of 46.5 Gy in 30 fractions, retreated 18 months later with a BED tolerance reduction of 10% due to high-dose chemotherapy. Re-treatment in 20 fractions of 1.9 Gy with around 0.1% risk.
2. Photon–proton: Initial photon dose of 47.5 Gy in 30 fractions. No adverse history. Proton re-treatment 18 months later by 23 fractions of 1.6 Gy (using

a variable RBE with a LET of 1.5 keV μm^{-1}); if a 1.1 RBE assumption had been used, the model suggests 24 fractions of 1.65 Gy. The second option would appear to confer a higher risk.

3. Proton–photon: An initial proton treatment delivered 39 Gy in 30 fractions to the optic chiasm at mid-SOBP as in example 2. The RBE was estimated to be 1.15 by the variable RBE model given in chapter 7. Re-treatment by photons 2 years later, with no adverse histories, is suggested as 30 fractions of 1.66 Gy.
4. Proton–proton: Here the LET is assumed to be, respectively, 1.3 and 1.8 keV μm^{-1} and a conservative factor of 10% was used to further reduce re-treatment tolerance. The initial treatment gave 38.5 Gy in 30 fractions to the spinal cord. Re-treatment 2.5 years later of 22 fractions of 1.67 Gy.
5. Carbon–carbon: Two carbon-ion treatment courses were required 2.5 years apart with respective LET values of 50 and 60 keV μm^{-1}. The initial treatment spinal cord dose was 10 Gy in 15 fractions. Re-treatment, using a conservative factor of 10% for adverse history, was estimated to be 11 fractions of 1.5 Gy.

The overall method is essentially conservative and can involve iterative processes to achieve a compromise between dose per fraction and the number of re-treatment fractions. Higher doses might be selected especially for small volume re-treatment by more confident clinicians, and in some instances doses may be further lowered in clinical situations that indicate a lower tolerance and higher risk, because of multiple surgical approaches, the magnitude of cytotoxic chemotherapy exposure and other concurrent medical conditions including age, etc. It is important to establish if the re-treatment is of radical or palliative intent. The duration of remission in re-treatments may be less than or greater than the original treatment, and as a rough guide should be proportional to the delivered BED.

Just as with treatment interruptions, also considerable care is required when attempting these compensations. A period of appropriate training and familiarity with all the concepts presented above is recommended.

References

Ang K K, Jiang G L, Feng Y *et al* 2001 Extent and kinetics of recovery of occult spinal cord injury *Int. J. Radiat. Oncol. Biol. Phys.* **50** 1013–20

Bese N S, Hendry J and Jeremic B 2007 Effects of prolongation of overall treatment time due to unplanned interruptions during radiotherapy of different tumor sites and practical methods for compensation *Int. J. Radiat. Oncol. Biol. Phys.* **68** 654–61

Dale R G, Hendry J H, Jones B *et al* 2002 Practical methods for compensating for missed treatment days in radiotherapy, with particular reference to head and neck schedules *Clin. Oncol.* **14** 382–93

Dale R G and Jones B 2022 Radiotherapy treatment delays in the UK during the COVID-19 pandemic *Radiat. Phys. Chem.* **200** 110214

Dale R G, Plataniotis G A and Jones B 2024 A generalised method for calculating tumour EQD2 values *Phys. Med. (Eur. J. Med. Phys.)* **118** 103294

Fowler J F, Denekamp J, Sheldon P W *et al* 1974 Optimum fractionation in x-ray treatment of C3H mouse mammary tumours *Br. J. Radiol.* **47** 781–9

Fowler J F, Harrari P M, Leborgne F and Leborgne J H 2003 Acute radiation reactions in oral and pharyngeal mucosa: tolerable levels in altered fractionation schedules *Radiother. Oncol.* **69** 161–8

Jones B, Carabe-Fernandez A and Dale R G 2006 Calculation of high-LET radiotherapy dose required for compensation of overall treatment time extensions *Br. J. Radiol.* **79** 254–7

Jones B and Grant W 2014 Retreatment of central nervous system tumours *Clin. Oncol.* **26** 407–18

Jones B and Hopewell J H 2014 Alternative models for estimating the radiotherapy retreatment dose for the spinal cord *Int. J. Radiat. Biol.* **90** 731–41

Jones B and Hopewell J W 2019 Spinal cord re-treatments using photon and proton based radiotherapy: LQ-derived tolerance doses *Eur. J. Med. Phys. (Phys. Med.).* **64** 304–10

Jones B and Dale R G 2020 Clinical and practical considerations in the design of appropriate compensation schedules following treatment interruptions *BJR|Open 2020* **2** 1

Kim J J and Tannock I F 2005 Repopulation of cancer cells during therapy: an important cause of treatment failure *Nat. Rev. Cancer* **5** 516–25

Moore J W, Woolley T E, Hopewell J W and Jones B 2021 Further development of spinal cord retreatment dose estimation: including radiotherapy with protons and light ions *Int. J. Radiat. Biol.* **97** 1657–66

Royal College of Radiologists 2008 and 2019 *Timely Delivery of Radical Radiotherapy: Guidelines for the Management of Unscheduled Treatment Interruptions* 3rd and 4th edns (London: Royal College of Radiologists)

Stewart F A 1999 Re-treatment after full-course radiotherapy: is it a viable option? *Acta Oncol.* **38** 855–62

Thames H D, Kuban D, Levy L B *et al* 2010 The role of overall treatment time in the outcome of radiotherapy of prostate cancer: an analysis of biochemical failure in 4839 men treated between 1987 and 1995 *Radiother. Oncol.* **96** 6–12

Withers H R, Taylor J M and Maciejewski B 1988 The hazard of accelerated tumor clonogen repopulation during radiotherapy *Acta Oncol.* **27** 131–46

Woolley T E, Belmonte-Beitia J, Calvo G F *et al* 2018 Changes in the retreatment radiation tolerance of the spinal cord with time after the initial treatment *Int. J. Radiat. Biol.* **94** 515–31

IOP Publishing

Quantitative Radiobiology for Proton Therapy

Bleddyn Jones

Chapter 13

Errors of Bragg peak positioning and their radio-biological correction

The correction of any significant error made in treatment delivery, whatever the cause, is inevitably more difficult for particle therapy than in the case of more conventional therapy, where the biological effective dose (BED) approach has been recommended. The additional difficulty is because not only may the linear energy transfer (LET) change, but also the dose per fraction, and each of these can change the relative biological effect (RBE).

Worked examples of such corrections, which contain assumed changes in LET and dose with resulting changes in RBE_{max} and RBE_{min} in BED equations, are given for particle therapy treatments. Some *in silico* random sampling studies of the extent to which tumour control may be reduced when random or systematic errors occur in Bragg peak positioning are provided. Errors in treatment delivery should be reduced as far as possible in particle therapy, which should have robust quality assurance systems.

13.1 Introduction

In charged-particle therapy (CPT), using protons and heavier ions, energy deposition occurs in an entirely different way from the x-rays/photons used in conventional radiotherapy. Particle Bragg peaks provide selective dose distributions, reducing collateral radiation to many important tissues, and so improve the results of radiotherapy. For this to be fully realised, it is essential to overcome two inherent difficulties associated with particle therapy:

1. Optimal prediction and confirmation of Bragg peak position within the body.
2. Improved knowledge of the relationship between the increased ionisation density within Bragg peaks (quantified as linear energy transfer, or LET) and biological effects. This is necessary in order to prescribe the best possible

tumour dose and restrict critical normal tissue doses to the safest possible extent.

It is important not to consider these factors as being entirely separate, since errors of Bragg peak positioning will lead to altered dose and LET simultaneously, with consequent non-linear effects on biological or clinical outcomes due to two causes.

This chapter uses the new simpler energy-efficiency model for predicting relative biological effect (RBE) from LET within biological effective dose (BED) equations, as given in chapter 2 onwards. The latter are useful in clinical practice and have been adapted for particle therapy. The new model requires only input of the low-LET α and β parameters and the Z number (nuclear charge) of any ion and is independent of further micro-dosimetry considerations, but relies on saturation and efficiency concepts. It can therefore be used as a second check for more complex models used at the present time, and for tentative radiobiological modelling. The model fits data from many classical particle beam experiments using different ions and at different doses or levels of cell survival.

Modelling the effect of erroneous dose delivery shows that particle therapies are more susceptible to a loss of tumour control than are x-ray-based treatments. Thus particle therapy demands greater attention to detail with best use of image guidance techniques. The importance of using the most correct RBE is emphasised, since if the RBE is incorrect, there is increased susceptibility to treatment-delivery errors.

A method for compensating unintended dose delivery errors, with worked examples, is presented. Changes in dose and LET (with resultant changes in radiosensitivity α and β values) are fed into BED equations, which are commonly used to correct errors in photon treatments. To implement these would be time consuming since three-dimensional LET mapping of patient imaging data is required; this is not routinely available at the present time. In principle the method provides a rational system for achieving outcomes close to what was originally intended.

Some further definitions for the terminology of the suggested corrective measures are given here.

13.1.1 Further abbreviations and definitions

1. For LET (assuming LET is an appropriate average):
    1. TL_I = intended tumour LET.
    2. TL_E = erroneous tumour LET.
    3. NL_I = intended normal tissue LET.
    4. NL_E = erroneous normal tissue LET.
    5. TL_C = tumour LET during corrective treatments.
    6. NL_C = normal tissue LET during corrective treatments.
2. For dose, which is assumed to be the physical dose and not the RBE-corrected dose at this stage:
    1. Td_I = intended tumour dose.
    2. Td_E = erroneous tumour dose.

3. Nd_I=intended normal tissue.
4. Nd_E = erroneous normal tissue dose.

13.1.2 Background considerations

Delivery of radiotherapy treatment can sometimes be inaccurate and unreliable even in the case of conventional (x-ray- or photon-based) radiotherapy, where systematic and random errors can occur for a wide variety of reasons. Incorrect dose may be due to accelerator output errors, dose calculation errors for complex treatments where dose is estimated using computer algorithms that may not necessarily take into account the true complexity of intervening tissue inhomogeneities, the effects of patient position variations and patient/tumour movement with time during and between treatment fractions, and other temporal changes in the tumour or patient anatomy during a fractionated treatment course. This error-proneness is potentially greater for particle therapy—the dose calculation may not be as reliable due to other factors inherent in the total system of treatment dose planning, including variations in beam delivery and particle range differences superimposed on the photon situation, which can result in marked changes in the intended highly selective energy deposition. This energy, when locally absorbed, is quantified in two ways: as LET on a microscopic scale, and as dose in the conventional way. The added difficulty is that LET and dose both influence the relative biological effect (or efficiency), often referred to as RBE. RBE is not required in the calculation of dose correction for errors made in conventional photon therapy, but changes in dose, and also in some instances LET, will each influence the 'correct dose' for a patient, not only in terms of tumour dose but also dose to the critical normal tissues.

The LET-containing radiation BED equations, which include the RBE limits termed RBE_{max} and RBE_{min}, can be used to estimate isoeffective fractionation schedules as well as to correct unintended treatment interruptions (Jones *et al* 2006). BED equations have been recommended as the method of choice to calculate dose corrections after errors of photon-based radiotherapy delivery (Jones and Dale 2008), but no general system has been described for calculation of treatment-delivery errors when using positively charged particle beams. The purpose of this chapter is to assess the potential impact of such errors and also describe how to compensate for them.

13.1.3 Brief description of methods

The radiobiological linkage between LET, dose and RBE is based on the linear energy-efficiency model already given in chapters 8 and 9. Any error in LET and dose will produce a deviancy of ΔL for LET and Δd for dose. For the sake of simplicity, here we assume a precise value of LET rather than in more practical situations where a spread of LET values over a specified range of energies is inevitably used in the treatment-delivery process, and which would complicate matters further.

The following approach briefly describes how to determine the change in BED due to any error. It is necessary to assume reasonable values of the low-LET α and β parameters. Then:

1. Estimate the effect of any change in LET initially and its effect on α and β. This can be achieved quite simply from the particle Z number, which determines LET_U.
2. Determine, from the changes in α and β, the changes in $\mathrm{RBE_{max}}$ and $\mathrm{RBE_{min}}$ and use these to estimate the change in BED due to the error.
3. From a new treatment plan, determine if LET is changed as well as dose. Use the same equations to determine any changes in α and β and so in $\mathrm{RBE_{max}}$ and $\mathrm{RBE_{min}}$.
4. Use these values of $\mathrm{RBE_{max}}$ and $\mathrm{RBE_{min}}$ within the BED equations to determine the dose required for maintaining the required tumour BED.

Reiteration of these final steps may be required to produce a final satisfactory or adequate compromise solution.

This overall procedure will be described in greater detail below.

It will be important to compare such a novel and relatively simple approach with those obtained by assuming the more complex micro-dosimetry systems quoted in chapter 8.

13.2 Model description

13.2.1 Biological effective dose equations

The BED (sometimes referred to as $\mathrm{EQD_0}$) is normally, for low-LET (1–1.5 keV $\mu\mathrm{m}^{-1}$) radiations:

$$\mathrm{BED} = D_L\left(1 + \frac{d_L}{\alpha/\beta}\right), \tag{13.1}$$

where D_L is the total dose and d_L the dose per fraction, the two being linked by the number of fractions N, where $N.d_L = D_L$, and α/β is a biological parameter which controls fractionation sensitivity for the control low-LET radiation, and has units of dose. For higher values of LET the equation changes to

$$\mathrm{BED} = D_H\left(\mathrm{RBE_{max}} + \frac{RBE_{\min}^2\, d_H}{\alpha/\beta}\right). \tag{13.2}$$

In this last equation, it is important to note that the α/β ratio here remains unchanged from that of the control low-LET radiation. The low-LET α/β ratio is effectively acting as a constant, but is modified by the presence of the two limiting RBE parameters.

Next, it is essential to link the RBE values to the prevailing LET value. This is necessary because the relationship between LET and RBE, although linear initially (when plotted on linear scales), becomes non-linear with a turnover point at a critical value of LET (termed LET_U), after which RBE decreases with LET down to a value of just above 1 in the case of beams used in medical applications. However, for these applications it is rare to experience LET values greater than the turnover point since treatment volumes are covered by a mixture of LET values from parts of individual particle beams, which have lower LET values proximal to the Bragg peak and higher values within and especially towards the end of the peaks.

The method follows some simple steps, each with numerical parameters given in chapters 8 and 9. In brief:

1. LET_U is obtained from $LET_U = 30.5 + S/k\ (1 - \exp[-k\ (z - 1]),$ $[S = 114.4,\ k = 0.51]$.
2. α_U is found from $\alpha_U = A/j\ (1 - \exp[-j\ \alpha_L])$. $[A = 10.6, j = 3.9]$.
3. β_U is found from $\beta_U = B/i\ (1 - \exp[-i\ \beta_L])$. $[B = 3.2,\ i = 40]$.
4. Values of α_H and β_H at any particular value of LET (LET_x) are found from the following:
   (a) A relatively simple equation representing efficiency changes between the control (megavoltage photon) radiation LET value and the LET_U value, as a change in radiosensitivity from α_L to be a larger value of α (α_H) at any higher value of LET (LET_x) up to a maximum possible value of α given by α_U. The same LET_U is also assumed for β (in order to preserve symmetry with dose). So, we obtain

$$\alpha_H = \alpha_C + \frac{LET_x - LET_C}{LET_U - LET_C} \cdot (\alpha_U - \alpha_C),$$

$$\beta_H = \beta_C + \frac{LET_x - LET_C}{LET_U - LET_C} \cdot (\beta_U - \beta_C).$$

   (b) A simple equation representing inefficiency for all LET values above LET_U, but converted into an efficiency equation, as

$$\alpha_H = \alpha_C + \left(1 - \frac{LET_x - LET_U}{LET_U}\right) \cdot (\alpha_U - \alpha_C),$$

$$\beta_H = \beta_C + \left(1 - \frac{LET_x - LET_C}{LET_U}\right) \cdot (\beta_U - \beta_C).$$

5. The RBE_{max} and RBE_{min} values can then be obtained.
6. For the RBE, corrected for dose per fraction, it is necessary to solve an isoeffect equation where $\alpha_L\ d_L + \beta_L\ {d_L}^2 = \alpha_H\ d_H + \beta_H\ {d_H}^2$ is solved for d_L, which is then divided by the d_H to give the RBE at any value of d_H. In terms of BED, this means solving the isoeffect equation BED of control radiation, which is equal to the BED of particle radiation, i.e.

$$nd_L\left(1 + \frac{d_L}{k}\right) = nd_L\left(RBE_{max} + \frac{RBE_{min}^2 \cdot d_L}{k}\right).$$

The RBE is then the solution of this equation for d_L, then divided by d_H.

Examples of this method to obtain RBE, fitted to various data sets, which include changes in dose (or surviving fraction), have been given in chapters 8 and 9.

13.2.2 Assessment of BED changes after an error

From estimates of the changes in α and β described above, the operative RBE_{max} and RBE_{min} in equation (13.2) above can be determined.

The intended, delivered and corrected BEDs can then be calculated providing the LET values and dose for these states are known. Any excess or deficit in BED is then obtained as the difference between the intended and delivered BEDs in both tumour and normal tissue. Any unintended overdosage or underdosage can then be compensated for by a new, modified dose to provide the originally intended tumour BED.

The above system applies to monoenergetic particles, or a small range of particle energies, which is reasonable for modelling purposes at this stage and could in principle be extended to a spectrum of LET values in accordance with energy ranges, by an averaging process.

With the above relatively simple to operate method for predicting changes in RBE due to changes in both LET and dose, it becomes possible to tentatively assess the clinical impact of changes in Bragg peak positioning during particle therapy, and for any ion species. For example, the intended BED at a LET of TL_I will be given by

$n\mathrm{Td}_I\ (RBE_{max} + RBE_{min}{}^2\ \mathrm{Td}_I/(\alpha/\beta)_L) = n\mathrm{T}d_I\ (\alpha_H/\alpha_L + (\alpha_H/\beta_L)\ \mathrm{Td}_I/(\alpha/\beta)_L)$. The values of α_H and β_H for the operative LET can then be obtained from the steps 1–5 in the list given in section 2.1 of this report.

For a different dose Td_E at a different LET value TL_E, the BED for n fractions is then

$n\mathrm{Td}_E(\alpha_H/\alpha_L + (\alpha_H/\beta_L)\ \mathrm{Td}_E/(\alpha/\beta)_L)$, which is the same as

$n\mathrm{Td}_E\ (RBE_{max} + RBE^2_{min}\ \mathrm{Td}_E/(\alpha/\beta)_L)$.

For example, consider protons, helium ions and carbon ions for an underdose of 50% of the intended dose. The plots shown in figures 13.1(a)–(f) show estimated changes in BED per fraction for a range of LET values up to the turnover point of the LET–RBE relationship. It should be noted that the lower range of these values pertain to clinical treatments, due to overlapping of Bragg-peak and non-Bragg-peak regions of the beams. It should be noted that the highest BEDs are found for the lowest α_L radiosensitivity parameter values, because of the greater relative change in α when α_L is small, which causes higher RBE_{max} values.

An International Commission on Radiation Units and Measurements (ICRU) matrix for particle beams has already been presented in chapter 4. This system should be borne in mind, since shifts in dose (and LET) from one ICRU sub-volume to another will be considered below.

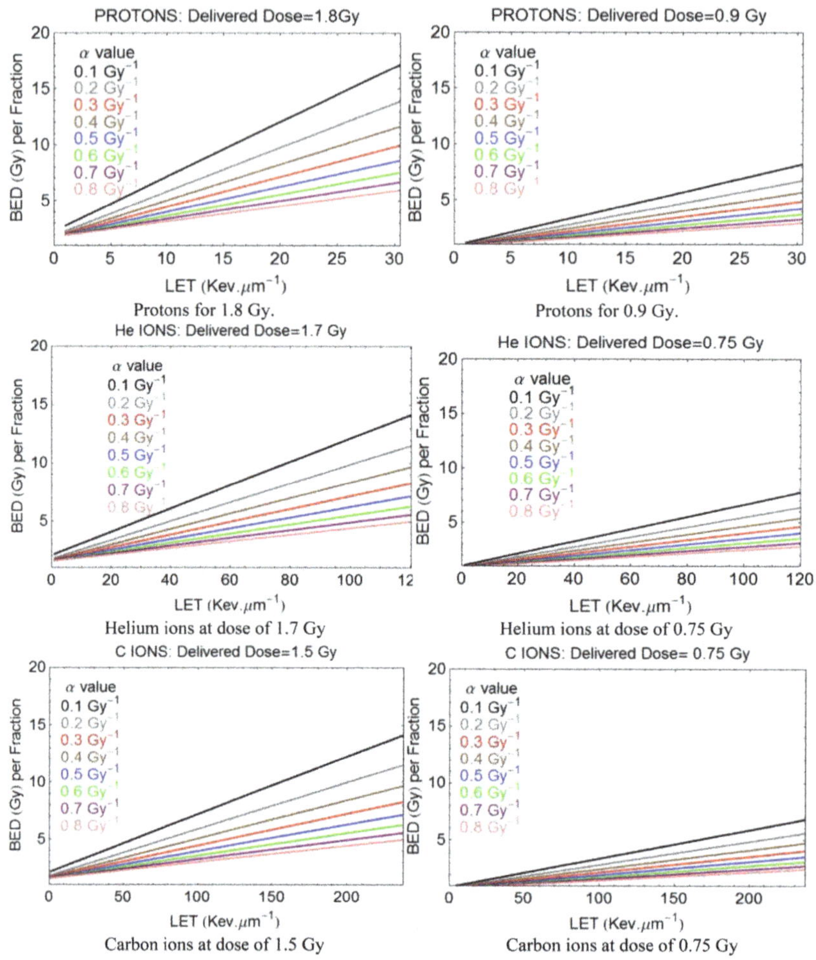

Figure 13.1. Plots (a)–(f) of biological effective doses (BED) for different values of linear energy transfer (LET) for different ionic species at two values of relatively low doses, with variations in the α_L radiosensitivity parameter, which is labelled as α in the graphs; β is kept constant in this study.

13.2.2.1 Simulations of treatment-delivery errors by modelling

Two simple modelling exercises, each for a population of 100 individuals, are shown below in figures 13.2(a) and (b). These show dose-response curves for tumour control probability (TCP) with increasing number of underdosed fractions ranging from three to 15 for intended 2 Gy photon fractions (solid lines) and the same for carbon ions (dashed lines). Figure 13.2(a) shows the situation where the same part of the tumour (10% of its volume) is underdosed to 0.6 Gy rather than 2 Gy (these doses being the physical doses used for both photons and carbon ions, for simplicity). It can be seen that the fall in TCP with increasing number of erroneous fractions is steeper for carbon ions than for photons. In figure 13.2(b), random underdosage is allowed, where 40% of the tumour volume is underdosed to the same amount.

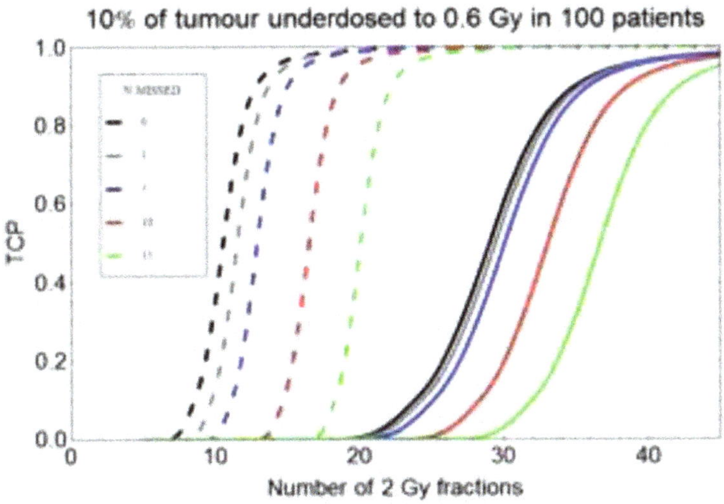

(a)

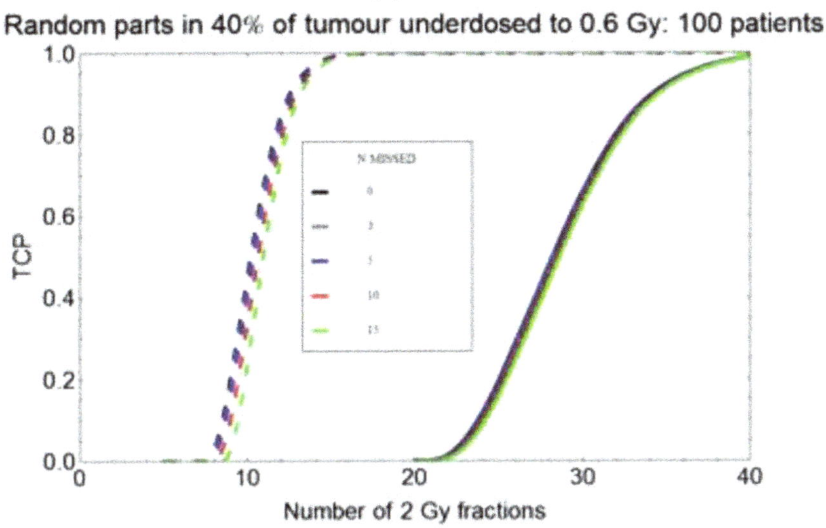

(b)

Figure 13.2. (a) and (b): Plot of TCP against number of 2 Gy fractions for variable numbers of erroneous treatments (solid curves photons, dashed curves carbon ions), where the same 10% of the tumour volume is randomly underdosed. Assumptions made: $RBE_{max} = 3$, $RBE_{min} = 1.25$, using random sampling for the α radiosensitivity parameter (mean 0.3 Gy^{-1}, with standard deviation 0.05 Gy^{-1}) for a tumour with 5×108 cells and a constant value of $\beta = 0.03$ Gy^{-2} (repopulation not included).

The falloff in TCP is not so significant in this case for both types of radiation, although the slope is again steeper for carbon. The steeper slope is due to a greater proportion of the curative dose being given in fewer fractions with carbon ions, so in such cases it is more important to avoid underdosage.

These two examples have not considered changes in LET. Changes in dose, LET and RBE are considered further below.

13.2.3 Worked examples of errors and their correction

Next some quantitative, though simplified, worked examples will be considered:

A. Half of the volume of a tumour is underdosed by 50% for three fractions, during which the average LET falls from 45 to 15 KeV μm^{-1}. The prescribed tumour dose was 70 Gy-Eq in 15 fractions using carbon ions.
   1. A squamous cell carcinoma where for megavoltage photons $\alpha = 0.35$ Gy^{-1}, $\beta = 0.04$ Gy^{-2} and the prescription RBE was 2.5.
   2. A prostate cancer where for megavoltage photons $\alpha = 0.18$ Gy^{-1}, $\beta = 0.035$ Gy^{-2} and the prescription RBE was 2.

Calculate compensatory doses to the underdosed half of the tumour for the remainder of treatment in order to maintain isoeffective tumour control.

B. What is the potential impact on a critical volume of normal tissue planned to receive a dose of 40 Gy in 15 fractions, with the assumption of an operative RBE = 2, which in the past has represented tolerance? Then, for three fractions the dose is erroneously increased by 50% with an increment in average LET from, say, 15 to 45 Kev μm^{-1}, assuming a 1% increase in serious complications per unit rise in BED above tolerance, and where for megavoltage photons $\alpha = 0.1$ Gy^{-1}, $\beta = 0.03$ Gy^{-2}?

13.2.3.1 Answers

The RBE_{max} and RBE_{min} can be found from the changes in α and β parameters with LET, which can then be used within BED equations together with the low-LET α/β value. An ultimate LET_U value of around 230 keV μm^{-1} is used for carbon ions, compatible with the data of Weyrather *et al* (1999) and the linear relationship between LET, α and β for values less than LET_U.

A.1 and A2

The results of calculations, using the equations provided above, which estimate the changes in the radiosensitivity parameters to provide RBE_{max} and RBE_{min} for the different LET values, are shown in table 13.1. These values are placed within the BED equations below where appropriate.

Note that the intended physical dose per fraction was 70/15 = 4.667 Gy-Eq, which when divided by the assumed RBE provides a physical dose of 4.667/2.5 = 1.866 Gy in example (1), but 4.667/2 = 2.33 Gy for example 2.

For worked example A1.

1. Proceed as follows, with $\alpha/\beta = 8.75$ Gy.
2. The intended tumour BED, with a dose per fraction of 70/2.5/15 = 1.867 Gy, was
3. $70/2.5(1.892 + 1.035^2.1.867/8.75) = 59.375$ $Gy_{[8.75]}$.
4. The BED after the three-fraction underdosage to the affected part of the tumour was

Table 13.1. Parameters for worked examples A1 and 2.

	A1: SCC ($\alpha = 0.35$, $\beta = 0.040$)	A2: Prostate ($\alpha = 0.18$, $\beta = 0.035$)
Ar LET = 45	$\alpha_U = 2.035$ $\alpha_H = 0.662$ $RBE_{max} = 1.892$ $\alpha_U = 0.0555$ $\beta_H = 0.0429$ $RBE_{min} = 1.892$	$\alpha_U = 1.402$ $\alpha_H = 0.406$ $RBE_{max} = 2.258$ $\alpha_U = 0.045$ $\beta_H = 0.037$ $RBE_{min} = 1.027$
Ar LET = 15	$\alpha_H = 0.454$ $RBE_{max} = 1.297$ $\beta_H = 0.041$ $RBE_{max} = 1.012$	$\alpha_H = 0.255$ $R_{BEmax} = 1.419$ $\beta_H = 0.0359$ $RBE_{max} = 1.0128$
Ar LET = 53	$\alpha_H = 0.780$ $RBE_{max} = 2.051$ $\beta_H = 0.0434$ $RBE_{max} = 1.04$	$\alpha_H = 0.447$ $RBE_{max} = 2.482$ $\beta_H = 0.0372$ $RBE_{max} = 1.031$

5. $3 \times 0.778\ (1.297 + 1.012^2.\ 0.778/8.75) = 3.855\ Gy_{[8.75]}$.
6. This means that 59.375 – 3.855 = 55.488 Gy is required from the remaining 12 treatments. The dose per fraction is then obtained from the solution of
7. $12\ d(2.051 + 1.041^2.d/8.75)$.
8. This gives $d = 2.01$ Gy.

For worked example A.2.

1. The intended tumour BED was $70/2(2.26 + 1.027^2\ 2.33/5.14) = 95.76\ Gy_{[5.14]}$.
2. The BED given after the three-fraction underdosage was
3. $3 \times 2.33 \times 0.5\ (1.42 + 1.01^2.\ 2.33 \times 0.5/5.14) = 5.78\ Gy_{[5.14]}$.
4. There is a deficit of $95.76 - 5.78 = 89.98\ Gy_{[5.14]}$.
5. This can be compensated for in the next 12 fractions, now with RBE parameters at a higher value of LET, by solving
6. $12\ d(2.48 + 1.03\ d^2/5.14) = 89.98$, where $d = 2.5$ Gy.

For worked example B.

1. For the critical volume of normal tissue, the megavoltage photon α of 0.1 Gy^{-1}, the relevant parameter changes are given in table 13.2.
2. The intended BED is 38.97 $Gy_{[3]}$, using a dose per fraction of 1.33 Gy, and this represents tolerance using the fixed value of RBE given. The 150% dose error will cause the dose per fraction to rise to around 2 Gy.
3. The excess BED over the three incorrect fractions, if uncorrected, would be

Table 13.2. Calculated parameters for worked example B.

Baseline parameters	Planned treatment (LET = 15 keV μm^{-1})	By error (LET = 45 keV μm^{-1})
$\alpha_L = 0.1$ (Gy^{-1})	$\alpha_U = 0.906$	$\alpha_U = 1.906$
$\beta_L = 0.033$ (Gy^{-1})	$\alpha_H = 0.15$	$\alpha_H = 0.249$
	$\mathrm{RBE}_{max} = 1.50$	$\mathrm{RBE}_{max} = 2.49$
	$\beta_U = 0.04$	$\beta_U = 0.04$
	$\beta_H = 0.0334$	$\beta_H = 0.0343$
	$\mathrm{RBE}_{min} = 1.007$	$\mathrm{RBE}_{min} = 1.02$

4. $3 \times 2\,(2.49 + 1.02^2.2/3) - 3 \times 1.33\,(1.50 + 1.01^2 \times 1.33/3) = 11.33\ \mathrm{Gy}_{[3]}$.
5. If toxicity increases by 1% per unit BED, then an 11.3% increase in toxicity might occur if no correction is applied.

The above steps are informative, and useful for teaching and research purposes, but there are many pitfalls within the process, more so than in the much simpler corrections sometimes necessary for errors arising in photon-based therapy.

13.2.4 The potential impact of erroneous fractions on tumour control

A further study is based on problem A1 above, but assumes that the same half of the volume of a tumour has been underdosed on one or more sequential fractions. This has been simulated in greater detail with estimation of tumour control probabilities (TCPs). Plots of the numbers of erroneous treatment against the expected TCP are shown in figure 13.3. Here several assumptions of different tumour RBE values have been made in addition to the RBEs predicted by the model described in this report (purple data points). Detailed inspection will show that the dose of 70 Gy in 15 fractions is very forgiving for treatment errors in the case of photons (the green data points). This is because the tumour can be cured with doses of around 40–45 Gy in 15 fractions, but the excess dose guarantees a high cure rate even when dose delivery is imprecise for up to 10 fractions. When the tumour RBE of 2.5 (as stated in the problem) is itself incorrect, as shown by the red data points, the physical dose has been excessively reduced, and even if all treatments are accurately delivered the TCP is reduced to around 0.4 (or a control rate of 40%), with a sharp falloff in TCP if only one or two erroneous treatments are made. For more than two erroneous treatments the TCP is effectively zero. For lower assumed values of tumour RBE, the prescribed dose is not so reduced, allowing increasing TCP and also improving the numbers of erroneous treatments that can be made before causing a significant reduction in TCP.

In reality, higher doses do oppose radioresistance regardless of cause, whether intrinsic (e.g. genetic) or acquired (e.g. hypoxia). This example is sufficient to demonstrate that higher doses are protective against at least some forms of error in dose misplacement during particle therapy. Such higher doses can only be permitted

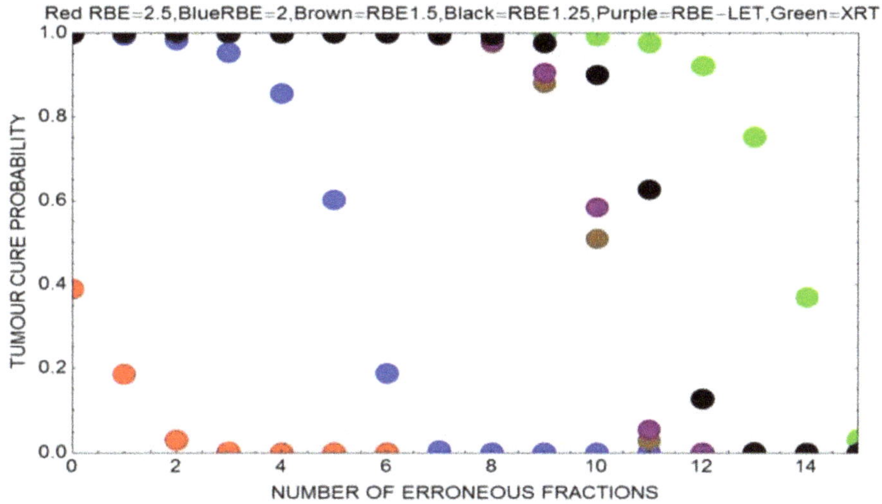

Figure 13.3. Plots of tumour cure probability against number of erroneous fractions where the same half of a tumour is underdosed by 50%. TCP is calculated using standard Poisson statistics with the same radiobiological assumptions as in question A1, with altered radiobiological parameters as in table 13.1, with 10^9 clonogens per tumour. No repopulation factor has been used since the overall time is constant and less than the approximately 28 day onset time of significant repopulation in a squamous cell carcinoma.

if normal tissue tolerances of smaller volumes of critical organs at risk are respected, for example if the planning target volume (PTV) includes normal tissue whose functional contribution can be lost, but without appreciable detriment in quality of life.

There are other situations in oncology, for example the treatment of radiosensitive childhood tumours, where dose escalation to very high levels may not be acceptable since normal tissue tolerances of nearby structures have to be respected, for example the eye or spinal cord. In the context of more radioresistant tumours, for example a craniopharyngioma where optic nerve and optic chiasmal structures may extend into the clinical target volume/PTV, dose escalation, if used at all, may have to be limited to a part of the tumour. In such situations, there is a risk that tumour underdosage may reduce tumour control, which justifies the use of detailed image guidance, especially if non-ionising radiation impacts on patient throughput.

Just as in airports, so in radiotherapy departments, delays occur due to a variety of reasons which are often connected with patient safety. Sometimes, interruptions during a treatment fraction occur due to accelerator malfunction or the beam delivery process during therapy, although this is infrequent. In practice, a failed quality assurance (QA) check before treatment has commenced leads to a delay in beginning or resuming treatments. Delays are sometimes simulated as having a Gaussian distribution, but they are naturally bounded at the lower limit (because of more serious causes of failure, which need much longer times to be corrected), so will tend to have a log-normal distribution. Interruption of a treatment fraction requires a much more complicated approach, as shown above. Only if the treatment interruption is less than 0.5 hr should the remainder of the dose be applied without specific radiobiological correction. This is because DNA is repaired rapidly (in the central nervous system the fast component repair has a half-time of 12 min and the slow component just over 2 hr; see chapter 2). The correction, if adopted comprehensively, will require input from physicists, clinical radiobiologists with an interest in modelling, and the responsible clinician.

The best that could be aimed for at the present time would be a 24 hr break in treatment, although longer intervals may be anticipated in some instances. There are convenient ways to overcome longer delays after erroneous treatments have been delivered, if these occur early in a treatment course of many fractions, since the usual fractionation can be continued a day later, leaving the correction of the erroneous fraction (or fractions) to a later time, towards the end of a treatment course. This would allow the 'correcting team' a longer time to consider the problem; this may avoid the situation where a rapid but incorrect decision is taken after an erroneous fraction has been partly or totally given. In situations where voxel-by-voxel compensations are attempted this would require automated computing, with input of the relevant radiobiological parameters and many reiterations to obtain a reasonable compromised solution.

Specific training in the clinical radiobiology area is required for several disciplines. Clinicians should be made more aware of the LET-dose-RBE issues and be encouraged to practice simple calculations with their physics and radiobiology colleagues.

This problem should be discussed in depth by the relevant bodies that govern the use of radiotherapy in each country. At the present time, full correction may take a physicist 4–6 hr and the clinician 1–2 hr to discuss; if the problem requires several iterations these times will be far longer, taking perhaps a whole day or more.

Should a treatment error not be corrected until after the intended overall treatment time has elapsed, then repopulation-related calculations may also be necessary, as described in chapter 12. This adds a further level of complexity where additional compromises will be necessary because the correct solution to preserve the same tumour control will not be the same as for normal tissue complications.

13.2.4.1 General discussion

The causes of failure in achieving local tumour control with radiotherapy are numerous, including intrinsic and acquired radioresistance, patient-related factors and dose delivery errors. At the present time, much attention is being given to QA measures regarding dose and the accuracy of its delivery for each treatment. Further measures which minimise potential errors, such as adaptive radiotherapy (ADR), are by now in routine use in some treatment centres (Schwartz *et al* 2012). In ADR, the radiation fields are checked (using one or more of a variety of imaging procedures) at either frequent exposures, or even at each exposure, and the treatment field directions/sizes modified to take into account changes in patient and tumour/normal tissue position and dimensions.

The Bragg peak position is dependent on the initial energy of the particle and its rate of energy loss with increasing tissue depth in the body; these parameters normally include some degree of variation, resulting in variations in the dose range. So, dose deposition consequently can be uncertain, especially if there are extremely non-homogenous tissue electron density variations in regions containing marked changes in chemical composition. CPT is consequently more sensitive in terms of changes in dose placement during therapy. Even loss or gain in patient weight during treatment, or daily setup errors, could influence particle range, causing simultaneous tumour underdosage and an increase in normal tissue dose compared to what was intended. Use of ultrasonic measurements of distances between skin and bone on a daily basis prior to entering the treatment room would help to reduce, for example, errors due to loss/gain in subcutaneous fat.

It is important to consider the potential effects of serial underdosage, even if this only affects part of a tumour volume and to study what the influence of this will be on tumour control following conventional therapy and CPT.

The results show that increasing numbers of repeated underdosage of the same section of a tumour can have deleterious consequences for tumour control probabilities.

Practical calculations should include the possibility of lower RBEs due to lower LET values in underdosed regions using the passive scattering technique. This would need to be done on a voxel-by-voxel basis, and is beyond the scope of the present study. A further important issue is the finding that for scanned beams, which allow intensity-modulated proton therapy, there can be higher LET values (and so RBE values) just outside the PTV, where dose is reduced (Grassberger *et al* 2011). Both low dose and higher LET will lead to a higher RBE.

Adequate QA and vigilance is required during radiotherapy to ensure that systematic underdosage does not occur. This could occur due to a variety of reasons ranging from dose/particle numbers and energy/ranges as well as errors due to scattering or scanning of the beam. Patient setup errors, tissue depth and density variations, tumour shrinkage and other effects such as tumour motion with respiration may all contribute.

These issues impinge on medical ethics: how much of the uncertainties in the physical and biological aspects of particle therapy should be discussed with individual patients as part of informed consent? Should full informed consent include these in comparison with photon-based techniques? Should more phase III randomised studies be done because of the influence of these uncertainties? Will patients who might develop disappointing results after particle therapy take legal action on the basis that they were not fully informed as a natural human right, encoded in European law?

The results presented are dependent on the validity of the linear quadratic model and the various assumptions made. It will be important to collect more data on errors or interruptions during particle therapy, the net effect on LET distortions and estimated RBE changes, their correction details, and to correlate this information with tumour control outcomes and also toxicity since overshooting of Bragg peaks may result in excess normal tissue dosage. A pan-European database could be developed for this purpose.

The computing support required for LET-based corrections of errors is considerable, with use of Monte Carlo systems which incorporate radiation transport data and which can interact with treatment-planning information such as differences in tissue composition. In the short term, the only means of achieving this would be to use certain reference laboratories that are capable of achieving this and which could work with the software divisions of treatment-planning companies. There should be at least one location in Europe and the USA that could be an advisory centre for treatment interruptions of any kind. The use of cloud computing will undoubtedly help in this area, although anonymity of patient data is a legal requirement which also makes patient data transfer difficult in some parts of the world. Written permission obtained from patients before treatment is commenced would probably be advantageous in this respect.

13.3 Conclusions

In order to achieve the best clinical outcomes following CPT, it is important to do the following:

- Eliminate errors of dose delivery where possible by optimised treatment planning, good beam QA, use of image guidance and, where possible, external confirmation of Bragg peak positions/dose distributions during particle therapy.
- Correct any significant errors by using rational strategies based on LET, RBE and BED to restore the intended tumour control following tumour underdosage, or to reduce normal tissue effects if they have been unintentionally overdosed.

The radiation oncologist/clinical radiobiologist and physicist must liaise closely in order to achieve these aims. The calculation of a corrective dose should involve BED (equation (13.1)) after detailed analysis of the original and erroneous treatment dose and LET distributions. A new system which links LET to RBE for clinical applications using any ion species (including protons) has been developed. At the present time there is no routine application of LET mapping in commercial software systems for routine proton treatment planning. LET maps leading to RBE maps and equivalent dose estimations, all in three dimensions, are now urgently required. In their absence, there is a need for academic studies where LET maps are generated for different field sizes and consideration is given as to how these might be changed after intentional laboratory-based 'errors' have been introduced. Such an increase in information would allow better rational compensatory calculations to be used. Such a development might, even in the absence of delivery errors, improve the clinical outcomes of routine particle therapy, since the clinician would be alerted about the risks associated with higher- and lower-LET areas and aid in risk determination, as discussed in chapter 10.

The methods presented in this report provide a relatively simple framework for achieving the corrections for errors in particle therapy treatment delivery, although they require many more steps and assumptions than is the case for similar protocol deviations in megavoltage photon therapy.

Ideally, a single reference centre (or virtual centre) in Europe (with shared costs), or in each individual country, should be able to handle difficult errors efficiently, until necessary training has been undertaken. More advanced training programmes for clinicians and medical physicists are required in this area; their present training does not include adequate time or development of competencies in this particular area, especially the radiobiological aspects.

References

Grassberger C, Trofimov A, Lomax A and Paganetti H 2011 Variations in linear energy transfer within clinical proton therapy fields and the potential for biological treatment planning *Int. J. Radiat. Oncol. Biol. Phys.* **80** 1559–66

Jones B, Carabe-Fernandez A and Dale R G 2006 Calculation of high-LET radiotherapy dose required for compensation of overall treatment time extensions *Br. J. Radiol.* **79** 254–7

Jones B and Dale R G 2008 Radiobiological compensation of treatment errors in radiotherapy *Br. J. Radiol.* **81** 323–6

Schwartz D L, Garden A S, Thomas J *et al* 2012 Adaptive radiotherapy for head-and-neck cancer: initial clinical outcomes from a prospective trial *Int. J. Radiat. Oncol. Biol. Phys.* **83** 986–93

Weyrather W K, Ritter S, Scholz M and Kraft G 1999 RBE for carbon track-segment irradiation in cell lines of differing repair capacity *Int. J. Radiat. Biol.* **75** 1357–64

Chapter 14

What remains to be done: including FLASH dose rates and conclusions

The eventual optimisation of particle therapy must include the potential criteria for dose escalation, followed by presentation of a framework for a better quantitative assessment of the 'sensitisation' of high- and low-linear-energy-transfer (LET) radiation by drugs and other agents, preferably using the biological effective dose (BED) approach so that normal tissue effects can be protected. A sensitivity analysis of the energy-efficiency LET-RBE model (presented in chapters 8 and 9) is given.

The pressing need for further systematic research on high-LET radiobiology at a single international laboratory is discussed. So many problems remain to be solved before particle therapy can be given with the same degree of confidence as photon-based therapy in some situations. Better knowledge of LET behaviour in relation to mixed non-coplanar fields given at different dose rates and with different time intervals between sub-fraction exposures are required, in addition to improved data on charged-particle beam ballistics and kinematics at lower energies to guide LET and relative biological effect (RBE) assessments near the Bragg peak and beyond it. Better estimates of LET_U at the LET–RBE turnover point positions should be sought since they will determine the overall efficiency of cell killing. Such projects, if using automated experimental systems which use much larger numbers of cellular exposures than used previously, should provide improved modelling parameter accuracy and provide an important resource for comparative assessments of different models in a panel of carefully chosen cell lines with a range of radiobiological characteristics. Such work cannot be done in a fragmented way in different countries and at such difficult economic times. It is time for biology and medicine to follow the example of high-energy physics and perform its fundamental research in a centralised laboratory, at least for proof-of-principle cellular-based experiments.

doi:10.1088/978-0-7503-6209-2ch14

14.1 Introduction

It is clear that there is ample scope to improve radiotherapeutics by using proton- and ion-beam therapy (PIBT); but in what situations may the impact be greatest, and what can be done to reduce some of the existing disadvantages?

In radical treatments, PIBT will only reduce collateral radiation effects in tissue at sufficient distances from the cancer, but which will be important for long-term survivors; it should have the most impact in tumours with expected low metastatic rates but achievable high local control rates, and where late vascular and fibrotic complications, if reducible, as well as the bonus of reduced malignant induction probabilities, will all contribute to quality-of-life expectations.

A balance has to be struck between these benefits and the detriments that could follow relative biological effect (RBE) and Bragg peak placement uncertainties, which both need to be minimised for optimal normal tissue and tumour outcomes. The first priority in medicine is to do no harm (*primum non nocere*). Consequently, adjustment of the dose to be within acceptable normal tissue limits, where retention of that issue function is important, has to be the first priority. In some clinical situations, further radiation dose escalation may not necessarily produce greater cure rates, because of the influence of dose-modifying and other adjuvant therapies, and even with photon-based radiotherapy the cure rate may be very high. It is especially important that any radiation technique should not allow underdosage (or 'geographical miss') of the cancer, and that the allocated RBE will not result in a lower than intended tumour dose. There may be special instances where a simpler PIBT technique will produce better dose distributions than any photon technique, as in cases where metallic bearing prostheses exist (Jones 2006), or to avoid the heart, or in many re-treatment situations, in palliative radiotherapy (where unpleasant side effects should be avoided as far as possible even if these are due to acute-reacting tissue) as well as in other situations where congenitally acquired anatomical changes, or malformations, complicate treatment planning.

The role of PIBT in palliative and/or re-treatment situations (the latter may be given with radical or palliative intent), is often neglected due to the assumed costs and the aim to obtain prolonged survival using radical treatments. Some new proton centres appear to report that up to 30% of patients belong in this category. After all, why should a patient receive a sub-optimal dose distribution using photons when a better PIBT alternative is available and with much lower expected morbidity, especially if the treatment can be given efficiently in a limited number of fractions? Consider some practical examples: treatment of (a) para-aortic nodes, or (b) bone metastases in the cervical spine. In (a) the photon-beam exit doses are considerable whatever photon-based technique is used, and the treatment volumes can be large so that standard fractionation may be required (1.8–2 Gy per day over 4–5 weeks typically), although more focussed techniques can allow hypofractionation but with a considerable 'dose bath' with resultant acute effects. In (b) the exit doses to the throat and upper oesophagus can cause a prolonged mucositis, severe pain on swallowing, which would not occur with carefully planned PIBT. Although some modern photon techniques can treat the metastatic tumour alone, with good initial response, there is often a need to re-treat within or near to the previously irradiated volume, or there may be several nearby areas that require treatment in an '*en-bloc*' fashion.

Obtaining the most correct RBE for any particular situation remains a difficult hurdle, although some guidance provided by careful modelling studies has probably improved this situation by at least providing clinicians with clear-cut caveats. In the future there may be further predictive assays which feed into RBE values beyond what is now possible by taking assumed α/β ratios (as used in standard clinical radiobiological modelling), or likely values of α and β, especially since gene-expression patterns and DNA methylation are markedly different after protons in comparison with conventional x-ray-based therapies (Girdhani *et al* 2013, Chaudhary *et al* 2014, 2015). More clustered DNA damage in Bragg peak regions influences cell killing and ultimately the RBE dose ratio. It is possible that indications for proton-beam therapy in certain tumour types may be altered on this basis in the future. It is also intriguing that the oxygen enhancement ratio may also be reduced in the Bragg peak regions and could be close to those for fast neutrons, since neutrons cause ionisation mainly by releasing recoil protons. This again makes a strong case for the high-linear-energy-transfer (LET) regions to be maintained in the gross tumour volume, and not in normal tissue regions. A further possibility is to increase particle therapy dose rate sufficiently to cause induced hypoxia and so increase normal tissue radiation tolerances, but only providing tumour control is not adversely affected or at least affected to a lesser extent than the change in normal tissue radiotolerance.

The remainder of this final chapter considers a miscellany of different novel approaches.

14.2 Dose escalation where circumstances permit

The possibility of increasing the prescribed tumour dose when it is judged that the degree of important normal tissue sparing (outside the planning target volume, or PTV) is good, but where dysfunction of the normal tissue within the PTV will not significantly influence subsequent quality of life. Here it is assumed that the main organ at risk outside the PTV is taken to close to its tolerance in order to increase tumour dose as much as possible. This strategy links with the optimum dose per fraction concept presented in chapter 6.

Tables 14.1 and 14.2 present estimated proton dose increases that may be possible for a radioresistant and a radiosensitive tumour, respectively, in the case of a 1.1 RBE and the variable RBE model, where X is the degree of sparing (only $X = 1$, i.e. no sparing, and $X = 0.8$, or 80% sparing, are considered). Four different fractionation schedules are used. It can be seen that the fixed 1.1 RBE can result in overdosage when small doses per fraction are used, but the normal tissue biological effective dose (BED) is kept to within the tolerance of the critical normal tissue outside the PTV with the variable model and which permits the use of the increased doses per fraction to the tumour target as shown. The modelling used here is the same as in chapters 6, 8 and 9, but with assumed values of $\alpha = 0.55\ \mathrm{Gy}^{-1}$ and

Table 14.1. Radioresistant example.

	All RBE = 1.1 (the present condition)			Dose Escalated variable RBE			
Dose (Gy) per #, *N* and *X*	NT BED (EQD-2) in PTV	NT BED (EQD-2) OTV	TUM BED (EQD-2) in PTV	NT BED (EQD-2) In PTV	NT BED (EQD-2) OTV	TUM BED (EQD-2) in PTV	Modified dose/#
2, 25, 1	108.61* (54.30)	N/A	63.90 (48.35)	100.0 (50.0)	N/A	58.92 (44.59)	1.71
2, 25, 0.8	N/A	80.38 (40.19)	63.90 (48.35)	N/A	96.99 (48.50)	77.09 (58.34)	2.09
2.75, 15, 1	102.18* (51.09)	N/A	58.85 (44.53)	97.97 (48.98)	N/A	56.61 (42.84)	2.43
2.75, 15, 0.8	N/A	74.36 (37.18)	58.85 (44.53)	N/A	94.58 (47.29)	73.89 (55.92)	2.96
4.8, 6, 1	95.34 (47.67)	N/A	50.47 (38.19)	97.92 (48.96)	N/A	51.66 (39.09)	4.44
4.8, 6, 0.8	N/A	67.28 (33.64)	50.47 (38.19)	N/A	93.55 (46.77)	67.95 (51.42)	5.39
9, 2, 1	90.32 (45.16)	N/A	42.07 (31.83)	99.0 (49.5)	N/A	45.57 (34.48)	8.63
9, 2, 0.8	N/A	61.7 (30.86)	42.07 (31.83)	N/A	93.46 (46.73)	61.05 (46.20)	10.43

Table 14.2. Radiosensitive example.

	All RBE = 1.1 (the present condition)			Dose escalated variable RBE			
Dose (Gy) per #, N and X	NT BED (EQD-2) In PTV	NT BED (EQD-2) OTV	TUM BED (EQD-2) in PTV	NT BED (EQD-2) in PTV	NT BED (EQD-2) OTV	TUM BED (EQD-2) in PTV	Modified dose/#
2, 25, 1	108.61* (54.30)	N/A	44.43 (41.41)	100.0 (50.0)	N/A	40.90 (38.13)	1.71
2, 25, 0.8	N/A	80.38 (40.19)	44.43 (41.41)	N/A	96.99 (48.49)	53.59 (49.96)	2.09
2.75, 15, 1	102.18* (51.09)	N/A	40.72 (37.96)	97.97 (48.98)	N/A	39.24 (36.58)	2.43
2.75, 15, 0.8	N/A	74.36 (37.18)	40.72 (37.96)	N/A	94.58 (47.29)	50.40 (46.98)	2.96
4.8, 6, 1	95.34 (47.67)	N/A	32.79 (30.57)	97.92 (48.96)	N/A	33.46 (31.19)	4.44
4.8, 6, 0.8	N/A	67.28 (33.64)	32.79 (30.57)	N/A	93.55 (46.78)	42.35 (39.48)	5.39
9, 2, 1	90.32 (45.16)	N/A	23.93 (22.30)	99.0 (49.5)	N/A	25.53 (23.08)	8.63
9, 2, 0.8	N/A	61.7 (30.86)	23.93 (22.30)	N/A	93.46 (46.73)	32.36 (30.17)	10.43

N/A = not applicable; NT BED = normal tissue biological effective dose; TUM BED = tumour biological effective dose; OTV = outside target volume.

$\beta = 0.02$ Gy^{-2} ($\alpha/\beta = 27.5$ Gy) for the radiosensitive category, and with $\alpha = 0.28$ Gy^{-1} and $\beta = 0.045$ Gy^{-2} ($\alpha/\beta = 6.2$ Gy) for the radioresistant category; in each case, the normal tissue had assumed $\alpha = 0.06$ Gy^{-1} and $\beta = 0.02$ Gy^{-2} ($\alpha/\beta = 2$ Gy).

14.3 Simultaneous 'sensitisation' effects by new therapies

The considerable advances made with descriptive molecular biology and its applications in cancer research provide new opportunities for molecular modification of radiation responses. These may be useful within the time frame of radiotherapy treatment courses, provided that any positive tumour effect exceeds any deleterious effects on key normal tissues. Quantification of such effects remains controversial, and in the context of using such approaches with charged-particle beams there are additional complexities due to issues with the RBE. The sensitiser enhancement ratio (SER) is defined as the radiation only dose required for the same biological effect (without the sensitising agent) divided by the radiation dose for the same effect when the sensitiser is present. It is analogous to the RBE definition, which utilises horizontal shifts of the cell-survival curves.

Following discussions with Prof. R. G. Dale, in order to find the vertical shifts in the cell-survival curves due to a sensitising drug, it is suggested that a BED approach is taken in order to accommodate the RBE and the SER. The theoretical cell-survival curves in figure 14.1 refer to the use of a drug (D) to sensitise (1) standard megavoltage photon therapy and (2) a high-LET therapy, e.g. using carbon ions.

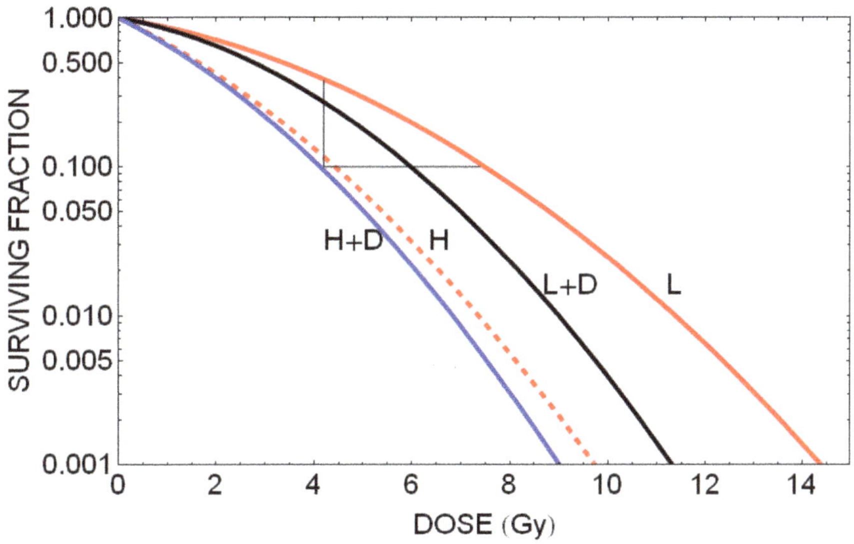

Figure 14.1. Cell survival curves for assumed parameters of $\alpha_L = 0.12$, $\beta_L = 0.025$; $a = 1.1$, $b = 1.3$; $A = 1.05$, $B = 1.2$; $=$ RBE$_{max} = 3$, RBE$_{min} = 1.2$. 'L' refers to the low-LET reference radiation, 'H' to a higher LET using carbon ions and 'D' refers to the sensitising drug. The horizontal line at a surviving fraction of 0.1 can be used to estimate the RBE and SERs. In contrast, the incremental BED ratio method described in the text reflects the vertical changes between the four curves, as represented by the vertical line at a dose of 4.2 Gy.

It is assumed that the drug sensitises the low-LET α_L and β_L values by factors of *a* and *b*, respectively, but the drug changes the high-LET radiosensitivities by factors of *A* and *B*. For example, the α_L becomes $A.\alpha_L$, which can be renamed as ${}_s\alpha_L$ (where the subscript s refers to the sensitised α at low LET), which will be the parameter measured by the cell biologist. The same terminology applies for β, and the process is extended to the high-LET state as shown in table 14.3, which gives the relevant equations for sensitisation, including the radiosenstivity changes and their BED equivalents for the purposes of future analysis.

In table 14.4, the (advantageous) incremental ratios of the BEDs due to sensitisation are shown for different radiation doses; this approach would be reasonable for the analysis of clinical results. Figure 14.2 shows the effective SERs achieved with the combined effects of the drug and the two classes of radiation as a function of dose. The form of these curves depends on the degree to which α and β are sensitised. In general it should be remembered that sensitisation of α (the dominant effect in high-LET radiations) has greater biological effects at low dose per fraction, but sensitisation confers more effects with increased dose per fraction.

A protocol for the analysis of low- and high-LET radiations with sensitising drugs is provided in table 14.5 using the same four cell-survival curves as described for figure 14.1. Such approaches, which may show striking advantages with respect to tumour cell killing must, of course, be repeated using acute- and late-reacting

Table 14.3. Lists of surviving fraction and BED equations for each category shown in figure 14.1, where the low-LET α/β ratio is now represented by *k*. The composite (upper) and measured (lower) radiosensitivities in each category are shown in column 2, with BED representations in column 3.

Radiation and drug category	$-\log_e$ (Surviving fraction)	BED
Low LET only	$N(\alpha_L.d + \beta_L.d^2)$	$D(1 + d/k)$
Low LET + D	$N(\alpha_L.a.d + \beta_L.b.^2d^2) = N({}_s\alpha_L.d + {}_s\beta_L.b^2d^2)$	$D(a + b^2d/k)$
High LET only	$N(\alpha_L.R_{max}d + \beta_L.R_{min}{}^2d^2) = N(\alpha_H.d + \beta_H.d^2)$	$D(R_{max} + R_{min}{}^2d/k)$
High LET +D	$N(\alpha_L.R_{max}Ad + \beta_L.R_{min}{}^2B^2d^2) = N({}_s\alpha_H.d + {}_s\beta_H.d^2)$	$D(R_{max}A + R_{min}{}^2B^2d/k)$

Table 14.4. BED increment ratios for four treatment conditions.

BED ratios	$d = 2$ Gy	$d = 4$ Gy	$d = 6$ Gy
1. High LET/low LET	2.54	2.29	2.13
2. (Low LET + SD)/low LET alone	1.27	1.37	1.43
3. (High LET + SD)/high LET alone	1.12	1.16	1.20
4. (Combined high LET + drug-sensitised)/low LET alone	2.83	2.66	2.55

SD = sensitisation drug.

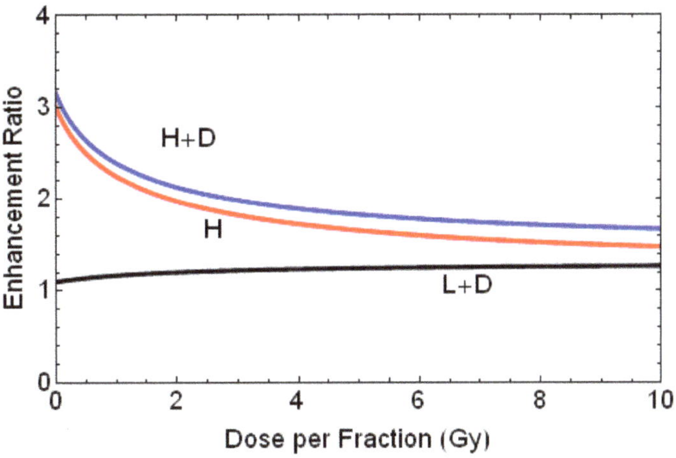

Figure 14.2. Plot of enhancement ratios changing with physical dose per fraction for three conditions of enhancement, where 'L+D' is drug with low-LET radiation, 'H' is high LET alone and 'H+D' is high-LET radiation plus a sensitising drug.

Table 14.5. How experimental data can be used to determine sensitisation parameters R_{max}, R_{min}, *a, b, A* and *B*.

Experimental data obtained	Output
Low- and high-LET radiation (both with no SD) cell-survival curves experiments provide α_H and α_L parameters	R_{max} ($=\alpha_H/\alpha_L$) and R_{min} ($=\sqrt{\beta_H}/\sqrt{\beta_L}$)
Low LET with SD provide ${}_S\alpha_L$ and ${}_S\beta_L$ parameters	a ($={}_S\alpha_L/\alpha_L$) and b ($=\sqrt{{}_S\beta_L}/\sqrt{\beta_L}$)
High LET with SD provide ${}_S\alpha_H$ and ${}_S\beta_H$ parameters	A ($={}_S\alpha_H/\alpha_H$) and B ($=\sqrt{{}_S\beta_H}/\sqrt{\beta_H}$)

normal tissue assays (not only acute-reacting tissues, as was the case with so many RBE studies in the past).

14.4 Sensitivity analysis of the energy-efficiency model

For the model presented in chapters 8 and 9, the dependency of the LET_U position and the degree of saturation of α and β with increasing LET will all influence the RBE estimates, as shown in figures 14.3(a)–(c) for reasonable shifts in the assumed values used in this book, which are the central values given. The changes, although small, can be of clinical significance, more so at low dose for the α-related shifts and at high dose for the β-related shifts and at lower doses for the LET_U position. It is important that the model input parameters are updated in accordance with new information. Further detailed research would be required to refine the precision of these parameters, as indicated below.

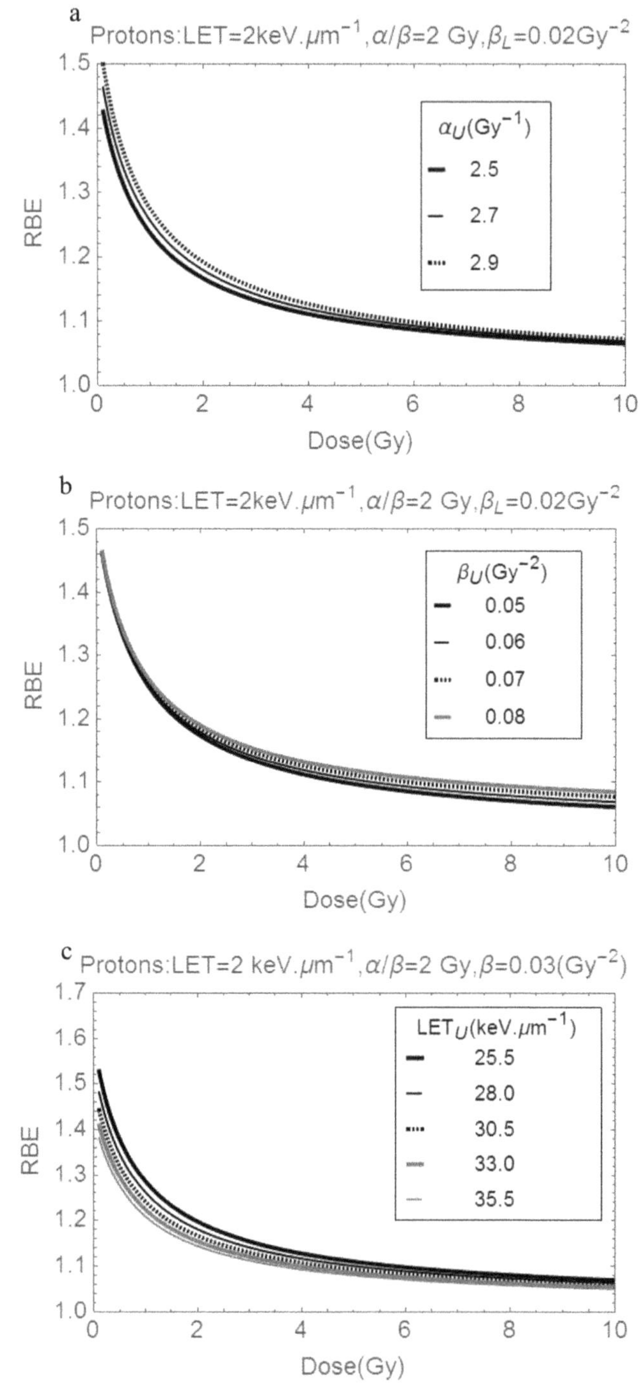

Figure 14.3. (a)–(c): Plots of RBE with dose per fraction showing sensitivity to changes of assumed a_U, β_U and LET$_U$, the maximum efficiency point LET$_U$, for $\alpha/\beta = 2$ Gy, where the LET is 2 keV mm^{-1}.

It is clear from the above graphical displays that small improvements may be possible and can only be achieved by appropriate experimentation. To find the true LET–RBE turnover points it is also necessary to determine both the α and β changes with LET, so that the entire model may be validated to greater accuracy and compared with other models. This might involve either a very large international collaboration, but preferably conducted in one laboratory under carefully controlled conditions with the capacity to study a range of ion beams at different energies and with delivery systems where the influence of inter-track distances on biological effects can be studied, where the tracks are in the same primary direction and with other geometrical combinations (e.g. orthogonal or opposed tracks) by varying the irradiation conditions, and introducing variations in time between exposures. Such mixed fields should also be tested at higher dose rates. Far more comprehensive data of spread-out Bragg peak (SOBP) placement positions at gradually increasing depths are urgently required for scattered beams as well as the introduction of deliberate changes in dose rate (including both increase and reduction of the dose rate) in scanned beams. It is paradoxical that so much work has been done to commission beams with respect to physical dose before clinical use, but so little preliminary investigation into the biological effectiveness.

Also required is a library of tabulated LET values for different field sizes and SOBP dimensions at perhaps three standard points within the SOBP (e.g. max, median and mean values) and/or their values at defined positions such as the entry, middle and end of SOBPs. It is surprising that such work remains to be done.

14.5 What could be achieved in a single international laboratory dedicated to high-LET radiobiology

The proposed Bio-LEIR project at CERN (Dosanjh *et al* 2013) was entirely capable of addressing all the above issues. This was meticulously planned and remains feasible, but unfortunately the CERN executives decided instead to fund detector and radionuclide projects instead. Just as in the case of the CERN Large Hadron Collider experiments, which confirmed the presence of all previously known sub-atomic particles during the first 6 weeks of energy ramp-up, before their later confirmation of the Higgs boson hypothesis (and impressively to a much greater level of parameter precision then achieved previously), so also could bioexperiments benefit from a carefully planned experimental programme to confirm previous phenomena, but provided with larger data sets to find robust and more accurate parameters for predictive modelling purposes. Some examples of what might be achieved are discussed below, although there could be many fringe benefits in other fields such as radioprotection and space travel as well as in radionuclide effects in medicine, etc.

14.5.1 Simulated experiments

Simulations have been performed of future experiments designed to determine the LET–RBE turnover point positions at LET_U (and for the underlying LET–α and

LET–β relationships) for protons and ions with different Z numbers. The methods are as follows:

1. Use random-sampling computer techniques with typical coefficients of variation for cell-survival studies to provide α and β values at the control and reference LET values. The number of different cell-survival experiments can be varied.
2. Then, vary the number of experiments for accurate estimation of the two linear gradients of α and β (separately) with LET for lines before and beyond LET_U, in order to determine their intersection position at LET_U with a high degree of accuracy for each Z number. The α and β parameters obtained may be combined to give an RBE value for each given dose.
3. Confirm if LET_U remains constant at three to four different dose levels, and for different cell lines, for each different ion (i.e. Z value).
4. Confirm and strengthen the precision of mathematical relationship between Z and LET_U, with Monte Carlo simulations of these.
5. Estimate the increased precision of the gradient of α and β with LET and determine their maximum values, α_U and β_U, at LET_U for each Z number and for different cell types, and correlate these with their reference radiation values (α_L and β_L).
6. Repeat the above in several typical beam-depth dose positions and for different incident energies.
7. Apply statistical goodness-of-fit tests to find the best of the existing LET-RBE models, or which models fit the data best in what situation, e.g. low/intermediate/high dose.
8. Estimate to what extent the better prediction of RBE would improve results of potential clinical applications.

Figure 14.4 shows an example simulation.

Four repeated simulations, using seeded random sampling, provide LET_U values of 29.6, 32.06, 33.73 and 27.64, yielding a mean of 30.75 ± 1.34 standard error of the mean (SEM) when there are 20 LET-RBE data points. The output of one such simulation is given in figure 14.5. The simulations were set up with an assumed real LET_U value of 30.5. This is a reasonably good result for medical purposes, but if the numbers of LET-RBE data points are reduced to 16 the estimate falls to 29.96 ± 1.24, and if further reduced to 12 the estimate becomes 31.5 ± 1.92. The last two examples were simulated with fewer repeat experiments leading up to the RBE determination (three repeats rather than four for each irradiation, and six points rather than eight on the reference radiation survival curve). Further reductions in the number of repeat cellular experiments required to produce each RBE data point show even more unreliable results. It follows that very large experiments are necessary to produce the most reliable data, although it is important at this stage to assess the clinical significance of an error in estimating LET_U. From geometrical considerations, an experimental LET_U result of, say, 28.8 or 31.8 keV μm^{-1} (instead of the assumed correct 30.5) would lead to an approximately 5% error in RBE estimation. However, by feeding this result into clinical isoeffect equations using the

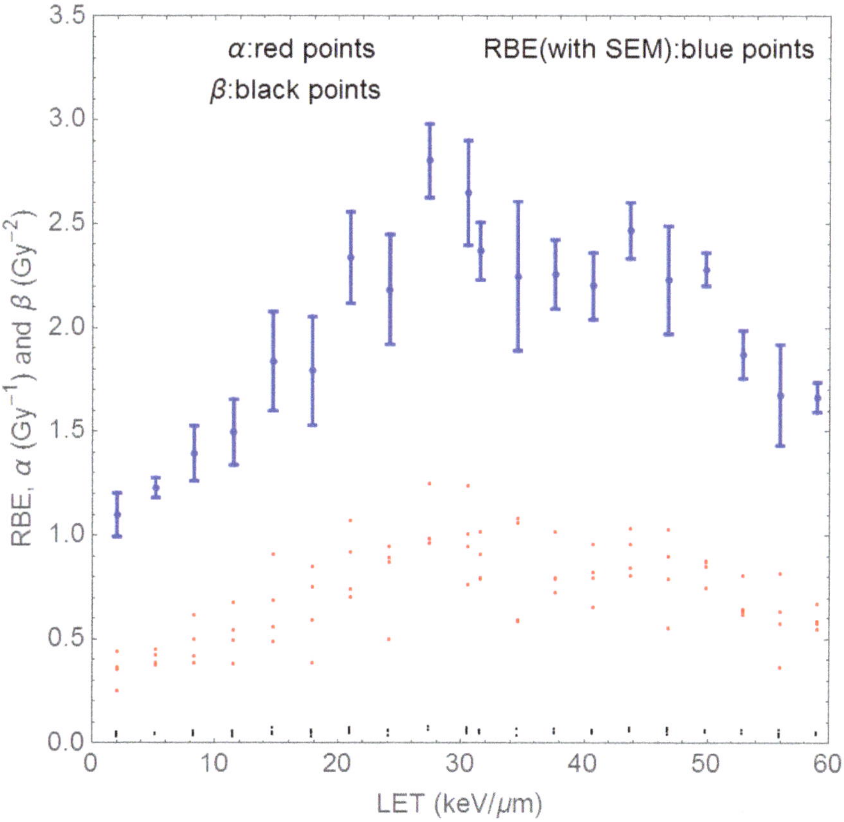

Figure 14.4. Example of a single Mathematica (Wolfram, USA) simulation of a LET_U determination experiment for protons, using variations in cellular radiosensitivities for cell-survival assays. Here 20 RBE data points are used. The LET_U value is obtained by obtaining the intersection point of the two upward and downward data linear regression fits. The expected LET_U is assumed to be 30.5 keV μm^{-1}, but the fitted value for this simulation is 27.64 (owing to a coefficient of variance of 20% for all radiosensitivity measurements).

BED concept, in which RBE is represented by its maximum and minimum limits at any specified LET,

$$\text{BED} = nd_H\left(\text{RBE}_{\text{max}} + \frac{\text{RBE}^2_{\text{min}} \cdot d_H}{(\alpha/\beta)_L}\right),$$

(as in chapter 2, equation (2.16)), where n is the number of doses given and the α/β ratio is that of the reference (or control) radiation modality, the change in the recommended dose for isoeffective neurological damage reaches a 5% difference when the estimated LET_U value falls down to between 25 and 26 keV μm^{-1} (around a 17% change in LET_U), when the local LET is as high as only 9 keV μm^{-1}, a value which can appear on proton therapy three-dimensional LET maps. So these estimates suggest that the magnitude of the error is not fully propagated in a

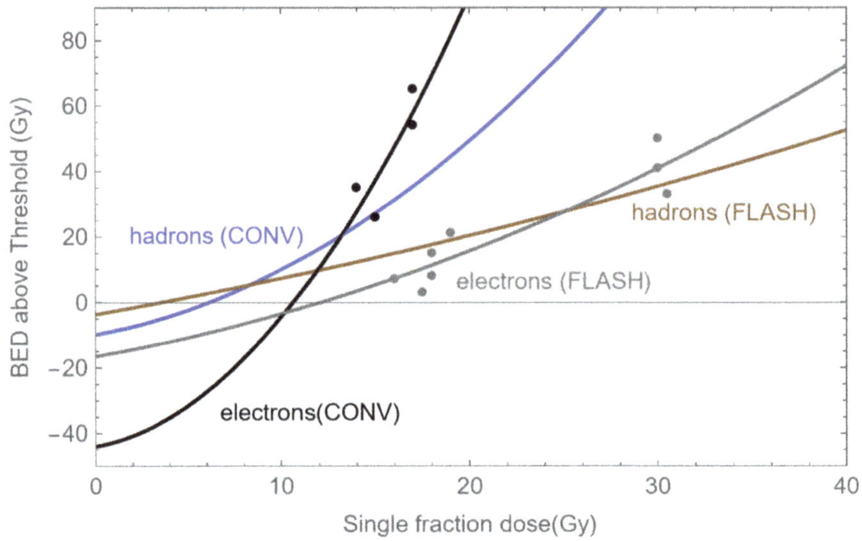

Figure 14.5. BED* and dose plots for electrons and hadrons and conventional (CONV = 0.03 Gy s^{-1}) and FLASH (60 Gy s^{-1}) dose rates, with BED transformed dose-reponse data published by Vozenin *et al.* (The assumed hadron RBE parameters are RBE_{max} = 4.5 and $RBE_{min}{}^{2}$ = 1.5. The original experimental data, transformed into BED here, is shown in this example only.)

practical clinical situation, where tissue is treated from multiple directions using pencil beams and where the LET values are not close to their maximum possible values. However, small deviations of dose beyond the already allowed International Commission on Radiation Units and Measurements (ICRU) dose variation of −5% to + 7% across a clinical target volume (consisting of the cancer plus surrounding normal tissue at high risk of harbouring infiltrating tumour cells) might also contribute to tissue complications. In general terms this would be at a rate of around 1%–2% per additional Gy, and so an additional 5% difference could mean up to 10% or more increased tissue complications and also possibly a reduction of tumour control if the error propagates as a dose reduction to the tumour, at around a 1% per Gy. These differences may seem small but could be of important clinical significance.

However, the situation is further complicated by the present clinical practice of allocating a constant RBE value of 1.1 for protons in all tissues regardless of dose and LET. Then, for a LET of 9 keV μm^{-1}, the discrepancies between the calculated and normally given dose (normalised to 100%) are 80.21% for use of the correct LET_U and 76.92% for an incorrect LET_U of 27 keV μm^{-1}. So a correct allocation of LET_U would make a further dose change of around 4.2% over and above the large difference due to a fixed versus flexible RBE allocation. This shows the considerable potential importance of using a variable LET-based RBE system with an accurate LET_U value. To change the present assumption of a constant proton RBE regardless of LET, dose, and cellular system would require a large series of careful experiments.

The same considerations would apply for heavier ions where the SOBP values of, say, carbon ions are normally at a LET which is around 20%–30% of the LET_U value, whereas the above proton example had a LET of up to 9 keV μm^{-1}, i.e. around 30% of the LET_U value. Much more detailed work is required to pursue these aspects further and for each ion species.

14.5.2 Uniqueness of LET_U for each ion species

The uniqueness of LET_U for each ion species is now considered further. This hypothesis can be addressed only to a certain extent from existing data (see Jones 2015), owing to there being relatively few reliable data points available (for heavier ions the turnover points are not so well defined due to data and range limitations, as can be visualised in the data-mining report of Sørensen *et al* 2011). Only by combining results from past experiments using different cell types and at different doses can the LET_U position be studied at the present time, but then such retrospective data cannot possibly be used to test many other hypotheses mentioned earlier.

Two such examples, for carbon ions and helium ions, are shown in table 14.6, where statistically significant differences in LET_U positions are obtained. Rigorous experimental proof of unique LET_U turnover points for each ion species would oppose many existing statements, that a LET value of around 110 keV μm^{-1} represents the maximum obtainable RBE for all ion species, as stated in many standard radiobiology textbooks, for example Hall & Giaccia (2011, 2019).

It was further argued in Jones and Hill (2019) that since the estimated LET_U of five different ion species (including protons) were all higher for increasing Z values in the case of protons, helium, carbon, neon and argon ions that the probability of this being due to chance was 1/5! (or 0.0083). Further LET_U estimations for ionic silicon and iron, again with LET_U being proportional to Z, provides a probability of 1/7! (or 0.00019), so this is a viable hypothesis which overturns the widely held previous assumptions of LET_U being invariant, despite the earlier views of Katz *et al* (1971) that Z^2 and relativistic velocity did determine RBE in some way (although without specific reference to the LET_U concept).

Further pragmatic experiments linked with theory could be performed, for example the following:

Table. 14.6. Some details of the experimental data sets for helium and carbon ions used for comparison.

Ion and data source	Cell type	Estimated LET_U (keV μm^{-1}) (mean, standard error)
Carbon ions (Weyrather *et al* 1999; GSI, Darmstadt, Germany)	CHO	145.81 ± 9.88
	V-79	159.05 ± 3.95
	Combined CHO + V-79 data	152.43 ± 4.29
Helium (Barendsen 1968; Netherlands)	Human T cells	124.24 ± 0.56

The locations of the combined carbon ion and helium data are significantly different (Mann–Whitney $p = 0.028$, t-test $p < 0.0001$).

- Investigate the reduction in RBE with depth reported in France (F. Megnin-Chanet's experiments reported by Calugaru *et al* 2011) with a greater number of data points and for different cell types and doses, and compare to Monte Carlo simulations. This is likely to require additional information beyond radiation fluence, kinetic energy released per unit mass (or KERMA), absorbed dose and LET, which are defined in one plane only: the possibility of quantifying the mean inter-track distance with depth needs to be considered, or by using a more volumetric interpretation of LET in the *x*-, *y*- and *z*-planes, due to increased Coulombic scattering with depth, especially in the case of protons but less so with heavier ions. Indeed, this might be found to be a proton-only effect, but it is vital to determine this as treatment-planning systems could incorporate such effects.
- The biological effects of nuclear fragmentation products can be separately studied.
- Establish comprehensive data sets for RBE_{max} and RBE_{min} values at different LETs for different ion beams in panels of cells with known genetic characterisation.

14.5.3 Priority in radiobiological experiments

The priority would be to establish the 'ground rules' for RBE determination but with greater precision and in a wider range of cellular systems. Later advanced experiments in collaboration with selected worldwide universities would inevitably follow, examining cellular signalling and damage-response mechanisms at the molecular level, and their modification. It is important to point out that during the more basic RBE experiments, some cellular material can be stored for analysis at other centres of excellence with great expertise in molecular mechanisms. Thus the experiments could provide data for several purposes, as determined by an overall controlling committee structure. Other universities are already aiming to sensitise/modify radiation effects, or personalise radiation by attention to genetic and proteomic screening, etc. Also, the capacity to do long, continuous low-dose-rate exposures for nuclear medicine and eventually the use of mixed-field radiations (i.e. combinations of ions), their modification by hypoxia and other molecular approaches would be of great interest. Any such experiments should be based on the secure foundation of more fundamental knowledge regarding LET and RBE, without which there is no secure basis.

Before radiobiology studies can commence, it would be essential to begin with beam characterisation work, sophisticated dosimetry and confirmation of dose in humanoid-tissue-equivalent 'phantom' structures, to confirm the numbers of particles, their ranges with depth and to translate the energy released and absorbed to the absorbed dose concept and determined to the quality standards demanded in medical practice and as approved by registered medical physicists. The experience gained would be invaluable and could be used to establish a dosimetry reference laboratory for particle beams working closely with national standards laboratories and international bodies such as the aforementioned ICRU and International

Commission on Radiological Protection. An entire range of diagnostic and dosimetry equipment would be necessary for routine dose monitoring and would present the opportunity for advanced detector research and development, using direct beam monitoring, detectors inserted in tissue-equivalent phantoms and remote detections of nuclear activation products.

14.5.3.1 Further studies using ultra-high or FLASH dose-rate effects

After comprehensive studies of the beam ballistics for the various ions, radiobiological studies would follow using the same experimental beam geometry, which can be made to simulate the human body and the typical dimensions of treatments in various anatomical sites. The relationship between inter-track distances (related to fluence and dose rates) and RBE needs investigation in detail, as suggested in chapter 1, with dose-rate equations given in chapter 2. Some preliminary modelling initiatives are considered here. The equations given in Jones (2022, 2023) can be modified to include RBE parameters. It was found that ultra-high (or FLASH) dose-rate *in vivo* data on a lung fibrosis experimental model used in Lausanne, Switzerland by Vozenin *et al* (2019) could be fitted by plotting the BED* (the excess BED beyond the threshold BED for the effect to occur). The fitted FLASH data curve had a different threshold dose and intercept BED, and was shallower, its gradients controlled by a much higher α/β ratio. The change in α/β ratio (from 3.4 for lung fibrosis at a dose rate of 0.03 Gy s^{-1} to become 32.74 Gy at a dose rate of 60 Gy s^{-1}), a factor of 9.63, due to the increased dose rate was closely approximated by the function

$$J = \left(\frac{R}{R_{\mathrm{ref}}}\right)^{0.3} = 9.78, \tag{14.1}$$

where R is the FLASH dose rate and R_{ref} is the dose rate of the reference radiation at standard dose rates of around 1–2 Gy $\min^{-1}$, and which is close to the cube root function implied by consideration of mean inter-track distances in a small volume and must also be related to the oxygen depletion rate. It follows that J not only modifies the α/β ratio but also is related to the change in dose rate, or time to deliver a specified dose. It is important to understand that for dose rates 1 and 2 (which appear in subscripts below), the S' (mean track distance separation in a volume), F' (the near instantaneous fluence rate), dose rates and exposure times (T) as introduced in chapter 1, are related as

$$\frac{S_1'}{S_2'} = \sqrt[3]{\frac{F_2'}{F_1'}} = \sqrt[3]{\frac{\text{dose rate}_2}{\text{dose rate}_1}} = \sqrt[3]{\frac{T_1}{T_2}},$$

provided that the same total dose is given in these respective times (since any dose $d =$ dose rate $\times\ T$).

These concepts can then be used within a BED framework. For further details, see Jones (2022), where the argument is presented for dose-rate intensification leading leading to enhanced micro-volumetric energy transfer (or MVET) and so modify radiosensitivity by increasing the efficiency of energy transfer (similar to the LET effect presented in chapter 8). At extremely high dose rates radiosensitivity may be reduced because of the overkill effect and also, though even before overkill may occur, concomitant oxygen depletion will cause reduction in radiosensitivities, affecting the β parameter to a greater extent than the α parameter, since theamount of oxygen depletion will cause radiosensitivity reductions, affecting the β parameter to a greater extent than the α parameter because their oxygen enhancement ratios (OER) differ, OER_β being larger than OER_α (Nahum *et al* 2003).

For a comparison of four different experimental conditions, the modified BED equations (using the high-LET BED equations derived in chapter 2) are as follows, where BED* is the BED above the threshold BED value for the experimental effect of lung fibrosis and the α/β ratio (of 3.4 Gy) is that found for the reference low-LET radiation (megavoltage electrons) from the data-fitting process:

1. The reference radiation (e.g. megavoltage electrons) at conventional dose rate:

$$\mathrm{BED}^* = d\left(1 - \frac{d}{(\alpha/\beta)}\right) - 44.0. \tag{14.2}$$

2. The megavoltage electrons at FLASH dose rates:

$$\mathrm{BED}^* = d\left(1 - \frac{d}{J(\alpha/\beta)}\right) - 16.55. \tag{14.3}$$

3. The proton or hadron with higher LET than the electrons used above at conventional dose rate:

$$\mathrm{BED}^* = d\left(\mathrm{RBE}_{\max} - \frac{\mathrm{RBE}^2_{\min} \cdot d}{\mathrm{RBE}_{\max}\,(\alpha/\beta)}\right) - \frac{44.0}{\mathrm{RBE}_{\max}}. \tag{14.4}$$

4. The proton or hadron with higher LET than the electrons used above at the FLASH dose rate:

$$\mathrm{BED}^* = d\left(\mathrm{RBE}_{\max} - \frac{\mathrm{RBE}^2_{\min} \cdot d}{\mathrm{RBE}_{\max} \cdot J \quad (\alpha/\beta)}\right) - \frac{16.55}{\mathrm{RBE}_{\max}}. \tag{14.5}$$

These changes include the fact that the ratio $\frac{\mathrm{RBE}_{\max}}{\mathrm{RBE}^2_{\min}} = \frac{(\alpha/\beta)_{\mathrm{HighLET}}}{(\alpha/\beta)_{\mathrm{ref}}}$, as explained in chapter 2, where this ratio is given as R_C. Thus dividing the $\mathrm{RBE}^2_{\min}$ term by $\mathrm{RBE}_{\max}$ effectively modifies the reference α/β ratio to be that of the high-LET radiation. The intercept terms (44 and 16.55 Gy) were the respective values of the data-fitted intercepts for conventional and FLASH dose rates using electrons. These values are divided by $\mathrm{RBE}_{\max}$, since they occur at near-zero dose where only α cell kill occurs, to provide modified intercept BED values for the higher-LET experiments.

Examples of some simulated experiments are shown in figure 14.5 for a source using a higher-LET and higher-RBE hadron (e.g. neutrons or carbon ions) and figures 14.6(a) and (b) for protons, which are compared with the original electron-based experiments with superimposed lung fibrosis data in figure 14.5. It can be

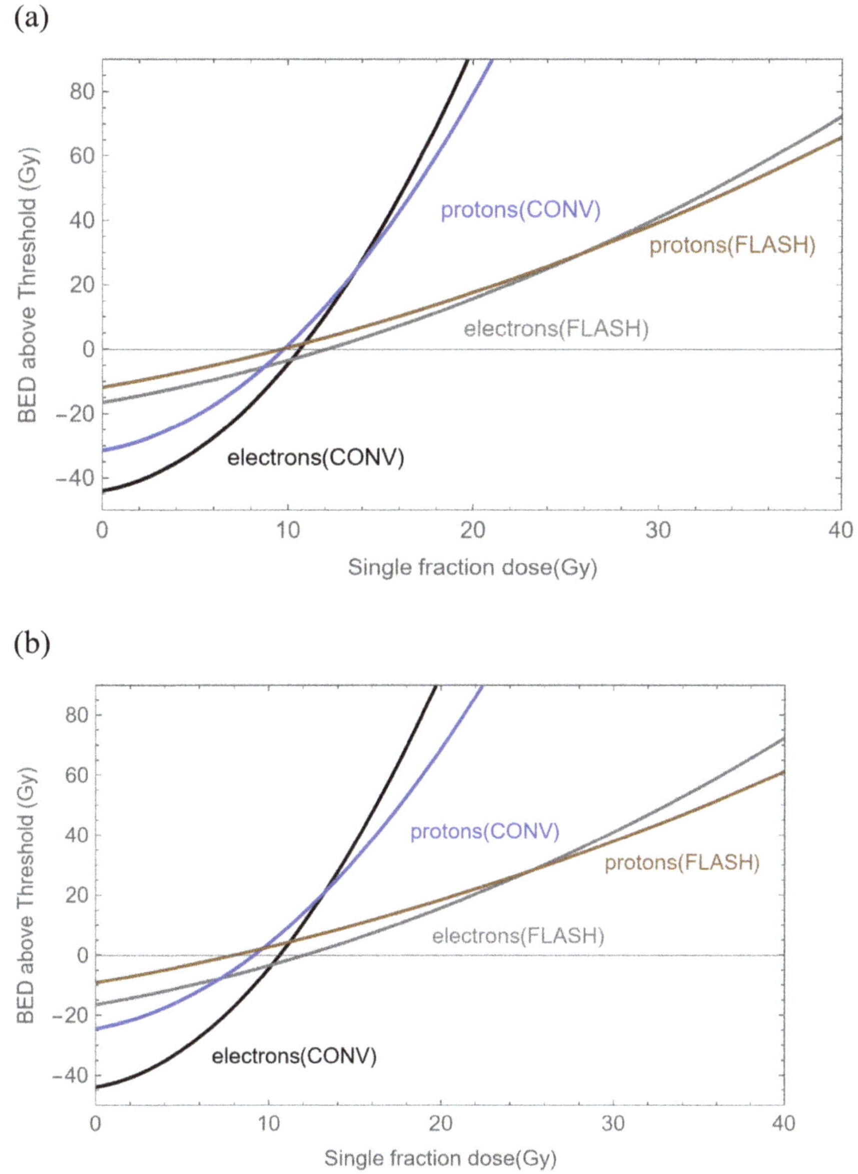

Figure 14.6. (a) and (b): Plots of the single fraction dose and the BED value for the observed effect above the threshold BED for that effect for electrons and protons and conventional (CONV) and FLASH dose rates. The assumed proton RBE parameters are $RBE_{max} = 1.4$ and$RBE^2_{min} = 1.08$ in 5(a), and $RBE_{max} = 1.8$ and $RBE^2_{min} = 1.12$ in 5(b). The α/β ratio is modified by the J operator.

seen that the transition to progressively higher LET (represented here by the RBE_{max} and RBE_{min} values) does influence the BED* curves, where at high doses some reduction in tissue effects occur if the same dose is given. For protons the change is relatively marginal, although dependent on the extent of increase in LET and RBE.

The modelled examples in figures 14.5 and 14.6 do not need to include the reduction in LET_U due to the increased dose rate (a speculation introduced in chapter 9), since the existing RBE parameters are now further modified by the change in α/β ratio, which will implicitly include such an effect as well as the radiosensitivity changes caused by very rapid oxygen depletion, which is sufficient to oppose oxygen rediffusion into pre-existing hypoxic sites. The presence of hypoxic areas in normal tissues may be surprising to non-radiobiologists, but normal tissue perfusion is phasic and tissue-invasive oxygen electrode studies, from the earliest times, have confirmed periodic hypoxia in many normal tissues, as well as more recent perfusion studies using dynamic magnetic resonance imaging (see Jones 2022). The effects on tumour sterilisation can be difficult to interpret. Modelling studies using BED equations where the dose rate ranges from very low dose rates of 0.1 Gy hr^{-1} to FLASH rates, by further adaption of the equations presented above, suggest that the therapeutic index may be best for radiosensitive tumours, but detailed experimentation is required to determine this. Also, the caveats listed in chapter 2 regarding naive extrapolation from tumour experiments in animals to humans should be heeded, since they include large differences in nuclear chromosome number, metabolic rate (and so oxygen consumption), oxygen diffusion distances from blood vessels, tumour hypoxia and re-oxygenation rates, cellular proliferation rates, growth fractions and overall radiosensitivities. For example, murine tumours usually require a dose which is around 3 times larger to achieve the same effect as in the human, and the optimum treatment duration for fractionated treatment is much shorter in animals, often by a factor of around 2 or more. Further examples can be found in standard radiobiology textbooks. It is not surprising that many radiobiological 'therapeutic advances' found in animal experiments have failed to produce clear-cut improvements in humans due to these factors and possibly others such as differences in mutational characteristics, which are beyond the scope of this chapter.

It remains to be seen whether protons and hadrons at ultra-high dose rates will be useful in the clinic owing to their use in single fractions, the associated difficulties with accurate dosimetry and the familiar question of if there are significant response differences between tumours and normal tissues, especially since some slower-growing tumour types have only slight differences in their physiology from that found in normal tissues.

There are also significant issues to overcome in accelerator technology in order to implement effective FLASH dose rates (Jolly *et al* 2020). This is a fast-moving area of research where radiobiology, physics and careful clinical applications will be required. The problems of clinical applications will be considerable, as FLASH effects require use of larger dose per fraction in order to cross critical thresholds and which will not be optimum in some tumour types.

14.6 Some untested situations

LET maps were fused with computed tomography scans over a decade ago (Grassberger *et al* 2011). These LET values are based on averaged LET values delivered from different angles to a target volume and at different times. It is not known how relevant they are, since there are possibilities that LET radiosensitising effects occur over very short durations of time (and are not as susceptible to enzymatic radiation repair); the fundamental radiation processes occur over short time windows and are complete within 2–30 ms (Wardman 2009). For the more clustered DNA damage which occurs with higher LET, it remains to be seen if a further dose given at an interval of, say, 5–10 min (consistent with gantry rotations and positioning checks) will result in an additive or non-linear survival effect, as well as on the yield of DNA and chromosomal breaks. This is an urgent question for experimental verification using cell-survival experiments where dose is given using such intervals.

14.7 Conclusions

There is considerable scope for experimental radiobiological studies to refine knowledge about the relationship between LET and RBE in protons and other heavier ions and how bioeffects can change with very high dose rates in different tissues.

This book has covered LET-RBE modelling based on a strong experimental evidence base that the maximum RBE for any ion will occur near to a specific LET value of LET_U, determined by a combination of kinematic parameters, beginning with protons, where at around 30.5 keV μm^{-1} the proton energy becomes insufficient to cross a cell diameter. Such ideas need to be pursued further and may offer a better starting point than many models based on DNA strand breaks within a cell and tissue structure, with all of their complexities, although some integration of various modelling approaches may be fruitful.

The aim must be to design experiments that will improve the predictive modelling associated with particle physics applications in medicine by addressing fundamental issues of how particle physics interacts with biosystems in a much more detailed way than previously attempted in order to obtain more accurate and reliable parameters than are available at the present time. The fulfilment of such a project would result in better-understood systems for all ion-beam therapies and provide guidance towards their optimal use.

Until that can be achieved, it will be necessary to make the best use of existing historical radiobiological RBE data sets, and to plead for greater research funding from governments to make particle therapies safer and more effective, either in some more fortunate countries or by cooperative large-scale international projects based at accessible, dedicated and reliable sites.

References

Barendsen G W 1968 Responses of cultured cells, tumours and normal tissues to radiations of different linear energy transfer *Curr. Topics Radiat. Res. Q.* **4** 293–356

Calugaru V, Nauraye C, Noël G *et al* 2011 Radiobiological characterization of two therapeutic proton beams with different initial energy spectra used at the Institut Curie Proton Therapy Center in Orsay *Int. J. Radiat. Oncol. Biol. Phys.* **81** 1136–43

Chaudhary P, Marshall T I, Currell F J *et al* 2015 Variations in the processing of DNA double-strand breaks along 60-MeV therapeutic proton beams *Int. J. Radiat. Oncol. Biol. Phys.* **95** 86–94

Chaudhary P, Marshall T I, Perozziello F M *et al* 2014 Relative biological effectiveness variation along monoenergetic and modulated Bragg peaks of a 62-MeV therapeutic proton beam: a preclinical assessment *Int. J. Radiat. Oncol. Biol. Phys.* **90** 27–35

Dosanjh M, Jones B and Myers S 2013 A possible biomedical facility at CERN *Br. J. Radiol.* **86** 1025–9

Girdhani S, Sachs R and Hlatky L 2013 Biological effects of proton radiation: what we know and don't know *Radiat. Res.* **179** 257–72

Grassberger C, Trofimov A, Lomax A and Paganetti H 2011 Variations in linear energy transfer within clinical proton therapy fields and the potential for biological treatment planning *Int. J. Radiat. Oncol. Biol. Phys.* **80** 1559–66

Hall E J and Giaccia A 2011 *Radiobiology for the Radiologist* 7th edn (Philadelphia, PA: Lippincott Williams and Wilkins) ch 6 and 7 pp 253–70

Hall E J and Giaccia A J 2019 *Radiobiology for the Radiologist* 8th edn (Philadelphia, PA: Wolters Kluwer) ch 7 pp 106–9

Jolly S, Owen H, Schippers M and Welsch C 2020 Technical challenges for FLASH proton therapy *Phys. Med.* **78** 71–82

Jones B 2006 The case for particle therapy *Brit. J. Radiol.* **79** 24–31

Jones B and Hill M A 2019 Physical characteristics at the turnover-points of relative biological effect (RBE) with linear energy transfer (LET) *Phys. Med. Biol.* **64** 225010

Jones B 2022 The influence of hypoxia on LET and RBE relationships with implications for ultra-high dose rates and FLASH modelling *Phys. Med. Biol.* **67** 125011

Jones B 2023 Modelled biological effectiveness comparisons of low, high and ultra-high (FLASH) radiation dose rates *Radiat. Phys. Chem.* **208** 110944

Jones B 2015 A simpler energy transfer efficiency model to predict relative biological effect (RBE) for protons and heavier Ions *Front. Oncol.* **5** 184 Erratum in: *Front. Oncol.* 2016;6:32

Katz R, Ackerson B, Homoyooufar M and Sharma S C 1971 Inactivation of cells by heavy ion bombardment *Radiat. Res.* **47** 402–25

Nahum A E, Movsas B, Horwitz E M, Stobbe C C and Chapman J D 2003 Incorporating clinical measurements of hypoxia into tumor local control modeling of prostate cancer: implications for the alpha/beta ratio *Int. J. Radiat. Oncol. Biol. Phys.* **57** 391–401

Sørensen B S, Overgaard J and Bassler N 2011 *In vitro* RBE-LET dependence for multiple particle types *Acta Oncol.* **50** 757–62

Vozenin M-C, Hendry J H and Limoli C L 2019 Biological benefits of ultra-high dose rate FLASH radiotherapy: sleeping beauty awoken *Clin. Oncol. (R Coll. Radiol.)* **31** 407–15

Wardman P 2009 The importance of radiation chemistry to radiation and free radical biology *Br. J. Radiol.* **82** 89–104

Weyrather W K, Ritter S, Scholz M and Kraft G 1999 RBE for carbon track-segment irradiation in cell lines of differing repair capacity *Int. J. Radiat. Biol.* **75** 1357–64

www.ingramcontent.com/pod-product-compliance
Ingram Content Group UK Ltd.
Pitfield, Milton Keynes, MK11 3LW, UK
UKHW051901100926
8556IPUK00005B/725

9 780750 362078